AVICENNA'S MEDICINE

"*Avicenna's Medicine* represents a breath of fresh air to those interested in the history of Western medicine. It is presented in a consistently clear and concise form that makes Avicenna's writings accessible to the English reader. In addition, a number of chapters at the beginning of the book act as a primer in the principles of Graeco-Arabic Medicine. *Avicenna's Medicine* is one of the most interesting and exciting volumes that has come my way in a long time. It provides insight into a medicine that is a historical part of the development of modern Western medicine and an ethnic traditional medicine that is still more or less practiced on the Indian subcontinent and in some parts of the Middle East. This may well serve to rekindle a resurgence of interest in Avicenna's medicine in the West; something it surely deserves."

PAUL HYSEN, PH.D., DOCTOR OF NATUROPATHY
AND CHIROPRACTIC

"Avicenna's *Canon* is not only the most important and influential single text in the history of medicine, it is also the main work of reference for a major traditional school of medicine that is still alive and has much to teach us today. The present translation, *Avicenna's Medicine,* is welcome not only because it makes many of the ideas of the *Canon* accessible in English but also because it deals with practical applications of its principles for those drawn to holistic or integrative medicine wherever they might be."

SEYYED HOSSEIN NASR, AUTHOR OF *SCIENCE AND CIVILIZATION
IN ISLAM* AND PROFESSOR OF ISLAMIC STUDIES AT
GEORGE WASHINGTON UNIVERSITY

"The next time you visit your physician, whisper a prayer of thanks to Avicenna, because many of the foundations of modern medicine—empirical observation, objectivity, and rationalism—surfaced through his towering genius a millennium ago. *Avicenna's Medicine* is a valuable link in medicine's rich history. As the authors make clear in this marvelous translation, Avicenna's relevance to our era has not been exhausted."

LARRY DOSSEY, M.D., AUTHOR OF
HEALING WORDS AND *ONE MIND*

AVICENNA'S MEDICINE

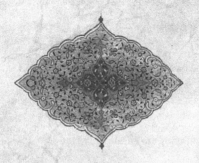

A NEW TRANSLATION
of the 11th-Century Canon with Practical
Applications for Integrative Health Care

MONES ABU-ASAB, PH.D.
HAKIMA AMRI, PH.D.
MARC S. MICOZZI, M.D., PH.D.

Healing Arts Press
Rochester, Vermont • Toronto, Canada

Healing Arts Press
One Park Street
Rochester, Vermont 05767
www.HealingArtsPress.com

Healing Arts Press is a division of Inner Traditions International

Note to the reader: This book is intended as an informational guide. The remedies, approaches, and techniques described herein are meant to supplement, and not to be a substitute for, professional medical care or treatment. They should not be used to treat a serious ailment without prior consultation with a qualified health care professional.

Library of Congress Cataloging-in-Publication Data
Avicenna, 980–1037.
[Qanun fi al-tibb. Kitab 1. English]
Avicenna's medicine : a new translation of the 11th-century canon with practical applications for integrative health care / Mones Abu-Asab, Hakima Amri, Marc S. Micozzi.
    p. cm.
Includes bibliographical references and index.
Summary: "The first contemporary translation of the 1,000-year-old text at the foundation of modern medicine and biology"—Provided by publisher.
ISBN 978-1-59477-432-4 (hardcover) — ISBN 978-1-62055-170-7 (e-book)
I. Abu-Asab, Mones. II. Amri, Hakima. III. Micozzi, Marc S., 1953– IV. Title.
[DNLM: 1. Medicine, Unani. WZ 290]
610—dc23

                                                                        2012046668

Printed and bound in the United States

10 9 8 7 6 5 4 3 2

Text design and layout by Virginia Scott Bowman
This book was typeset in Garamond Premier Pro and Gill Sans with Caslon and Garamond used as disply typefaces

To send correspondence to the author of this book, mail a first-class letter to the author c/o Inner Traditions • Bear & Company, One Park Street, Rochester, VT 05767, and we will forward the communication, or contact the authors directly at **monesaa@yahoo.com** for Mones S. Abu-Asab, **amrih@georgetown.edu** for Hakima Amri, and **marcsmicozzi@gmail.com** for Marc Micozzi.

*To the continuum of people who have kept alive
the quest for knowledge over thousands of years*

*To my father, Mohamed Salah,
and my mother, Warda*
—Hakima Amri

Avicenna links ancient physicians with modern medicine. His devotion to the search for truth set the standard for all times. The cultures of both East and West are indebted to this great physician and philosopher.

RICHARD DEAN SMITH, "AVICENNA AND THE CANNON OF MEDICINE: A MILLENNIAL TRIBUTE," *WESTERN JOURNAL OF MEDICINE* 133 (1980): 367–70

Contents

FIRST ART

Definition of Medicine and Its Topics

SECOND ART

Disease, Causes, and General Symptoms

THIRD ART

Health, Disease, and the Necessity of Death

FOURTH ART

Aspects of Treatments according to General Diseases   333

♦

In Defense of Medical Tradition

Alain Touwaide

One millennium ago Abū Alī al-Husain ibn Abdullāh ibn Sīnā (980–1037), more commonly known as ibn Sīnā or Avicenna according to the medieval adaptation of his name, was in Gurgan, near the Caspian Sea. As he wrote in his autobiography, he had devoted himself "to studying the texts—the original and the commentaries—in the natural sciences and metaphysics, and the gates of knowledge began opening."

His lifetime was an extraordinary period for knowledge. After the Arabic Empire was created, it laid down the foundations of a new science and scientific culture by assimilating the legacy of all the surrounding polities, not only Byzantium, India, and Persia but also the mosaic of the many others in the vast area ranging from China in the East to Andalusia in the West. During the last decades of the tenth century, corresponding to ibn Sīnā's youth, scientists in all disciplines in the Arabic World had already produced new works that not only assimilated their heritage but also led it in new directions.

ibn Sīnā was not different. As he stated in his autobiography, after he assimilated many other scientific disciplines he "sought to know medicine and . . . read the books on it." He quickly "excelled in it in a very short time, to the point that distinguished physicians began to read the science of medicine" under him. He did not limit himself to theoretical study and teaching, but he also "cared for the sick" and acquired knowledge of "medical treatments that cannot be described and can be learned only from practice."

He then started to write down what he knew. This resulted in the *Qānūn*, which he began to compile one millennium ago. Corresponding to the description he himself made of his activity, the *Qānūn* is not a theoretical manual that exposes all the medical knowledge available at that time. Rather, it presents available medical theories and also—if not above all—submits them to a critical analysis that is not only theoretical but is also informed by his personal experience and observations from treating patients.

ibn Sīnā's way of working recalls his years of learning. He didn't read only the texts, as he stated, but he also read the commentaries on the texts, which is the critical evaluation of received knowledge. This is the method in the *Qānūn*, which brings together available knowledge and its analysis through clinical experience.

The work had an extraordinary *Fortuna*, certainly resulting from its merging of received knowledge and personal analysis. It diffused all over the Mediterranean in manuscript form before printing; it was translated into Latin in the thirteenth century;* it circulated widely in the Late Middle Ages; and it was printed as early as 1472 (Book 3) with no less than fourteen different editions by the end of the fifteenth century. Even the Greek medical texts—of which the *Qānūn* was the heir—were not printed before 1499 (Dioscorides, *De materia medica*) and even 1525 (Galen, *Opera omnia*). In Medieval universities, the *Qānūn* was a core text, and it remained so until late in the sixteenth century, even in the midst of the strong revival of Greek medicine actively promoted by the Ferrarese physician and classical scholar Nicolao Leoniceno (1428–1524). At the most prestigious university of Montpellier, for example, the *Qānūn* was used until the 1540s and was

---

*Gerard de Sabloneta possibly did the Latin translation, rather than the famous Italian translator of many scientific Arabic works Gerard of Cremona (ca. 1114–1187), as scholars thought for a long time.

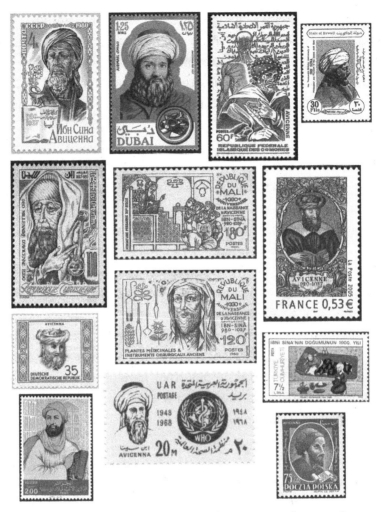

Avicenna's far-reaching and enduring influence is evident in these stamps from around the world, commemorating Avicenna's millennial birthday in the 20th century. From top left: Union of the Soviet Socialist Republics, Dubai, Republic of the Comoro Islands, Kuwait, Tunisia, Mali, France, Germany, Turkey, Algeria, Egypt, and Poland.

replaced by Greek textbooks only after the bishop protector of the university brought Greek texts back from Venice, where he had been the Ambassador to the French king François I.

A brilliant polymath, ibn Sīnā was considered as al-Shaikh al-Ra'is—the *Prince of Philosophers*—in his own lifetime. He summed up all available medical knowledge, submitted it to scrutiny through careful and repeated clinical observations, and duly recorded, compared, and studied resulting data in order to distinguish recurrent facts and correlations. When necessary, he departed from received knowledge, which he did not credit with special authority because of its antiquity, the prestige and aura of its author, or any other reason. However he did not reject received knowledge *en bloc*, as did Theophrastus Bombastus von Hohenheim, better known as Paracelsus (1493–1541), who threw out all books of medical authorities—including the *Qānūn*—in a spectacular auto-dafé.

Since then, the medical heritage of the past has often been dismissed and is now almost forgotten. Returning to one of this era's major accomplishments and reading it with a critical eye is what the authors of the present translation of the *Qānūn* offer here. They provide a new way at looking at a well-known work that may seem to have nothing to offer present medicine and the medical world. Just like Avicenna, the authors read the text in its original language, without being caught in the fallacies of available translations. They have perused its many commentaries and studies and have submitted the teaching of the *Shaikh* to a careful medical examination in light of the most advanced knowledge of present day.

The results of this new reading—which unlocks ibn Sīnā's proposals with the keys of contemporary, cutting-edge medical knowledge—will probably surprise. But one should think about the Fortuna of the *Qānūn* and reflect on the meaning of its tradition through the centuries, the languages, and the populations that used it as a basis for their medicine—and still do so in several areas of the world—and question apparent certainties, exactly as ibn Sīnā did. Tradition, particularly in the field of medicine, is a sign of efficacy in spite of Paracelsus.

ALAIN TOUWAIDE is the cofounder and scientific director of the Institute for the Preservation of Medical Traditions. For four decades he has researched the Mediterranean medical traditions from antiquity to modern science, with a special focus on the Greek, Latin, and Arabic traditions. He has visited all major and less-known libraries preserving collections of medical manuscripts worldwide and has been affiliated with the Smithsonian Institute for ten years (2002–2011). His pioneering work has been supported by the National Institutes of Health and has been recognized in recent years with the 2003 Award for Achievement in the Behavioral Sciences granted by the Washington Academy of Sciences, his election as Fellow of the American Association for the Advancement of Sciences in 2009, and his election as Overseas Fellow of the Royal Society of Medicine of the United Kingdom in 2011.

Preface

Many have long come to admire and appreciate Avicenna's medicine because it offers a wealth of clinical solutions as well as a most comprehensive pharmacopoeia of herbal remedies. Further, in our own original work of translation we find his explanations of biological and medical concepts, as well as the theoretical basis of medicine, to be among the best features of his writings. This aspect of Avicenna's work has never been emphasized before.

Among the goals we set for this book was to provide a fresh translation of Avicenna's *Canon of Medicine,* directly from the original Arabic script, that preserves the true spirit and accuracy of the book. For this reason, we carried out a translation of the original Arabic text by using two editions of his first book, the Cairo (1294 AH*) and Rome (1593 CE) editions. By adding our own explanations and commentaries, we aim to elucidate the concepts and terminology of the Unani medicine, or Greco-Arabic-Islamic medical system, as we can come to understand them in light of modern sciences and as physicians as well as scientists—a distinction that Avicenna frequently and explicitly points out in his work. In so doing, we do not shy from identifying what may be seen as "outdated" terminology regarding such terms as *spirit* and *spirits,* as well as the lack of other features, such as organ differentiation.

The presence of conceptually rich and sophisticated content in Avicenna's *Canon of Medicine* is not surprising since he was a

---

*The acronym AH stands for anno hegirae, the Hijri year of the Islamic Calendar. It marks the Hijra (هِجْرَة), or emigration, of Muhammad and his followers to the city of Medina in 622.

well-rounded "Renaissance man" (even before the Renaissance in Europe), knowledgeable of all the sciences and philosophical systems of his time. His medical writings aimed to rid medicine of superstition and base it on empirical observation, objectivity, and rationalism. Readers will come to discover how fascinating are his explanations of biological phenomena, such as those on aging in relation to hydration and energy, which are in total congruence with our modern scientific knowledge. When seen in proper translation, it is often stunning how Avicenna and Greco-Arabic-Islamic physicians before him, such as Hippocrates, Galen, and Rhazes, reached such superb understandings of biology with little technical instrumentation and no molecular biological knowledge.

Nonetheless, the rational, sophisticated synthesis and integration of basic science and organismal biology show Unani medicine, as described by Avicenna, as a true systems biology paradigm that also serves as a model for the practice of truly individualized medicine. Chapter after chapter, the reader will be amazed by the comprehensiveness and organization of the topics and by the consistent emphasis on prevention of disease and preservation of health.

Another important aspect of Avicenna's work will strike readers of this book, particularly those who follow progress in medicine. In many cases, only after the expenditure of millions of dollars, using the finest, cutting-edge technologies, modern biological sciences have ultimately reached the same conclusions that Avicenna and other ancient scientists were able to reach thousands of years ago. For example, one of modern biomedicine's latest conclusions, that cellular energy, as generated by the mitochondria, is a main key to the proper functioning of tissues and the health of the organism, can also be seen as a major theme throughout Avicenna's *Canon*, when properly translated and understood.

This book also addresses how physicians such as Galen and Avicenna employed keen observation to formulate general explanations, even in the face of a lack of any data at a biochemical level. In these particular situations the genius of Unani physicians was revealed in producing (or formulating) the most sophisticated hypotheses. Take for example the concept of spirit (*rouh* [Arabic]), explained later in the book, and theory of humors, among the most controversial in Unani medicine. Avicenna gives the spirit a purely physical definition as a lightweight entity and rejects any metaphysical circumscription of it.

Unani's theoretical and practical knowledge is based on humors. Throughout the *Canon*, Avicenna invokes the humors as real entities responsible for health and sickness. Many of the writers who had dismissed the humoral theory, or consigned it to the scrap heap of medical history, simply did not understand what is meant by the humors; for example, they erroneously assumed that the humors are meant as blood constituents or substitutes, but they are not. They are simply nutrients that provide the building blocks of the blood. Our new understanding of Avicenna's humors, as presented in this book, reveals that the humors can now be seen as the biochemical classes known today as proteins, lipids, and organic acids. And humors are the macromolecules of the food we eat after they have been absorbed from the stomach and the intestines and gone into the bloodstream. Meanwhile, modern biomedicine has still not identified thousands of the biomolecules that exist in the blood,* and scientists working on identifying blood proteins using mass spectrometry tell us that nearly half of all the compounds from human specimens have not yet been identified! So, perhaps there is a need for the ancient understanding of Avicenna's humors as a timeless, empirical, functional, and holistic basis for human health, while modern medicine still struggles to make sense of the whole while hunting down (and still searching for the many missing) individual parts.

Another aspect that exists in Unani medicine, but is missing in our current Western medical system (WMS), is evaluation of the actual **quality** of the biological compounds present in the bloodstream, not just measuring the presence and levels of biochemicals. In WMS the focus is on measuring the quantity of biomolecules; however, Unani theory and practice deals with **both** quality and quantity. You will find this point to be well illustrated throughout the book, where the description of humors and treatments addresses their harmful physical forms (i.e., their quality) as well as their quantity or concentrations. To

---

*Berman, *Beginning and the End*, 84.

our knowledge, there are no similar criteria in the WMS; it is about time that the **qualitative** aspects of biomolecules be considered in the assessment of health and prevention of disease as done in Unani and other traditional medical systems for millions of people over thousands of years.

In addition to presenting this fresh look at Unani medicine, which is of vital contemporary interest and importance, the reader will also gain insight into the medical knowledge and practice of the eleventh century, understand the centrality of prevention for a healthy lifestyle, expand awareness of the interplay of medicine and biology, and better understand the human body and its management.

Above all, the reader will recognize that the Unani model of individualized medicine is both a way of thinking and a framework of practice, see it as an art that once dominated the clinical relationship between the patient and the physician, understand that such a model is desperately needed now, and realize that individualized medicine can be brought back with knowledge already at hand.

INTRODUCTION

Why Revisit a
Thousand-Year-Old Book?

Why would three twenty-first-century medical scientists from well-known institutions want to write about the state of medicine in the eleventh century? To many practitioners of complementary, alternative, and integrative medicine, as well as open-minded scientists and physicians, there are very good reasons for revisiting Avicenna's works. What yet have we have missed and should still come to know from the Canon? How will the knowledge of Avicenna help us live healthier lives?

For scientists, one important aspect is to know how the integrative medicine of Avicenna's time can now be interpreted and applied in light of our twenty-first-century knowledge. The *Canon* is not merely a medical history of its time, but rather a basis for understanding human health and disease in an integral, panoramic approach. In our era of reductionistic medicine and thinking, the need for an integrative medical model, to balance the reductionistic modern medical paradigm, cannot be overstated.

One of the major reasons to have embarked on this work is our attempt to add to the discussion about the current state of medicine in the twenty-first century by bringing into focus the medical philosophy of Avicenna. His philosophy of individualized medicine is different from what is promoted today as such. He recognized the patient as a whole being rather than a collection of separate parts.* Today's severely exaggerated concept of individualized medicine is not about understanding the individual pathophysiological disease process of the patient, but rather about tailoring of drug treatments for "disease management," not personal health management.

Although there remain many admirers, modern critiques of Avicenna's medicine are tainted by distortions and misinterpretations of his medical concepts. The repeated dismissal of these concepts has cast a distorted light, and a dark shadow, on ancient medical knowledge. We can help to set the record straight by elucidating the key concepts that are considered the backbone of Avicenna's medicine. We present in this book the original words of Avicenna, as well as our current interpretations of them. In so doing, we show that the Unani medical system is sound. For example, and as we show in detail later, Avicenna presented a well-developed concept of disease. His system of pathology was based on figuring out the causes of illness, not focusing on the symptoms or the end-stage appearance of damaged tissues, as modern allopathic medicine emphasizes.

He treated patients by eliminating the causes of illness in a safe, nonharmful way. Even when it came to infectious diseases, he attributed the effects of microorganisms (he called them malicious bodies; we called them germs) to the body's weakness and its receptivity to infection, or "host factors."

But the biggest controversy in Avicenna's system was generated by attacks on the humoral concept of body fluids. Most recent writers and critics of the humoral theory of disease seem to be confused about what the humors really are, and may not have read any original descriptions of them.† In this regard, there are questions that beg to be asked: Why did all the seemingly brilliant physicians of the past accept the humoral theory? How were these physicians able to successfully diagnose and treat patients on the basis of humoral imbalance? Today Unani as well as ayurvedic physicians are still successfully treating

---

*Gruner, "Avicenna's *Canon of Medicine*," 239–48.
†Arikha, *Passions and Tempers*, 376; and Nuland, "Bad Medicine," 12.

patients using humoral diagnosis!* If the theory is totally wrong, how did it survive for thousands of years?

AVICENNA'S LIFE AND CONTRIBUTIONS

As if predicting his future fame, Avicenna recorded his autobiography from early on, and later the task was taken up by his student and follower for twenty-five years, Abd al-Wāhid Jūzjānī.†⁴ There are more details available about Avicenna's life than any other ancient physician or philosopher. He is called the al Sheikh al-Rais, or the *Chief Teacher*. Avicenna was born Abu Ali Al-Husain ibn 'Abd-Allah ibn Hasan ibn 'Ali Ibn Sīnā in August 980 in a large village near Bukhārā called Kharmaithan (the Land of the Sun). His father was from "the glittering" city of Balkh (بلخ; Bactra in Greek, home of the Bactrian camel, in today's northern Afghanistan), an important commercial, cultural, and political metropolis. It was also a center of religious and intellectual life where ancient Zoroastrianism, Buddhism, Manichaeism, Nestorian Christianity, and early Islam coexisted.

Avicenna spent his formative years in Bukhārā, where he showed early signs of talent; he had memorized the Qur'ān, as well as most of the Arabic poetry he had read, by the age of ten years. He learned Indian arithmetic (calculus and algebra) from the neighborhood grocer and studied Islamic jurisprudence on his own. Abu 'Abdallāh an-Nātelī, a leading philosopher of his time, educated Avicenna in the sciences and advised the father to encourage him to concentrate on learning. After Nātelī, Avicenna studied sciences on his own with the help of commentaries; he read Plato, Aristotle, and Ptolemy. He took up medicine at the age of thirteen years under Abu ibn Mansur and Isā ibn Yāhā, read available books, and did not find it to be a difficult subject. He was sixteen years old when he started visiting and treating patients.

At age seventeen, Avicenna was called to help in the treatment of the Samanid amir (emir) of Bukhārā, Nuh ibn Mansur, who was gravely

---

*Graz, "Prognostic Ability of Practitioners"; and Chisti, *Traditional Healer's Handbook*, 385.
†Afnan, *Avicenna: His Life and Works*.

ill and whose physicians had abandoned all hope for his recovery. To the astonishment of the other physicians, Avicenna was able to cure the amir. The amir rewarded him by appointing him as a court physician and gave him permission to use the dynastic library, which at the time contained one of the world's best collections of manuscripts and books. His scholarly work was done by night because during the day he was busy with the amir and had no time.

Upon the death of his father, Avicenna, then at the age of twenty-one years, left Bukhārā and went to Gurgān. There he started on the first book of his *Canon* and finished it later while in Isfahān. In Hamdān, every night at his home, Avicenna held a circle of study where his pupils read one part of the *Canon* and one part of *Kitāb al-Shifā* (*The Book of Healing*), which is the longest of his extant works.

Some sources attest to Avicenna's handsomeness and striking physique. Although he was praised for his knowledge, he was neither modest nor endearing and had great self-confidence and a flaring temper. He demanded quick wit and perfection from people around him and was known to go over his writing several times.

Of the two hundred books attributed to Avicenna, half are considered genuinely authentic, and fortunately the most significant of them survived. With the documentation of his student, Jūzjānī, we are able to construct the chronology of his writings. He wrote mostly in Arabic and only a few books in Persian. His style was discursive rather than assertive, more lucid than other scientists', and he is also credited with the development of a new philosophical style and terminology. He also introduced more precision in the use of Arabic terms. Sixty-eight of his works are on theology and metaphysics, eleven on astronomy, philosophy, and physics, four on poetry, and sixteen on medical sciences. His second most famous book is *Kitāb al-Shifā*, which is an eighteen-volume philosophical encyclopedia dealing with almost every conceivable topic. Avicenna's medical works earned him the title Prince of Physicians.

The *Canon* is still in print and is actively used at the Unani medical schools of India and Pakistan. His book *al-Adwiyah al-Qalbīyeh* (*The Heart Remedies*) was the first ever written on psychopharmacology.

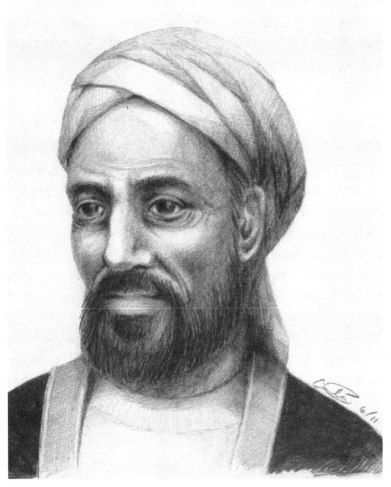

Abū Alī al-Husain ibn Abdullāh ibn Sīnā (980–1037), more commonly known as ibn Sīnā or Avicenna. Portrait by Coco K. Tang, 2011.

Some of his other medical works are *The Book on Psyche, Relationship of Body and Mind,* and *Origin of Grief and the Interpretation of Dreams.*

The conflict between reason and divine revelation dominated Avicenna's time and shaped his philosophical contributions. By seeking refuge from pure Aristotelian reason and from religious dogma, he arrived at a synthesis that placed him at the helm of philosophical thought.

For a physician, his death came in the strangest of ways. While on a military mission with the amir of Isfahān, he developed a severe colic and treated himself with excessive rectal injections. The side effects of the treatment hurt his intestine, and he died in 1037 CE of the complications of an ulcerated and perforated intestine.

TRANSLATIONS AND TREATISES OF THE *CANON*

Avicenna wrote his *Canon* in Arabic, the dominant language of science at that time, and since then, there has not been an English translation of the *Canon of Medicine* directly from the original source.* All the English translations were done from other translations—into Latin, Urdu, and Farsi—but these translations have failed to capture the spirit of the book. As native Arabic speakers (M. S. A.-A. and H. A.), we are in awe of the elegance of the original text. One of our colleagues suggested that all students of science should read the *Canon* to learn good scientific writing and expression.

Avicenna was successful in introducing precision in the use of Arabic terms. Before him, al-Kindi and al-Farabi[†] had attempted to do so, but their efforts had taken the form of aphorisms according to Soheil M. Afnan[‡] (see footnote 8 in Afnan's book). Avicenna's thought and writing are characterized by his passion for classification; his intricate subcategorizing surpassed that of any Greek author, and it is where the medieval European philosophers learned the method.

It is important to point out that any translation and interpretation of Avicenna's *Canon* is also a reflection of the understanding of the translators. A literal translation of some parts of the *Canon* is pragmatically difficult for the reader to put into proper context, and some concepts are hard to grasp without a broad knowledge of biology.

---

*Gruner, *Treatise on the* Canon, 612.

†Abū Yūsuf Ya'qūb ibn Ishāq al-Kindī (Arabic: أبو يوسف يعقوب إبن إسحاق الكندي), known to the West by the Latinized version of his name, Alkindus (ca. 801–873 CE); Abū Nasr al-Fārābī (Arabic: أبو نصر محمد الفارابي), known in the West as Alpharabius (ca. 872–950 or 951 CE).

‡Afnan, *Avicenna: His Life and Works.*

Therefore, we attempt to clearly phrase Avicenna's work as it makes sense to us and to interject our own explanations where we feel that they will be useful for the reader.

Avicenna's career and writings are particularly inspiring for his collection and synthesis of knowledge from the entire known world, his emphasis on the practical application of medical principles (the need to apply knowledge to heal the sick), and his preservation and dissemination of learning to take medicine forward.* Modern advances in the new sciences of molecular biology, biochemistry, physiology, and pharmacology have not replaced or diminished the basic tenets of Avicenna's system; to the contrary, they have revealed to us the need to explain them in light of contemporary knowledge and to find a way to reconcile the two. Actually, the WMS may benefit from taking a fresh look at Avicenna's medical concepts, for they appear to be supported by modern scientific knowledge.

For over a thousand years, Avicenna's *Canon* has been recognized essentially as the authoritative encyclopedia on the Greco-Arabic-Islamic medical system. As a comprehensive body of work that encompasses theory and practice, it follows the teachings, interpretations, and writings of Hippocrates, Galen, Dioscorides, Rhazes, Tabari, and Almajusi.† Beyond this, the elegance of its language and precision of terms, as well as the logical classifications and discussions of the topics, propelled the *Canon* to surpass other medical books. There is a plethora of scholarly commentaries and books on the *Canon,* many confined to the first book, containing the fundamental theories and problems of medicine.

---

*Gordon et al., "Avicenna Directories," 9–11.

†Dioscorides is the author of *De Materia Medica;* Abū Bakr Muhammad ibn Zakariyā Rāzī (Arabic: أبوبكرمحمد بن زكريا الرازي; Latin: Rhazes or Rasis) was a chemist, physician, philosopher, and scholar. Rhazes was born in Rayy, Iran, in the year 865 CE (251 AH) and died there in 925 CE (313 AH). Rhazes' two books are *Alhawi* and *Almansuri fi Altib.* Tabari authored *Firdaus Alhikma,* and Al-Majusi authored *Almaliki (Kamil Alsan'a).*

Reader's Note on the Books of Avicenna's *Canon*

Avicenna's full *Canon* is comprised of 5 volumes or Books:

Book I: General Matters of Medicinal Science

Book II: Single Drugs

Book III: Diseases Specific to Organs

Book IV: Diseases Not Specific to a Single Organ; The Cosmetic Art

Book V: The Formulary and Aqrabadhin

For this book, we have translated the first volume only (Book I). Within our exact translation of Avicenna's text, Ibn-Sina frequently refers to his other books, mentioned above.

In the Middle East, known abridgements of the first book are Fakhr al-Din Razi's (d. 1209) *Sharuh Razi* and Qutb Aldin Shirazi's (1236–1311) *Al-Tohfa al-sa'diya*. Comprehensive commentaries on the *Canon* are Ibn Nafis's (d. 1288) *Sharh AlQarshi* and Hakim Ali Husain Gilani's (963–1014 AH) *Sharh Kulliyat-I Qanun*.

In the Western world, the earliest documented encounter with the *Canon* was during the twelfth century through a Latin translation carried out by Gerard of Cremona (1114–1187), or possibly by Gerard de Sabloneta.* Gerard, an Italian who traveled to Toledo, in Islamic Spain, is considered the father of European Arabism and was the most prolific of all translators of Arabic books. An Uzbek translation of all five volumes, but without commentary, was published in Tashkent (in the former *Union of Soviet Socialist Republics*), from 1954 to 1960.† The ophthalmology section was published in German in 1902.‡ Later in the twentieth century, Dr. Oskar Cameron Gruner translated into English the 1st Book of the *Canon* with the help of the Latin editions of 1595 and 1608, and published it in London in 1930 under the title *Treatise on the* Canon. Gruner attempted to correct many of the mistakes of

---

*For more on the controversy of Gerard's identity, see the foreword by Alain Touwaide.
†Shah, *General Principles*.
‡Hirshberg, *Die Augenheikunde de Ibn Sina*.

the Latin version, but some *tibb* (Unani medicine) practitioners did not like his free translation style of blending philosophy, medicine, physics, and mysticism, and accused him of not conveying the true spirit of the *Canon*.* The Latin translation was the only European translation of the entire *Canon*. A better attempt at producing an English translation was carried out by Dr. Mazhar M. Shah, whose freestyle translation from Arabic, titled *General Principles*, relied heavily on Urdu translations. Most recently, Laleh Mehree Bakhtiar combined the translations by Gruner and Shah of the first book of the *Canon* and added the parts on anatomy in her *Canon of Medicine*. However, her introductory comments are devoid of any scientific basis.

THE DISEASE CONCEPT IN AVICENNA'S MEDICINE

One of the most interesting concepts of traditional medical systems, whether Chinese, Ayurvedic, or Unani, is their nearly identical disease concept as a unifying principle for all these large and ubiquitous medical systems. It should be obvious to us now that, wherever these medical systems may have fallen short on detail, they compensated by elaborating comprehensive, coherent, and useful general concepts that remain a source of strength and a reason for their survival. Not only have their concepts stood the test of time, but modern medical science also now lends support and validation to many of them.

As Avicenna elaborated, the disease state starts by *dystemperament,* which is a change in the normal temperament of an individual, or of an organ, to a new temperament that is outside the range of normal. The temperament is a product of the mixing of the four physical states: warmth, coldness, wetness (or dampness), and dryness. Therefore, a change in one will produce a change in the others. Prolonged dystemperament imbalances the body fluids, the humors, not only in quantity but also in quality. Thus, the state of disease in Unani medicine is based on dystemperament and humoral imbalance.

As Shah stated in his translation of the *Canon,* the temperaments

---

*Gruner, *Comprehensive Glossary.*

are real. We are aware now that a lack of warmth (i.e., the necessary normal range of temperature) disrupts homeostasis, as does a lack of sufficient moisture or hydration within the cells and tissues (dehydration). Differentiated cells require a constant supply of energy to maintain their proper function; a dip in the supply, whether as free heat or adenosine triphosphate (ATP), will bring down the specialized functions of a cell, and a tissue, and in severe cases, the damage will be irreversible. Not only cold exposure will produce such effects, but also infections and poisons. Excessive warmth is also produced by infections of microorganisms.

Temperament is an easier concept to grasp than humors; the subject of humors will be dealt with in the next section, starting on page 65. The three major traditional medical systems mentioned above (Chinese, Ayurvedic, and Unani) are based on the temperament and humoral concepts, which makes one wonder how such concepts evolved independently among the three systems and survived for thousands for years, and how physicians used them, and are still using them, to successfully diagnose and treat patients.

In WMS, the temperaments are considered obsolete and therefore are rarely invoked as the causal agents of a disease. The humors have been replaced by precise molecules such as cholesterol, hemoglobin, and dozens of other measures that appear today on any routine blood work. So, the general health or sickness profile of the Unani concept, based on either dystemperament or humoral imbalance, or both, has been replaced by a series of single, isolated indicators as the basis for diagnosis and treatment. It is exactly here that the modern physicians fail to connect the details supplied to them by the remarkable achievements of modern science. And here the medicine of Avicenna offers a rationalization that is currently missing in modern medicine. We have seen physicians who take the route of using recent technology to translate technical data into the Unani medical paradigm for the diagnosis and treatment of illness. These are by far the superior physicians.

Ancient and contemporary practitioners of humoral medicine worked with classes of bodily fluids rather than single components. It seems that lumping similar biomolecules together did not affect the outcome, and since the instrumentation and knowledge of that time did not permit such precise identification, they had to find a practical way of practicing medicine.

Furthermore, while modern scientists are still debating the causes and the particulars of cancer and its development, Avicenna has speculated on the causes, classified the origins of tumor and cancers, prescribed when to apply surgery to remove a tumor or to leave it undisturbed, and recommended special diets for individuals with cancers. As we have been discovering, all of his hypotheses and observations are in line with recent discoveries about cancer.*

Whether one agrees with all, some, or none of Avicenna's tenets, there is no doubt that his disease concept in Unani is a sound·one. It is truly amazing that an eleventh-century physician could have had this incredible power of observation, understanding of biological nature, and ability to synthesize and communicate his science. This truth logically makes one wonder whether we really need to expend all the trouble, time, and expense on the latest state-of-the-art technologies to effectively diagnose a disease!

THE HUMORS: ARE THEY TRULY THE ENIGMATIC FLUIDS OF THE BODY?

There is not a more misunderstood concept in the history of medicine than the humoral theory. One of the large misconceptions is that the humoral theory started in Greece in the fifth century BCE with the works of Hippocrates and was expanded on by Galen. Such complete attribution to the Greeks is very common in the Western literature since most writers do not bother to check pre-Greek resources nor do they have access to non-Western literature. However, the Western humoral theory dates back to the ancient Egyptian and Mesopotamian physicians. The ancient Egyptians had a well-developed four-humor theory in practice when the Greeks had only three. It was Thales of Miletus (ca. 640 BCE–546 BCE) who studied medicine in Egypt and

---

*Mamtimin, "Plasma Metabonomic Analysis with ¹H Nuclear Megnetic Resonance," 111–15.

added the fourth humor, black bile, to the Greek medical system to bring it into line with the Egyptian.*

The word *humor* is derived from the Greek word *chymos* and its equivalent in Latin, *humor*. Its literal meaning is "fluid," so the common interpretation of humors is that they are bodily fluids that are essential for its proper function. However, the Arabic term for humors as used by Avicenna and others is akhlāt (أخلاط, singular khālt, خلط), which has a different meaning than "fluid." Akhālt means "mixtures," and although Avicenna defined them in general as "liquidy substance," this may not apply well to black bile humor and some other abnormal humors. The Arabic meaning of temperament (mizāj, مزاج) is the "qualitative mixture" built from the elements (hot, cold, wet or damp, and dry and their combinations) and confers the elemental characteristics on the body. The humors in the body according to Avicenna originate from the digested food, and their characteristics and actions depend on the nature of the ingested food, the digestive processes, their physical form (i.e., quality), and their interactions within the body. So in a modern interpretation, the humors are not the blood components, as some have interpreted, but rather the chemical classes derived from food such as carbohydrates, proteins, lipids, organic acids, and their intermediates, which replenish the body with nutrients carried in the blood. Abnormal humors result from the incomplete breakdown of these classes of molecules in the bloodstream, or their aggregation (polymerization) and precipitation.

There are four major humors: blood (*dām*), phlegm (*bālghām*), yellow bile (*safrā'*), and black bile (*sáudā'*). The characteristics of each humor, like temperaments, are associated with those of one of the physical elemental qualities (hot, cold, moist, and dry). Thus, blood humor (*dām*) is hot and moist, phlegm (*bālghām*) humor is cold and moist, yellow bile (*safrā'*) is hot and dry, and black bile (*sáudā'*) is cold and dry. The proper balance of the humors within the body determines the health state of the body and mind, that is, the humors determine the physiological state of health.

---

*Osborn, "Greek Medicine."

Avicenna wrote an elaborate description of the humors, which we explain in detail in the Fourth Lesson of the First Art. The humoral concept is not as simple as some critics of the system may lead us to believe; there is a sophisticated classification of the humors that divides them into normal humors (the good balanced humors) and the abnormal imbalanced ones, and there are subtypes under each of these types. According to Avicenna, humors originate in the body by the digestive processes of ingested food that take place in the stomach, liver, blood, and tissues. He views digestion as a cooking process that breaks down the food into various components where the conditions of digestion determine the physical characteristics and quality of the end products. Therefore, the humors are the available (or resulting) products of four digestive processes that take place within the body. Digestive conditions and food composition determine the proportions of the food that will be converted into each humor. For example, moderate digestive heat is conducive to the generation of blood humor from moderate food (neither hot nor dry), black bile forms if the food was heavy, dry, and especially hot, and yellow bile is generated from slightly hot and sweet fatty food through prolonged digestion, while underdigestion (i.e., insufficient breakdown) produces phlegm from heavy, moist, viscous, and cold foods.

Galen and Avicenna recognized that water is the milieu in which the humors are suspended, as they also recognized that blood is also the carrier of the breath pneuma (in Greek), or rouh (in Arabic), but did not attribute the presence and circulation of breath to any of the humors. One can interpret the last point to mean that their view of the humors was strictly related to nutrients circulating in the blood, or simply that it was beyond their knowledge at that time to speculate on the interaction of the blood or humors with breath.

Matching Avicenna's description of the humors with our current knowledge of biochemistry, one may conclude:

• Blood humor is homologous to peptides (small proteins made of amino acid, the building blocks of proteins).

- Phlegm is homologous to macromolecules of peptides and proteins.
- Yellow bile is homologous to fat.
- Black bile is homologous to all other residual macromolecules such as nucleic and organic acids and other byproducts of metabolism such as lactic and uric acids.

Avicenna also explained the transmutability of some of the humors from one form to another; for example, phlegm may become blood humor with proper digestive heat, the breakdown of three of the humors by excessive heat transforms them into black bile, and the four humors may give rise to their own abnormal and harmful forms when the proper conditions that are favorable to good health (fresh clean air, food, and water, movement and rest, sleep, etc.) are inadequate.

AVICENNA IN THE TWENTY-FIRST CENTURY

It is important to keep in mind that our current Western medical system is an extension of the Greco-Arabic-Islamic system. Not only were the Latin translations of Arabic medical books pervasive throughout Europe, but Avicenna's *Canon* was also a standard medical textbook in several prominent medical schools as Leipzig, Louvain, Montpellier, and Tubingen. The medical curricula at the Universities of Vienna and Frankfurt-on-Oder were structured according to the *Canon*. Many leading Western Renaissance physicians were influenced by the Unani tibb system—for example, Jean François Fernel (ca. 1497–1558). His "crowning work," *Universa Medicina,* composed of three parts, the *Physiologia,* the *Pathologia,* and the *Therapeutice,* uses the classical Unani principles as the basis of his medical philosophy. Fernel, like Avicenna, used the elemental attributes to explain the body's temperaments, humors, powers, and faculties in a holistic approach that we may now call systems biology.*

We are aware that Avicenna's work, albeit based on observation

---

*Welch, "Fernel's 'Physiologia,'" 446–47.

and analysis, was not perfect; however, when viewed as a functional system, it is certainly a sound one. It still has a lot to offer humanity that may well benefit from its application to daily life, for health preservation, and for treatment of medical problems. The biggest challenge now posed is to understand this system according to the way its masters originally intended. The mindset of tenth-century scientists and physicians is different from that of their twenty-first century counterparts, and thence lies one challenge in the interpretation of Avicenna. Nothing illustrates this challenge better than the differences in the Unani disease concept and approach to treatment in comparison with those of modern medicine.

Avicenna, like Hippocrates before him, wrote about medicine in order to bring objectivity to medicine and remove superstition from medical theory and practice. He clearly defined "spirits" as light objects and not as some mysterious entities that defy definition, which we now can see as the oxygen in the air. He predicted the presence of microorganisms and attributed some illnesses to the "malicious bodies" (germs) that can move into the body from soil and water and corrupt its functions.

Other attributes that make the *Canon* interesting reading are the summary statements that Avicenna inserted throughout the book. He summarized the relationship of heat and water to life in one statement: "Life is sustained by heat, and grows by moisture." One can recognize within the *Canon* some of the broad theoretical blueprint for research topics in modern biology. The search for the "spirits" lead the scientists of the eighteenth century to discover oxygen, which later elucidated the process of respiration. The French chemist Antoine-Laurent de Lavoisier stated, "Respiration is a slow combustion of carbon and hydrogen, similar in every way to that which takes place in a lamp or lighted candle and, in that respect, breathing animals are active combustible bodies that are burning. . . ."* This line of investigation ultimately developed into the field of cellular energetics during the first half of the twentieth century. The first decade of the twenty-first

*Lane, *Power, Sex, Suicide*, 71.

century has witnessed the revisiting of cellular energetics to explain issues with cancer, degenerative disease, and drug toxicities. The focus of this trend is to determine the role of the cell's powerhouse, the mitochondrion, in health and disease. Over the last three thousand years, the ancient Egyptians and Mesopotamians, then Hippocrates, Galen, Rhazes, Avicenna, and others have been pointing us in the direction of body energetics as a major factor in health preservation and disease. However, only recently have modern biomedical researchers taken this concept seriously to begin working on its molecular and signaling pathways. Perhaps they are finally on their way to reaching the same conclusions that are in Avicenna's *Canon*!

At this point, it is appropriate to quote Gruner, who wrote, "Advances of modern sciences in molecular biology, biochemistry, physiology, and pharmacology have not replaced or diminished the basic tenets of Avicenna's system; to the contrary, they have revealed to us the need to explain them in light of the new knowledge and find a way to reconcile the two."* Finally, Avicenna's *Canon* brings an uncommon universality to medicine in both theory and practice that he himself may never have imagined. As Afnan elegantly put, "As many like to claim Avicenna, he proves over and over that he is universal."†

---

*Gruner, "Avicenna's *Canon of Medicine*," 239–48.
†Afnan, *Avicenna: His Life and Works.*

CHAPTER 1

Concepts of Unani Medicine

A Primer

Although the predecessors of the current Western medical system (WMS) descended from antecedents within the Unani tradition, the WMS certainly does not presently resemble the classical Unani medicine in any aspect—not even in the concepts that form the bedrock of Unani theory and practice. The two systems now are so different in theory and practice that they appear to have evolved from two different origins. As it evolved from its predecessors, the WMS medical community slowly abandoned the theoretical frameworks represented in Unani for what it thought would be more precise markers of disease.

Instead of using the classes of humors as indicators for health assessment, the WMS has now adopted a long list of single blood markers (or individual blood markers, i.e., glucose, cholesterol, triglycerides, C-reactive protein, etc., referred to as laboratory tests in the clinical jargon). This shift from the historic emphasis on changes that can be observed within a class of markers (i.e., the humors) to that of only single, isolated, biochemical markers has helped transition the WMS to a new reductionist framework of disease diagnosis and management, as well as one-drug-fits-all treatments that differ from the fundamentally preventive and personalized care of Unani medicine.

The blood markers of clinical tests today are mainly used to confirm the presence of illness. They are not used as a preventive tool and do not emphasize population variations, let alone individual specificity. A given disease may often arise through different pathways (a process described as heterogeneity), which gives rise to several subtypes; therefore, single biochemical tests of "biomarkers" are not good indicators of the disease process or its subtypes. In the WMS, what is labeled as a disease, pathologically, is based on the abnormal appearance of tissue cells under a microscope. When the dynamic homeostatic processes of the body are disrupted, creating functional complaints (which can be observed empirically as in the Unani tradition even before the result is biomedically defined as "disease"), the tissue cells eventually respond by becoming abnormal, losing their normal appearance. There are only a few ways that the cells can change in response to disease processes, and standard tissue "pathology" appears relatively late in the process, after the tissues have exhausted their energetic and metabolic means of responding (or reacting) to the disease and trying to maintain homeostasis and "normality."

Additionally, other available biomedical tools have been unable to clearly discern molecular variations and define the boundaries of the disease process to predict its course. Furthermore, the WMS tests cannot be used for early detection of serious illnesses like cancer since they are poor markers of early disease transformation.* Thus, the WMS physician must work without time-tested theories and tools to help make an independent assessment of health status, and has now become a "manager" of disease who must primarily or solely rely on expensive testing machines to diagnose and assess recovery and progress. Physical examination and diagnosis of the WMS patient have been replaced by reading test results, which, in any case, are already delayed messages from a point past where the patient is now.

The effect of the current WMS paradigm on the pharmaceutical industry turned out to be catastrophic (for the patient). The rash of drug recalls that has been beleaguering the pharmaceutical industry in the last twenty years is a direct manifestation of drug design based on an incomplete and often incorrect biological and clinical paradigm.

---

*Abu-Asab et al., "Biomarkers," 105–12.

Why has the pharmaceutical industry not been capable of producing new drugs that are safe and without severe side effects, that would represent true "therapeutic breakthroughs," like we were used to seeing in the middle of the twentieth century? Why are the "blockbuster" drugs of recent decades not the safe, therapeutic "breakthroughs" our parents had come to trust in?

The unfortunate fact, coming out of the side effects of many drugs, is that they damage the mitochondria, the energy generators of the cells, thus, in the timeless terms of Unani medicine, "extinguishing the innate heat of the affected organ."* As the reader will discover in this book, problems that affect the mitochondria are the basic cause of disease; as Avicenna long ago stated in the 3rd Lesson, 2nd Art, "When the organ function becomes abnormal, then there is a problem with its energy, and a problem with organ's energy causes a disease in the organ."

The conceptual framework of Unani medicine encompasses universal principles. Avicenna *repeatedly* asserts and highlights in his *Canon* that these principles are borrowed from the relatively sophisticated physical sciences of his own era. And that the physician does not need to prove their validity because it is the scientists' duty to do that, and not the physician's. That also implies that in understanding biological function and metabolism we should be able to use physics as the basis for chemistry, inorganic chemistry as the basis for organic chemistry, organic chemistry as the basis for biochemistry, biochemistry as the basis for molecular biology and cellular physiology, cell physiology as the basis for biology and physiology, and biology and physiology as the basis for medicine. Instead each of these fields of study, while required, is isolated from the others and does not compute in terms of the concepts and terminology (jargon) of one another. Anyone who has gone through premedical, medical, and postgraduate medical training struggles in vain to discover any underlying concepts and principles that universally apply. Instead, studying each part is like starting over, studying a new language, and often with a new alphabet!

---

*Dykens, *Drug-Induced Mitochondrial Dysfunction.*

As quaint as it may seem, in our modern medical "tower of Babel," the consistent concepts of Unani medicine include the elements, temperaments, humors, "spirit," and innate heat. Avicenna accepts these concepts as axioms since according to him they have been proven by the scientists (whom he calls the natural philosophers, as we in the West did until the nineteenth century; scientists in those days were still called philosophers).

As we discuss in several places in this book, the Unani concepts have stood the test of time, and they are on solid ground from a scientific point of view. The theory of evolution provides a modern framework for biological sciences, where explanations of biological phenomena are compatible with evolutionary biology (called Darwinian medicine and evolutionary medicine). The same compatibility may be applied to Unani concepts; the medical practice and its pharmacology are functional within this conceptual framework.

Readers who are knowledgeable in the theory of evolution will also realize that Unani principles are compatible with the evolutionary framework. Take, for example, the Unani emphasis on innate heat as the measure of health; it is an extension of the fact that symbiotic evolution of the eukaryotic cell provides a better supply of energy to the cell and enables it to carry out differentiation and specialized functions. Without adequate energy production in the cells (i.e., innate heat), cells do not function properly, and that is the Unani definition of disease (see 3rd Lesson, 2nd Art).

Drawing on the above argument, we are listing and discussing in this primer brief descriptions and interpretations of Unani concepts and a few important terms that are used and repeated in the 1st Book of the *Canon*. We aim here to facilitate the reading and understanding of the translated original text.

NOTE ON THE CURRENT TRANSLATION

The current translation is of the 1st Book of the *Canon*, which is largely considered among the best on the theory of Unani medicine. In addition to the theoretical issues, the book encompasses many procedures for disease prevention and health preservation. We have kept the style, as much as possible, close to the original by aiming for clarity. The original writing style of Avicenna is precise, consistent, accurate, and scientific; he has been known to rewrite and edit his work several times before sharing it with his students. Where the knowledge was not supported by clear evidence, or he himself did not have direct experience, Avicenna uses "may be" to denote that, as you will see in the text.

We have adhered to the original organization of the book. However, we have opted to keep out the part on anatomy because we felt that it does not add to the understanding of Unani principles, and it has been superseded by existing (or modern) publications on the topic. The Arabic and Farsi (Persian) names and terms have been placed next to the English translation to facilitate for researchers comparison with the original text. The scientific names of plants have been added after the English names to lessen the ambiguity about the exact plants that Avicenna had listed. Terms and names as well as other Arabic or Farsi words are listed in a glossary at the end of this book. We believe such a glossary is helpful to those who like to refer to the original text or plan on working on similar books (or works).

TERMINOLOGY OF ELEVENTH-CENTURY SCIENCE

The state of knowledge and the lack of sufficient scientific instrumentation in the eleventh century were limiting factors for the resolution of many issues of the time. To compensate for such shortcomings, the scientist of that time resorted to deductive reasoning, observations, and descriptions to fill the void. Such an approach produced occasionally ambiguous terminology that broadly defined phenomena, concepts, and processes. Despite some ambiguity, the terminology was mostly accurate and reflected a wide consensus of the scientists of the time, and even that which extended over a period measured in hundreds or thousands of years. Although old terms like *spirit, humor,* and *elements* seem to us as inaccurate generalizations that do not stand the scrutiny of today's scientific rigor, a closer analysis tells us that they are descriptive terms for the unknown of that time, for now we can translate them as follows:

- *spirit* as referring to oxygen (in fact, *inspiration* can describe taking a breath or being filled with spirit—a connection among mind-body-spirit that the ancients understood better than we do today)
- *humors* as referring to classes of biochemical compounds in the human body, and
- *elements* as referring to the physical states of matter and their corresponding characteristics.

There are more such terms in Avicenna's writings. In this primer we are focusing on the elucidation of some Unani concepts and terms that may become problematic when casting them into the same current usage of the terms, in order to bring out their original meanings as intended by Unani physicians.

CONCEPTS IN UNANI TIBB: MODERN EXPLANATIONS

The Elements: The Four-Element Concept

The well-known cliché about the elements that is repeated over and over is that the ancients thought that all matter is made of four elements. This is actually a blithe distortion of the real meaning of the term and its intended applications. Traditionally, the English translations of the term had ignored the other terms that are actually more informative, as is discussed in the introduction of the 1st Art in this book (page 43).

There are a number of terms listed by Avicenna, such as *origins* and *basics*, that denote that these objects can not be divided into smaller units retaining the same characteristics. The eleventh-century scientists were aware of elements such as iron, copper, gold, silver, and such as elements in our modern sense. However, the four-elements concept is a different system of classification of matter than is our periodic table of elements; it is based on the physical state (solid, liquid, gas, energy), acceptance or rejection of moisture (wet, dry), acceptance or rejection of heat (hot, cold), and relationship to other elements (inner, middle, outer, mixed). Why is such a classification needed? The answer is simple: because it is compatible with the biological nature of living organisms. The physical state, heat, and water are three criteria that can describe the conditions of a biological entity—organs, structures, biochemical compounds, liquids, and such. The combinations of the three physical characteristics of the four elements give rise to the temperaments.

THE TEMPERAMENTS

The temperament (mizaj, الـمـزاج) is a concept and a method by which physicians assess the deviation of the body or any of its organs from normal homeostasis in comparison to the patient's population, race, and species. Simply, it is the expression that Unani physicians use to tell whether the whole body or one of its organs has the right temperature (colder or warmer) and has the right amount of moisture (wetter or drier).

There is no absolute temperament, that is, there is not one universal temperament to which we compare the health of an individual. Also, there is not one temperament that is the best or the optimum for all types of geographical locations. In modern terms, these insights from Avicenna represent the important roles of ecology and environment in the adaptation of the individual through homeostasis and the role of evolution in the adaptation of populations to maintain homeostasis. The temperament of an individual is population-specific based on the evolution of the population within a particular geographic location. The normal population temperament, which is basically the upper and lower limits of the normal range, is the narrowest of temperaments. The population temperament range is a subtype within the larger range of temperaments, and the latter is a subtype with the human species temperament range. Genders differ in their temperaments' ranges. Also, organs of the body vary according to variations listed above.

Abnormal temperament, called dystemperament, occurs when the body or its organs deviate in one or two of the temperamental qualities. Here is where the Unani physician has to determine the qualitative deviation (i.e., which quality is affected, the heat or the hydration) and amount of deviation (the quantity). The physician's assessment of deviation will determine the types of medication to use and their potency.

THE HUMORS

The humors (akhlat, الأخلاط), as Avicenna defines them, are the soluble substances produced from food and drink by the various digestive processes in the mouth, stomach, intestines, blood, and organs. Avicenna follows the traditional Unani classification of humors that includes four major types of humors (blood, phlegm, yellow bile, and black bile). These four humors correspond to the major classes of the biological molecules that we know today:

- Normal proteins fall under blood humor.
- Unassimilated and incompletely digested proteins fall under phlegm humor.
- Fats and lipids fall under yellow bile humor.
- Other classes, such as organic acids, nucleic acids, and metabolic byproducts fit within black bile humor.

Normal humors may change in their quality and quantity and become abnormal humors. Take for example the low-density lipoprotein (LDL), which currently has a bad reputation due to its statistical association with coronary artery disease and the supposed formation of atherosclerosis in arteries. In the context of Unani, LDL is a blood humor, a protein that solubilizes fatty acids and carries the cholesterol molecules across the arterial wall, a normal and beneficial process; however, for unknown reasons LDL polymerizes and precipitates on the inner arterial wall, forming plaques that obstruct the blood flow, leading to cardiovascular disease and death. The polymerization of LDL transforms it from a beneficial blood humor to an abnormal phlegm humor that requires maturation to correct the abnormality. The humoral imbalance in quality and quantity is the trigger for increasing the susceptibility to illness, or it could be indicative of an existing illness.

Critics of the humoral theory argue that the humors are undefined and that no one has demonstrated their presence in the body; others think that humors must be constituents of the blood itself. Unfortunately, such erroneous conceptions dominate the public discourse and have made their way into the print media, becoming the prevailing contemporary viewpoint on humors.

Sadly, these opinions are also prevalent even among those who are open-minded about the use of traditional medicine. Those who claim such misconceptions have not read the original texts on humors, such as that of Avicenna, or if they have, they have not understood them. There are thousands of unknown compounds in the human body that have not yet been identified, and their abnormal qualitative and quantitative changes that contribute to disease have not yet been explored.

Therefore, we are still faced with the same dilemma (albeit to a lesser degree, since we have now some blood parameters to work with) that the physicians of the eleventh century had to deal with; that is, how to spot the early signs of illness, diagnose, and treat when the exact chemical composition is unknown. Now that we know the general chemical classes of the humors, the question becomes, Would a humoral explanation in conjunction with modern blood and serum indicators give us a better preventive and diagnostic advantage? The readers should try to answer this question for themselves.

RAW HUMORS AND THEIR MATURATION

Throughout the *Canon,* there are many references to raw, unripe, and immature humors. Explaining this concept is important to understanding the disease mechanism according to Unani medicine because susceptibility to illness and disease development is tied to the accumulation of raw humor in the body (see the example on LDLs on page 24).

Raw humor is a quality issue that has to be dealt with; the **quality** of the humor, or a metabolite in our modern biology, is an important factor in health preservation, a fact that is rarely given attention when merely measuring the **quantity** of a biomolecule. In a Western-type clinical environment, the physician or nurse may not be aware of this issue since all blood indicators they deal with are quantitative and only measured in the blood, the assessment and treatment is based on whether the test results show above or below the normal range. According to Avicenna, in many instances the raw humor may be higher in concentration within the organ, and not within the vessels, and its effect is local rather than systemic. Ironically, the difference in measuring levels in blood versus organs is well known in the practice of toxicology and forensic pathology—so that modern medicine applies these distinctions to understanding what killed someone, but unfortunately does not use this understanding to help care for the health of living patients!

In Unani medicine, many of the treatments by diet, drugs, or manual procedures target the raw humor to loosen and mature it, which will lead to its conversion to a normal humor or get it ready for evacuation. Maturation of a raw humor is a process that involves digestion of undigested material of the humor or the breakdown of its abnormal aggregation and viscosity. The same process is applied to the waste byproducts in the body to dislodge them and get them out of the body.

WATER IS NOT A HUMOR

Water is an essential part of biological systems, and Unani medicine considers the state of hydration as an integral part of the four temperaments. However, the watery fraction of the blood and other substances is not a humor because it does not nourish but is necessary to soften the food and facilitate its absorption (see the discussion of humors in the 1st Art). Water assists in taking out waste in urine. An excess of water thins the humors and may cause some health problems like nosebleed and loose bowels. Loss of the water fraction from a humor causes its precipitation or combustion, according to Avicenna's terminology (see pages 70 and 73).

THE "SPIRIT" AND "SPIRITS"

Avicenna uses the Arabic term *rouh* (روح), which we translate to its closest analogy in English—spirit. However, we place the term "spirit" in quotation marks throughout the book because rouh as used in Unani medicine is not exactly equivalent to spirit (from Latin spiritus, meaning "breath"), which is actually the equivalent to the Arabic term nāfas (نَـفَـس). The term rouh remains for many people among the most enigmatic and confusing terms, and our interpretation of its use strictly follows the definition that is given by Avicenna. According to Avicenna, rouh as used in Unani medicine differs from the use of spirit in that it denotes an actual physical entity or material that exists in the air, which we have interpreted as oxygen (see page 37).

The confusion about rouh is cultural because it is used to confer a noncorporeal connotation. In classical Arabic, there is a distinction between soul (nāfs, نَـفْـس) and spirit (rouh, روح), however, the two are used interchangeably all the time. The Greek physicians of Unani medicine used the term pneuma, which means breath. In the Arabic and Islamic cultures the term *rouh* is used for the "soul."

The meaning of *rouh* in Unani medicine mirrors similar homologous concepts in other ancient traditional medical systems such as the traditional Chinese medicine and ayurvedic medicine. In traditional Chinese medicine, there is *qi*, and in ayurvedic medicine there is *prana*. The four terms, *rouh, pneuma, qi,* and *prana,* are homologous; they explain the same concept, which is more or less the breath taken in during respiration. However, we now know that within that breath there is the oxygen that is needed to complete the respiratory process within the mitochondria and that without it no organism made of eukaryotic cells would remain alive. Thus, we interpret Avicenna's *rouh,* and the other three terms, to be oxygen.* As you will see, substituting "spirit" for the word *oxygen* throughout the book will make perfect sense, especially for readers who are knowledgeable in biology.

Some erroneously attribute to Avicenna the idea that the heart is the producer of the "spirit," which is a mistaken translation of

---

*Amri, "Physiology of Qi."

Avicenna's writing. His exact statement is that "the heart is starting place of the spirit." This is supported by his assertion that "there is a consensus that the brain and the liver accept nutrients, heat, and 'spirit' from the heart" (see the 5th Lesson, 1st Art). Here he concurred with his predecessors that the heart is, in fact, the universal distributor (we now know through the circulation) of oxygen (through the blood) to all other organs. As we have stated above, Avicenna and others before him were aware that the "spirit" comes from air, that it becomes mixed with the blood in the lungs, and that it then gets distributed, or circulated, to the rest of the body by the heart.

The reason the term "spirits" is used sometimes rather than "spirit" is that the Unani theoreticians thought that there were several types of "spirits," namely, "the 'spirits' of the functions," and that each organ has its own "spirit" responsible for the specialized function of the organ. Therefore, the organs' functions were not attributed to their tissue differentiation but rather to their differences in temperaments (i.e., their energy level). Since we equate the "spirit" with oxygen, then it is axiomatic that there is only one "spirit." However, the Unani ranking of organs from hottest to coldest (as an index of innate energy) cannot be dismissed, since we know now that organs vary in the number of energy-producing mitochondria of their cells and that the shape and size of each organ's mitochondria are specific to that organ.

THE INNATE HEAT

The innate heat (harārā ghareziya, الحراره الغريزيه) is also referred to as vital heat, natural heat, or *calidum innatum,* in Latin. The term describes the heat produced within the body by the respiration within the mitochondria, which should be within a normal population range for each individual. Heat is one of two factors to which Avicenna attributes the existence of life; he states, "Life is sustained by heat, and grows by moisture." He attributes health preservation to the maintenance of the normal level of innate heat, senescence to its weakness, and death to its extinction. Innate heat of the body and its organs is also described as a temperament on a scale between hot and cold in comparison with the individual's population of origin.

The relationship between the innate heat and drug treatment is reiterated in several places within this book. Avicenna explains the interaction between the medication and the body in terms of the effect of the drug on the innate heat; he states that for a drug to work "its effect within the human body [should] produce warmth or coldness unlike those of the human body" (see the 1st Section, 3rd Lesson, 1st Art).

In addition to innate heat, there is sometimes the "abnormal heat" (harārā ghareba, حراره غريبه) that is generated due to toxins, hypoxia, or weakness of the innate heat, and results in putrefaction. The abnormal heat is a state where the innate heat is not strong enough to carry out the normal functions to their completion. According to Avicenna the innate heat ripens, digests, and turns nutrients into normal humors, while abnormal heat corrupts and ruins them. Putrefaction changes the food and nutrients temperament (moisture and heat) without converting them to normal humors (i.e., prevents them from normal assimilation). Thus, it further encourages the formation of anaerobic environments and incomplete digestion and maturation of nutrients. According to Avicenna, "If the innate heat is strong it will enable nature to mediate its action on moistures by maturation, digestion, and preservation of health, therefore, the moistures act in the proper functions and do not follow the influence of abnormal heat, thus produce no putrefaction."

CHARRING

Charring, or burning, as used by Avicenna is analogous to the burning of food on top of a stove when the evaporation of water leaves charred remains. Avicenna uses the Arabic words *ihtiraq* (إحتراق) and *harq* (حرق) to describe the process. The concept of charring is invoked by Avicenna to explain some abnormalities such as mental problems (epilepsy, melancholy), excessive fatigue (see the section on the effects of sleep and wakefulness: 13th Section, 1st Statement, 2nd Lesson, 2nd

Art), some types of swelling, black urine, and black feces. According to Avicenna, the charring process affects the humors and turns them into unusable waste. There are three causes for the charring of humors: excessive heat and dehydration, the overloading of black bile, and hypoxia.

Excessive heat causes the separation of the light part from the thick in humors; this process is also accompanied by dehydration (see the section on humors in the 1st Art). Avicenna writes that charring is "where the light part disintegrates and leaves the thick part" (see the 13th Section, 3rd Lesson, 2nd Art). He also adds that it usually involves the settling down of charred material since "burning is the separation of the wet material by dispersion from the dry one by precipitation."

Furthermore, Avicenna explains charring as the overloading of black bile that leads to the destruction of the tissue. He writes, "The excretion of the original black bile is an indicator of excessive charring and the disappearance of moisture." Because most black bile is acidic (organic acids), the increase of acidity alters the cell functions, and its continued increase may destroy the cells.

A third cause of charring is hypoxia. It leads to reduction in oxidative phosphorylation, thus the decrease in the innate heat and water production as well as the accumulation of lactic acid (a black bile substance). Continued hypoxia leads to the breakdown of cellular organelles such as mitochondria and the accumulation of black bile products in the cells.

The following quotation explains the various types of heating that take place: "*Heating without burning takes place often and does not cause putrefaction, and may happen before putrefaction since putrefaction stays after the dissipation of the factor that caused the initial heat; putrefaction acts on the moist humors by altering their moisture content and their normal functional temperament without converting them to any of the normal qualitative temperaments. Normal warming may prepare and change the wet heat from a qualitative temperament to another that is called digestion and not putrefaction. However, burning is the separation of the wet material by dispersion from the dry one by precipitation. Simple warming is the increase in the temperature of the wet material without changing its temperament to another"* (see the 2nd Art, 2nd Lesson, 2nd statement, 1st Section).

STRENGTH

Strength (Al-quwa, القوه) as used by Avicenna mostly refers to the metabolic functions in relation to respiration and oxidative phosphorylation, which produce ATP, the energy fuel of the cells. It also may refer to the health of the body as a whole or to an organ.

HEALING CRISIS

The Arabic term for healing crisis is *bahran* (بحران). It is defined as the sudden change in the condition of the patient suffering from acute fever, which is usually accompanied by excessive sweating and rapid decrease in temperature. The abnormal heat of fever acts on the maturing of the superfluous matters so that they can be dealt with by the body. It is also described as a detoxification process.

AGING AND DEATH

Avicenna proclaims that the initial temperament the individual is born with determines his or her longevity, and he uses the temperamental health to explain the inevitability of death. Aging and dying are still enigmatic on the molecular scale to modern sciences. However, Avicenna had the broad concept figured out, and his explanation is congruent with our recent knowledge, and with new facts at hand we now can explain his reasoning at the cellular and biochemical levels. Avicenna states, "After the period of youth heat starts to diminish due to the decline in moisture, and in agreement with the internal innate heat and support of physical and psychological actions that are needed, therefore, in the absence of a natural reversal, all bodily functions reach their end" (see the 1st Art, 3rd Section, Temperaments of Ages and Gender).

This statement summarizes the aging process that takes place in the body. The novel concept in this statement is that it ties the aging process to cellular respiration and hydration. As we explain on pages 117 and 118, the hydration of the cell is a by-product of respiration, which produces water as well as energy (any chemical combustion process combines carbohydrate with oxygen and converts it to carbon dioxide and water).

Moisture in the cells and tissues does not come only from the water and liquids that we drink. Actually, the water that we drink may not effectively moisten all of the tissues, or it may take a very long time to reach them and moisten them. The primary source of hydration in the cells and tissues comes from these respiratory processes, such as the breakdown of glucose (through glycolysis and the tricarboxylic acid cycle), fat, and lipids, as well as amino acids, to water and carbon dioxide, in addition to the formation of ATP, the energy currency of the cell. This type of water hydration needs oxygen in order to be formed in the mitochondria, the cellular organelles that are the power generators of most of the cellular energy.

Mitochondria, the energy-producing cellular organelles, are responsible for carrying out the cellular respiratory process, thus the number of mitochondria and their health status are directly correlated to overall health and longevity.

◆

DEFINITION OF MEDICINE AND ITS TOPICS

6 Lessons

Life is sustained by heat, and grows by moisture.

Avicenna

Avicenna starts the *Canon* by defining medicine—its components, the theoretical components of the naturals (tabie'iat, طبيعيات), and the causes of disease (mousabibat, مسببات). The theory of the naturals is a unifying explanation of humans and nature that explains the shared natural building elements of the universe and of humans and classifies the normal constituents and functions of a healthy individual. This 1st Lesson in the Canon is a concise explanation of the reasoning for selecting such components for the medical system. Here is the Lesson in Avicenna's own words. To help distinguish Avicenna's text from our commentary, the translation appears in a different font than our explanations and remarks.

CHAPTER 2
Topics of Medicine

First Lesson of the First Art: Topics of Medicine

- First Lesson (2 sections)
- The Theoretical Basis of Unani Medicine
  (authors' commentary)

FIRST LESSON OF THE FIRST ART

Topics of Medicine
(2 Sections)

FIRST SECTION

Definition of Medicine

I say that medicine is a science through which we figure out the states of the human body, what makes it healthy and what takes away health, so that to preserve the health when present and restore it when gone. One may say that medicine is divided into theoretical and practical, and I have made it all theoretical by saying it is a science. I then answer by saying that some professions may be theoretical and practical, and some logic is theoretical and practical, and it is said some of medicine is theoretical and practical; and it is meant that the theoretical is different than the practical; however, there is no need to explain the difference except in the case of medicine. It is unlike what many think, that one part of medicine is learning and the other is working. It is important for you to know that what I meant is something different and that each of the two sections of medicine is a science, where one is the science of the basics of medicine and the other is the science of practicing medicine. The first concerns the theory, and the second concerns the practice. The theory in the first encompasses the basics as axioms without explaining their mechanisms, such as saying that fevers are of three types and that temperaments are nine. And by practice we do not mean the actual applications of modalities, but the section of medicine where learning leads to an opinion. This opinion is directly connected to explaining the mechanism of action. For example, it is said in medicine that the hot swellings should be approached initially with a repercussive, a coolant, and an exposit,* followed by a mixture of repercussives and softeners, and toward the decline, only decomposing softeners should be applied—except in swellings that are produced by major organs. Such learning gives you an opinion on the mechanism of action; therefore, if you carry out these two parts you get a scientific knowledge and a practical science even if you do not perform the practical part.

No one should say that the states of the body are three: health, disease, and a third state in between the first two, and that I have limited them to two, because if one thinks about it they find that this trinity is unnecessary, but I have not disturbed it. So, if this trinity is a must, then I say that the absence of health is sickness, and the third state does not fall within the healthy. The healthy state produces the proper functions, and these can be defined as wanted and needed. Therefore, the discussion about the third state is not beneficial for medicine, and instead should be carried out by the field of logic.

---

*To exposit is to bring the cause of the hot swelling to the outside.

SECOND SECTION

Topics of Medicine

Medicine is concerned with the human body's healthy and diseased states, and the reasons for sickness. There are reasons for health and sickness, and these may be obvious or hidden. The latter may be figured out from the symptoms; therefore, we should know the symptoms of health and disease. In real sciences, knowledge of a subject happens by knowing its causes and origins, if these were missing then by its symptoms and characteristics. There are four types of causes: physical (maddiya, مادیه), active (fa'ilia, فاعلیه), formative sorriya (صوریه), and functional (tamamiya, تمامیه).

The physical causes are the objects that affect good health and disease, the closest object [within the body] is an organ or breath, and a distant one is a humor, and more distant are the basics [the four elements]. The last two are classified according to their composition and possibly transformation, and each is considered as a unit within a class that forms either the temperament or the structure (haia, هیئه). They form a temperament through transformation or form a structure according to the composition.

Reader's Note

Throughout the book we are using "spirit," breath, or respiration as a translation of روح (rouh), which in Arabic means "spirit." Until the discovery of oxygen in the eighteenth century, the exact entity was a mystery, and it was thought that there were different types of "spirits" in the air, each responsible for the function of a specific organ. *Breath* in Arabic is called *nāfas* (نَفَس), which is different from its close homonym *nāfs* (نَفْس), which means "a soul or being," and may be used to refer to humans and animals. There is a great deal of confusion in the interpretation of these two words, especially among nonnative Arabic speakers.

Active causes are the ones that change or preserve the conditions of the human body, such as air, food, water, drinks, retentions and evacuation, habitat, residency, movement and rest—both physical and psychological, sleep and wakefulness, age changes, sex differences, occupations, habits, and objects that come in touch with the human body that are natural or unnatural.

Formative causes are the temperaments, faculties, and structures.

Functional causes deal with faculties and their functions, and the "spirits" of the functions, as we will show later.

As to complete the topic, for preserving health and eliminating disease, there are other subjects depending on these two conditions. There are the management by food and drink, choice of air quality, alternating between movement and rest, treatment by drugs, and physical manipulation. These are applied to three categories of healthy, diseased, and in-between—although they are not really in the middle.

And if we look in more detail, we have gathered that medicine examines the basics [the elements], temperaments, humors, simple and compound organs, "spirits," natural vital and psychic faculties, functions, states of health and disease and intermediate, as well as the causes arising from food, drink, air, water, habitats, residencies, evacuation and retention, professions, habits, physical and psychological movements and calmness, age, race, and unnaturals that may affect or enter the body, as well as management of health by food, drink, selection of ventilation, choice of movement and calmness, and treatment with drug and manual applications to preserve health and treat a disease. In some of these matters the physician should develop a synthesis for a working idea that is compatible with real science. However, the physician should initially accept the basic principles of the physicist and should prove their validity in his own practice. Some of these basic principles are axiomatic and their proofs can be reached with other sciences, and in such ways basic principles are elevated to the first wisdom that is called metaphysics. If some demand proofs of the elements, temperaments, and what follows them, which is the subject of physical sciences, then they err by bringing issues into medicine that do not belong to it, and they err to think that they can prove the principles, and then they find out that they cannot prove anything. The physicians should trust what they can see and learn from the effects of what they cannot see, and in general the questions should be: Which of the elements and what are their quantities? Which of the temperaments, the humors, and the faculties, and how much? Which of the "spirits," how much, and where?

A change from one state to another and its duration occurs due to a cause; these causes are as above. However, organs and what benefits them can be realized through [observational] faculties and dissection. What the physician needs to theorize and prove are the particular causes of disease and their symptoms, how to remove disease, and how to preserve health by proving what is hidden in detail, measure, and comprehension. If Galen has attempted to prove the first part [i.e., the naturals], he should not do it as a physician but as a philosopher versed in natural science. When a Muslim scholar tries to prove the rightness for absolute consensus, it is not because he is a scholar but for being an orator, therefore, the physician as a physician and the scholar as a scholar cannot carry out any verification; otherwise a quandary will ensue.

AUTHORS' COMMENTARY

The Theoretical Basis of Unani Medicine

Unani medicine, widely known in the Middle East as tibb, is a comprehensive health system that encompasses theoretical knowledge and practical applications (see figure 2.1). It rests on the universal laws as understood by ancient Egyptians and Greeks, as well as Arabs and non-Arabs of the Middle Ages. They produced a coherent and interrelated medical system where science and philosophy were employed simultaneously to create a comprehensive understanding of health and disease. Tibb is recognized by the World Health Organization as one of the alternative systems of medicine (see www.who.int/medicines/en/; accessed December 10, 2012). The system's origins can be traced back to ancient Egypt and Mesopotamia (Iraq), however, the earliest surviving complete works are those of the great Greek physicians

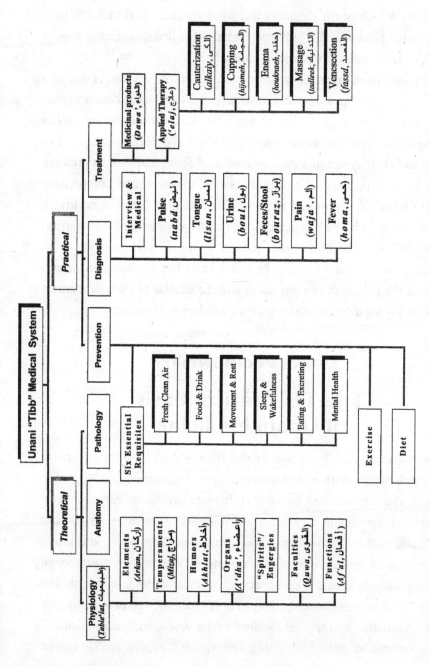

Figure 2.1. Avicenna's Canon is based on the Unani "Tibb" medical system. This ancient system dates back to the Egyptians and combines science and philosophy simultaneously to create a comprehensive understanding of health and disease.

Hippocrates (ca. 460 BCE–370 BCE) and Galen (ca. 129 CE–199/201 CE), who both studied medicine in Egypt. Although the works of Hippocrates and Galen were available in Aramaic (a Semitic language widely used in greater Syria), Arabic translations did not become available until the seventh and eighth centuries. Arab and Muslim physicians such as Rhazes, Avicenna, and Avenzoar further enriched Unani medicine from their own experience and pertinent observation. Avicenna also incorporated Chinese and Indian (ayurvedic) medical knowledge.

Like other traditional medical systems, Unani follows a holistic approach to health maintenance, diagnosis of illness, and restoration of health. As a holistic system, it recognizes all factors that contribute to a healthy body, it promotes the natural recuperative power of the body, and it avoids harming sound parts of the body when pursuing treatment options for a disease.

In an arrangement that mirrors the ancient philosophers' understanding of the evolution of life on Earth and its relationship to the universe, tibb's theory encompasses seven sets of hierarchically related concepts called the naturals (tabie'iat, طبيعيات); the elements, basics, or origins (arkan, أركان); temperaments (mizaj, مزاج); humors (akhlat, أخلاط); organs (a'dha', أعضاء); "spirits" and/or breath (arwah, أرواح); faculties (quwa, القوى); and functions (af'al, أفعال). On the other hand, Unani practice follows the theory of causes (mousabibat, مسببات) for identifying the causes of illness and the theory of signs '(ala-mat, علامات) to define diagnostic symptoms.

THE ESSENTIALS OF LIFE: HEAT AND WATER

As will become evident throughout this book, there are two factors intertwined with the theory and practice of Unani (as well as other traditional medical systems); these are heat and moisture. Ancient philosophers adhered to these two characteristics of matter because they are always fixed to the matter (the elements) and can be felt and measured in a comparison between two objects. Additionally, to understand their significance in all forms of life, one needs to know where and how life evolved hundreds of millions of years ago and how without these two factors life as we know it would not have appeared on Earth.

According to the latest hypothesis, early forms of life, called pro-karyotic organisms, such as bacteria, formed in the ocean's waters around thermal vents spewing hot water. Water provided the milieu where the biochemical reactions took place, and heat was the cata-lyst that supplied the energy of activation to propel the chemical com-ponents to enter into compounds through the formation of chemical bonds.

The ample free energy (i.e., heat, referred to in scientific litera-ture as delta-G [ΔG]) around the oceans' thermal vents produced large quantities of macromolecules, and they became the basis for a more complex form of organization that produced the early forms of self-replicating macromolecules and later bacteria. This scenario started over four billion years ago. Many millions of years later, the unicellular bacteria gave rise to a more sophisticated cell form, the eukaryotic cell. This cell differed from bacteria in having compartments with spe-cific functions. For example, the eukaryotic cell has a nucleus where its genetic material is located, and it has a specialized powerhouse, the mitochondrion, which supplies the free energy and biochemicals needed for its functions. The theory of symbiotic evolution explains the eukaryotic cell's appearance as being due to the engulfment of one bacterium by another where the two were in a symbiotic relationship benefiting from each other.

The new eukaryotic cell that formed with its own energy genera-tor contained within its membrane did not need to remain around the thermal vents of the ocean to stay alive or replicate; its own power generator—the mitochondrion—gave it an advantage that allowed life to expand into all possible niches. Each eukaryotic cell has hun-dreds of mitochondria, which are under the biochemical control of the nucleus.

Although the eukaryotic cell offered new life-forms that were endowed with differentiation and multicellularity, its system was not perfect. Understanding the function of the mitochondria within the eukaryotic cell opens a window for us to understand the vulnerability of the cellular system and the susceptibilities to disease of higher organisms such as humans.

Complex animals, including mammals, birds, and humans, maintain the proper functions of their bodies through established physiological parameters such as controlled temperature and environment, termed *homeostasis*. Sustaining homeostasis within human cells and tissues is a prerequisite for the proper functions of the body and health preservation.

Homeostasis requires the proper temperature and acidity ranges, as well as sufficient water content or hydration. Most of the biochemical reactions of the cell will take place only within the proper narrow ranges of temperature and acidity. For example, the cellular enzymes that are responsible for catalyzing all biochemical reactions are the most sensitive to changes in temperature, acidity, and hydration.

The levels of metabolic chemicals must be maintained in very narrow ranges to be compatible with life. Therefore, disorders and diseases are measured by very small but significant differences in these levels, within narrow ranges.

The importance of heat and hydration for a biological system cannot be overemphasized; these are the primordial prerequisites of life from its simplest to the highest forms, and therefore, these are the two aspects of matter that the traditional medical systems have emphasized for explaining the characteristics and effects of elements, bodily fluids, and treatments with drugs and other modalities.

THE ELEMENTS: A BIOLOGICAL INTERPRETATION

It is worth mentioning here that the Western translations of traditional medical systems have always referred to the basic constituents of biological entities as the elements, however, in the tibb system they are termed the basics, origins ('ousoul, أصول), or phases, and never as elements. It was the Greek-Sicilian philosopher Empedocles (ca. 450 BCE) who termed the elements the four "roots" (*rhizōmata*, ῥιζώματα)—a very close term to the Arabic term for origins. Plato seems to have been the one who introduced the term *element* (stoicheion, στοιχεῖον). We are using the term *elements* here because it is ubiquitous in the literature and used to refer to the same concept in Chinese traditional medicine and ayurvedic medicine.

Although the ancients' concepts of elements among several civilizations (Greek, Arabic, Indian, Chinese, and others) are mostly identical, there are some differences in generalization to the modern concepts of biochemical elements if one follows a strict interpretation of the ancient concepts. In its practical usage, the Unani elements theory uses abstract symbols for quantifying energy and water. There are many today who dismiss the classical elements theory of the ancient systems as inaccurate and as being in conflict with our current understanding of elemental physics, however, as we will try to demonstrate in this book there is not a real conflict and understanding the Unani elements in a modern biological and biochemical context makes good sense. We will attempt to place this concept within its proper context, provide its relevance within the biological and medical paradigm, and explain how the elements became an integral part of the theoretical and practical basis of the Unani medical system.

Although the elements concept is universal, transcends all fields of knowledge, and can be viewed as a unifying theory, this concept is presented here within a health and medical framework and not as the purely physical classification of elements. Bear in mind that the majority of chemical elements do not exist in their elemental state within biological systems but rather as biochemicals in various compounds and organic matrices. Therefore, the Unani medical system considers the biological effects of elements on health in their relationship to heat and hydration. The physicians and philosophers of traditional medical systems were aware of the physical nature of chemical elements such as iron, arsenic, and others as well as their characteristics, but they still used the four-element concept for its relevance to explaining medical and biological phenomena.

The Unani elements also represent the known physical states of matter (solid, liquid, and gas) and energy (fire), and Unani attributes two qualities to each element (hot or cold, and dry or moist). The states of elements are perfectly congruent with our modern physics.

Such classification of elements is dynamic and permits a panoramic gross examination and understanding of the biological system by considering its homeostasis in an observable manner in real time. It will become obvious to the reader that the Unani medical system demands well-trained practitioners who are capable of real-time assessment of system deviations from normal ranges on the basis of bodily fluids and organs as well as their attributes. The practitioner has to understand that the basis of organization and differentiation within the body is the physical states of the matter combined with their qualities as expressed in the concept of the four elements as the temperaments.

CHAPTER 3

The Unani Elements

· · · · · · · · · · ·

The Basics or Origins
(ʿOusoul, أصول)

Second Lesson of the First Art: The Unani Elements

• On Elements (1 section)

The classical concept of elements in Unani medicine recognizes four elements as the major components of all living things. These are earth, water, air, and fire. Each of these elements has two characteristics in relation to heat and moisture. Earth is cold and dry, water is cold and wet, air is hot and wet, and fire is hot and dry. Additionally, earth and water are called heavy elements, while fire and air are light elements. Heavy elements are characterized as being strong, negative, passive, and female, while light elements are weak, positive, active, heavenly, and male.

The earth element in Avicenna's words is "a simple motionless heavy object that occupies the center in a group of elements. It helps life-forms attain cohesiveness, shape, and stability." He also described the elements in relation to each other, writing, "The water element engulfs the earth, and the two are surrounded by air," and he considered the fire element as the connector between the other three elements (see figure 3.1) and attributed to it bringing the earth and water from their elemental states into compounds by reducing their inertia. His description of the fire element is compatible with the modern description of free energy. Furthermore, he considered air and fire as constituents of the life's energies (the "spirits," see "On Elements," page 48).

Continuous change within the human body is produced by the interaction of the four elements. Because the elements must exist in equilibrium to maintain health (homeostasis), any change in the elements is monitored to assess the health status of each part of the body. This concept necessitated the development of a monitoring classification called the temperaments.

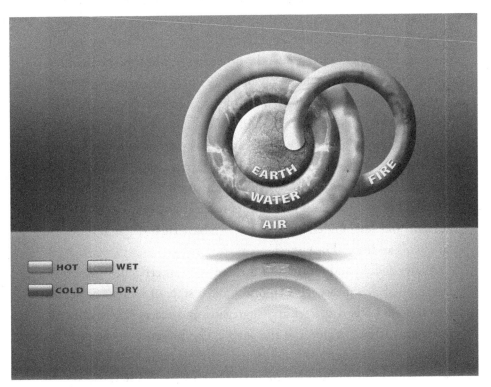

Figure 3.1. The classical concept of elements in Avicenna's medicine recognizes four elements as the major components of all living things. These are earth, water, air, and fire.

The Unani Elements
The Basics or Origins

FIRST SECTION

On Elements

The basics are simple objects that form the essential parts of the human body and others [figure 3.1]. They cannot split into other parts that differ from them in their characteristics; they are also produced by the breakdown of compounds, and their mixing produces all the various species. The physician must take from the physicist that they are only four; two of them are light, and the other two are heavy; the light ones are the fire and air, and the heavy ones are water and earth.

Earth is a simple body that naturally occupies the center of the other elements. It is stationary, and others move to it because of its heaviness. It is cold and dry in nature, and without any other affecters it shows coldness and dryness. Earth's existence in living beings is beneficial for firmness, stability, and preservation of shapes and appearances. Water is a simple body, and its natural position is surrounding the earth and surrounded by air if the two have their original states and the water's additional heaviness.

Water is cold and moist, and if there is no interference from other affecters it shows measurable coldness and a state of moisture. Because of its nature, water disperses and aggregates and accepts the shape of its container without preserving the shape. The presence of water in living organisms facilitates the appearance of their parts in shape, outline, and modification; although a moisturizer leaves as easily the malleable forms as it is accepted, a drying substance is hard to be absorbed or released by malleable forms. From the unity of the moist and dry, the dry accepts the moist and becomes expandable and malleable, while the moist is strongly shaped and modified. The porosity of the dry invites the moisture, and the latter adheres to the dry because of its liquidity.

Air is a simple body that naturally occupies a position between water and fire, and that is due to its additional lightness. Its nature is hot and moist in relation to what we had mentioned [of other elements]. Its existence in organisms produces porosity, amelioration, lightness, and separation.

Fire is a simple body that is positioned above all the other elemental bodies; its place in nature is due to its absolute lightness at the concave surface of the edge of the universe's orbit (الفلك) where the universe and sky end [at the outer limit of the universe; this follows an Aristotelian notion of elemental distribution with the "outer space" occupied by fire being spherical]. The nature of fire is hot and dry. Its existence within organisms brings about ripeness, amelioration, and unity; it runs through organisms by the action of the essence of breath ["spirit," pneuma, rouh, روح].

By engulfing the two heavy cold elements, fire ends their elemental state and brings them into mixtures [i.e., the temperaments]. The heavy elements assist in organ formation and stability, and the lighter ones assist in the formation and movement of "spirits" and organ movement. These are the basics.

CHAPTER 4

The Theory of Temperaments (Amzijeh, الامزجه)

Third Lesson of the First Art: The Theory of Temperaments
- **First Section: On Temperament**
- **Second Section: On Temperaments of Organs**
- **Third Section: On Temperaments of Ages and Gender**

The temperament in Arabic is called *mizāj* (مِزَاج) or *mazāj,* (مَزَاج), which literally means a state of mind or body (mazāj, مَزَاج) and mixture (mizāj, مِزَاج) however, in tibb it is used to describe the quality or qualities of the elemental mixture that constitutes the human body. The temperament here is the net quality as produced by the actions and reactions of the opposite physical qualities of the four elements (earth, water, air, and fire) and their qualities (hot, cold, wet, and dry). A temperament can be used to describe the quality of the body as whole, a single organ, or the totality of the metabolic processes and behavioral and mental profiles of the individual. An individual's temperamental phenotype is acquired; it changes during the various stages of life and is largely affected by the interactions of genotype, environmental effects, and lifestyle choices.

Understanding the theory of the temperaments is important for the practicing tibb physician for several reasons. As we explain in the section on diagnosis, certain disease conditions are associated with certain temperaments (i.e., dystemperament is a disease type; see the introduction to the Second Art on the disease concept in Unani), people vary in their temperaments and normal signs of one temperament are abnormal in others, and the choice of treatment and dose of medication is determined by the individual's or organ's temperamental phenotype. Unani physicians practice individualized medicine, an idea that has just started to take hold in modern medicine but is without solid practice yet.

The four basic temperaments are hot, cold, wet, and dry. However, these four always appear in distinct combinations that raise the total number of temperaments to nine. Other tibb physicians have argued for a higher number of temperaments; for example, Al-Antākī* mentioned seventeen in his book *Tādkerat*. Although Avicenna mentioned nine, his classification of temperaments was more comprehensive because he attributed differences in temperament to species, age, geographic habitat, race, gender, and other factors. The nine temperaments are classified into eight *unequables* and one *equable* (balanced). Unequables are products of the inequality of the opposite qualities; they are comprised of four single temperaments: hot, cold, wet, and dry; and four composites: hot and dry, hot and wet, cold and dry, and cold and wet.

Temperaments form a dynamic system because they are constantly interacting, therefore, the normal temperament is a range and not a strict point. A normal temperament is the most appropriate proportion of the primary qualities in the body or its parts under normal conditions. Humans have a body temperament range that differs from animals, age groups and geographic races have their own ranges, and healthy ranges are different from ranges of illness. Additionally, each organ has its own temperament with ranges of heat and cold, as well

---

*Dā'ūd ibn 'Umar al-Antākī (Arabic: داود بن عمر الانطاكي) died in Mecca in 1599 CE, or 1008 AH.

as wetness (or moisture, to stay consistent) and dryness. For example, the hottest organs are breath (Avicenna calls many body parts *organs*), blood, liver, flesh, and muscles; the coldest are phlegm humor, hair, bones, cartilage, and ligaments; the wettest are phlegm humor, blood, oil, fat, and brain; and the driest are hair, bone, cartilage, ligaments, and tendons.

Avicenna's 3rd Lesson of the 1st Book of the *Canon* on temperaments is elaborate and complex. He defined the healthy temperament as having the optimal mixture of the initial qualities (the elements) that allows the individual to have the best health under the environmental system that the individual lives within. Therefore, Avicenna rejected the existence of a universal optimal temperament and advocated that the human species has a wide-range temperament that is specific to its species, and that within the normal range of this temperament there are subtemperaments for races and populations. Even within a population, the individual has his or her unique temperament that differs from that of another individual. Each subtemperament has its normal range of upper and lower limits (i.e., maximum and minimum temperature values and maximum and minimum moisture values) where the individual is healthy. Avicenna also gave the body organs their own temperaments and stated that the brain, for example, is colder than the heart or liver. The boundaries of a temperament are always in relation to a related group and never as an absolute; the human species has its own temperament in comparison to other species; the same for members within a population of the same species or for an organ.

Avicenna's assessment of biological heterogeneity among humans at all levels from species, through race, population, individual, to organ, reads like a modern course in population biology. This recognition of heterogeneity at all of these levels is a concept that is just emerging in modern medicine, mainly to explain the complex heterogeneity of high-throughput biological data (such as mass spectrometry of serum and gene-expression microarrays), difficulty in finding disease biomarkers, and the failure of targeted treatments of cancers. Avicenna's temperament classification asserts that individualized medicine is the basis of

Unani tibb, as can be seen in this lesson, from the recognition of biological variation of temperaments in the "On Temperament" section.

Drug temperament is an important concept in Unani tibb because it determines what drug to use, its effective dose, its therapeutic effect, and its targeted individual. Avicenna explained that a drug used in the treatment of a patient has a temperament, which is not absolute but is described in relation to its effect on the human body after it has interacted with it. A drug is said to be hot or cold if the effect it produces in the human body is hot or cold, respectively. The same drug may have varying effects in different individuals.

The Theory of Temperaments

(3 Sections)

FIRST SECTION

On Temperament

Temperament is the quality produced from the interaction of opposing qualities that stabilize at a certain point. It is even present in the smallest components as the majority of their parts are in maximum contact with each other. When the qualities interact on their own, the result would be a similar quality: the temperament. The initial qualities mentioned in the Origins (The Elements, 2nd Lesson, 1st Section) of hot, cold, wet, and dry become lost in corrupted bodies. As measured by the absolute ratio distribution, temperament falls into two types. In the first type, the temperament is equitable for all primary qualities [they are equal in quantity and quality], and the resulting temperament quality is the actual median. In the second type, the temperament is not the absolute median but tilting toward one, or both, of the opposing qualities between the hot and cold and between the wet and dry. However, in medicine, the deviation from balance is neither of these two types. The physician must accept from the physicist that these two types should not exist to start with, let alone be the temperament of a human or an organ, and should know that the *balanced* [equitable, moderate] *temperament,* which the physicians use in their reasoning, is not derived from quantitative equality but rather from fairness in distribution, and that is, when in the body of a healthy individual (moumtazij, ممتزج) the temperament components have the optimum quantity and quality for a human temperament at the best distribution and ratio. This optimum human temperament mixture may be close to the first type [equitable for all four qualities as mentioned previously], and this optimum balanced temperament varies according to the types of peoples' bodies when compared with others with different temperaments. Optimum balanced temperament has eight groups according to (1) the species (nou', نوع) compared with an outgroup that differs from it, (2) the variation within the species, (3) a race [or population] within a species in comparison with other races of the same species, (4) the variation within the race, (5) the individual within a race compared with outgroups from his race and species, (6) the individual in comparison with his own conditions, (7) the organ in comparison with other organs within the same body or outside it, and (8) the organ in comparison with its own conditions.

The **first group** represents the human temperament in comparison with other creatures [species]; it has a range but without a strict boundary [i.e., a wide range between the upper and lower limits], however, if it goes outside the upper and lower limits it will cease to be a human temperament. The **second group** represents the median of the broad human temperament, which occurs in an individual of extreme balance from a race of extreme balance in an age of completed growth (hopefully not close to the first type, which makes its existence impossible). Even if this is not the first type as mentioned earlier in the section, still this temperament or individual rarely exists; this person approaches the true balance not by equality but by the balancing and neutralizing effects of the hot organs like the heart, cold like the brain, moist like the liver, and dry like the bones. If we consider each organ as independent by itself, except for the skin (it is described later), and in comparison with the breath ("spirits") and main organs, there cannot be a true balance but rather a tilting toward heat and moisture since the initiation of life is in the heart and the breath ("spirit"), and they are both excessively hot. *Life is sustained by heat, and grows by moisture; heat is supported by moisture and feeds on it.* [In this way, Avicenna's concepts can be likened to the Chinese five-phase system of medicine.]

The main organs are three, as we will illustrate later; the cold one is the brain, and its coldness does not neutralize the heat of the heart and liver; and the dry one or close to dryness is the heart, and its dryness does not neutralize the wetness of the brain and liver. However, the brain is not that cold, and the heart is not that dry, but the heart in comparison with the other is dry, and the brain in comparison with the others is cold.

The **third group** is narrower than the first group temperament [i.e., the species temperament] and has a valid temperament; this is valid for a race of people in relation to a geographic location or climate. For example, the Indians have a temperament that suits them, and the *ṣakalibah* [Eastern Europeans: Russians, Ukrainians, Belarusians, Serbians, etc.] have a different temperament that makes them healthy, and each temperament is balanced within the race but imbalanced for the other races [according to Mafaheem Encyclopedia*]. If an Indian develops the *ṣakalibah's* temperament they become sick and die, and *vice versa*. Therefore, every individual on this Earth has a specific temperament that is suitable for their climate, and this temperament has a range with upper and lower limits.

The **fourth group** is the median of the climate temperament, and this has the most balanced temperament for the group. The **fifth group** is the individual's temperament. It is narrower than the first and third groups, and it is necessary for a living healthy individual to have upper and lower limits. Each individual should have their own temperament that is specific and not similar to that of others. The **sixth group** is the optimal median of a personal temperament. The **seventh group** is the organ temperament that is specific to each organ. For example, the balance for bone is more dry and for the brain more moist, and the heart is warmer than the nerve. This temperament has a range with upper and lower limits and narrower than the early ones. The **eighth group** concerns the organ's balance so that the organ would be at its optimal condition, and it is the median of its temperament range.

If you compare all the species, the human species is the closest to real balance. However, if you consider the races, the one that has the most balanced temperament is the one located at the equatorial day zone, that is if there were not any territorial effects from mountains or sea; the closeness

---

*See in Arabic at www.elazhar.com/mafaheemux/15/19.asp (accessed December 11, 2012).

of the sun does not upset the balance because the fixed position of the sun has less effect on the air quality, and therefore, they enjoy a stability of environment and temperament—and I wrote a manuscript on this topic to correct misconceptions. After the race of this zone, the inhabitants of the fourth zone [region] are ranked as the second balanced.* This is because they are not constantly burned by the sun since it moves away periodically as in the second and third zones; and they are neither washed nor raw like those of the fifth zone or distant zones because of the sun's constant distance. Among individuals, it is the individual from the most balanced race from the most balanced species.

Among organs, it has been shown that main organs are not very close to real balance; you should know that the muscles are the closest to it, followed by the skin. The skin hardly reacts to water that is equally mixed from boiled and frozen; it also has balanced circulation to cool down nerves and does not react to an object that has an equitable mixture of the hardest and runny materials. It is known that the skin does not react to what it does not feel or to objects similar to it, and that objects with similar elements but opposite qualities react to each other since the object does not react to others of similar qualities. The most balanced skin is the hand's, and of the hand, in an increasing balance, are the palm, the fingers, the index, and first digit. This explains why the distal digits are feelers of an object's characteristics. Therefore, the judge has to be balanced on the two issues [heat and moisture] to be able to feel the deviation from balance and fairness [see Avicenna's definition of fairness above]. You should know in addition what we mean when we say that a drug is balanced, because we do not mean that it is equitable in reality because this is impossible, and also it is not similar to human balance since this is the human temperament itself, but we mean its quality after being conditioned by the body's innate heat. Therefore, if the drug quality is not different from that of the human body, then there would not be an effect from the drug. So, if I say that

---

*According to Al-Khwārizmī's weather zones; Abū ʿAbdallāh Muḥammad ibn Mūsā al-Khwārizmī (Persian/Arabic: أبو عبد الله محمد بن موسى الخوارزمي; ca. 780; Khwārizm, ca. 850).

the drug is hot or cold that does not mean that the drug essence itself is hot or cold, or that it is hotter or colder than the human body because otherwise the equitable would be like human's temperament, but rather we meant that its effect within the human body produces warmth or coldness unlike those of the human body. Therefore, the drug may be cold to the human body and hot to the body of the scorpion, and hot to the human body and cold to the snake's body. Furthermore, the same drug may be hotter to the body of one individual than to that of another individual. For this reason, physicians do not insist on using a drug if it fails to alter the temperament.

We have completed the explanation of the equitable temperaments and now to the inequitable. The **inequitable temperaments**, whether you consider them in comparison with species, race, individual, or organ, are eight in comparison to the equitable. These eight are produced by simple deviation in one quality or by compound deviation of two qualities together at the same time. The **simple with one deviated quality**, if it is in the active quality, produces two types: it may be warmer than it should be but not moister or dryer than it should be, or may be colder than it should be but not moister or dryer than it should be. But if it is in the reactive quality, then it has two types as well: it may be drier than it should be but neither warmer nor colder than it should be, or it may be wetter than it should be but neither warmer nor colder than it should be. However, these four are unstable and do not last for a long time since the warmer-than-usual makes the body drier than usual, and the colder-than-usual makes the body wetter than usual with strange wetness, and the drier-than-usual makes the body colder than it should be, and the excess wetness is faster in cooling it down than the drier; if it is in moderation it may preserve it for a longer time but it will eventually make it colder than it should. You understand from this that balanced temperament (or health) is more suited to warmth than coldness. These were the four simple (single) ones.

The compound temperaments have deviation in two qualities at the same time such as when the temperament is warmer and wetter together, or colder and wetter than it should be, or colder and drier together. The temperament cannot be warmer and colder together, or wetter and drier together. Each one of these eight temperaments could take place with a substance (humor, khalt خَلْط, maddeh مادَّه), which may happen when the temperament alone produces a condition that the body cannot react to due to the influence of a dominant humor that affects the body, for example, hectic fever (humma al-madkouk, حُمّى المَدقوق), the coldness of the waist region, or frostbite. Or, these eight temperaments may be accompanied by a substance that affects the body's reaction due to the presence of a nearby dominant humor such as the coolness of the human body because of vitreous or glassy phlegm (belghem zoujaji, بلغم زجاجي) or the warming of the body by leek-green bile (Safra kerathi, صفراء كراثي). You will find in the 3rd and 4th Books examples for each of the sixteen temperaments. Note that the temperament with a substance could translate into two conditions, one where the organ benefits from it due to its beneficial wetness and the other harmful due to its congestion in the channels and cavity of the organ that may cause enlargement. This is our discussion of the temperaments, so the physician can take from the physicist what he cannot figure out by himself.

SECOND SECTION
─────────────────

On Temperaments of Organs

Know that God has given every animal and every organ the temperament that is most suitable and beneficial to its functions and states as permissible. Verifying this truth is the mission of the scientist and not the physician. Additionally, God has given the human being the most balanced temperament in this world that is suitable to his active and reactive functions. Also given for each of the organs is its suitable temperament, thus are some organs warmer, some colder, some drier, and some wetter.

The **warmest** in the body are the "spirit" and the heart, which is the starting place of the "spirit," followed by the blood, which, although it originates in the liver, benefits from its contact with the heart's heat, which is lacking in the liver because it resembles hardened blood. The lung comes next, followed by flesh, which is colder than the lung because of the nerves going through it; muscle is colder than flesh because it is mixed with nerves and ligaments; the spleen is next because of blood residues; kidneys because they do not have much blood and layers of throbbing vessels, not due to the nerves' presence, but rather by the effect of their blood and "spirit"; layers of calm vessels because of blood alone; and finally, balanced palm skin. The **coldest** in the body is the phlegm [humor], followed in descending order (less cold) by fat, hair, bone, cartilage, ligament, tendon, nerve, spinal cord, brain, and skin.

The **wettest** in the body is the phlegm [humor], followed by blood, soluble fat, fat, brain, spinal cord, breast, testicles, lung, liver, spleen, kidneys, muscles, and then the skin. This is Galen's classification. However, you should know that the lung in its essence and nature is not very moist because every organ is similar in its temperament to what goes into it and similar in its opposite temperament to what remains in it. The lung is supplied by the warmest of the blood that is rich with yellow bile—this is from Galen's teaching. The lung may also accumulate a lot of moisture from other parts of the body and whatever comes down from catarrh (nazalet, نزلات).* Based on this, the liver may be moister than the lung in its innate wetness, and the lung far more accepting to wetness, and that its continuous wetness makes it moister in nature. Therefore, you should understand from the states of the phlegm and blood that the moisture of the phlegm is mostly wetness and that the moisture of the blood is part of its essence. However, the naturally watery phlegm is very moist, but the blood loses a lot of moisture that comes to it from naturally watery phlegm when it matures and converts to blood humor. You will learn that the natural phlegm originates from blood humor.

The **driest** part in the body is the hair because it forms from the

---

*Catarrh (pronounced "kə'-tar") is an inflammation of the mucous membranes. It may produce a thick exudate of mucus and white blood cells caused by the swelling of the mucous membranes in the head due to an infection. It is usually associated with the common cold and chesty coughs, but can also be found in patients with infections of the adenoids, middle ear, sinus, or tonsils. The phlegm produced by catarrh may either discharge or cause a blockage that may become chronic.

disintegration of smoky moisture* (bukhar dukhani, بخار دخاني) when it loses its vaporous humor and smokiness settles in. Bone follows hair because it is the hardest of the organs, and it is harder than hair since it forms from blood and it dries the natural moisture and holds on to it. This explains why the bone is nutritious to many animals but the hair is not or rarely is, since it is thought that bats digest it and like it. If we take equal weights of bone and hair and we distill them in the alembic and cucurbit, the bone would release a lot of water and fat and the remaining material has less weight, therefore, the bone is moister than hair. After the bone in dryness are the cartilage, ligament, tendon, fascia, arteries, veins, movement nerves, heart, and the feeling nerves. The movement nerve is colder and drier than the balanced, while the feeling nerve is colder and not drier than the balanced but may be close to it and far from the skin in coldness.

THIRD SECTION

On Temperaments of Ages [Al-assnan, الاسنان] and Gender [Al-ajnass, الاجناس]

Ages are four: age of growth (also called age of youth and renewal [Al-hadathe, الحداثه), and it is close to thirty years; age of maturity (age of strength [Al-shabeb, الشباب]), up to thirty-five or forty years; age of decline (middle age [sin al-muktaheleen, سن المكتهلين]) with preservation of vital strength, up to sixty years; and age of decline with loss of vital strength (age of senility [sin al-shoyukh, سن الشيوخ]), up until death.

The age of growth is divided into (1) infancy, the newborn is not yet ready for movement and standing; (2) boyhood, after standing up and before developing strength and teeth have not completed replacement; (3) growth; (4) adolescence lasts until facial hair appears; and (5) youth lasts until the cessation of growth. The temperament of boys from infancy until the age of growth has balanced heat and is moister. However, some

---

*Ancient authors associated "smoky" nature with ammonia, and we interpret it as referring to protein, however, in other areas it refers to carbon dioxide.

former physicians differed on the variation in hotness between boyhood and youth; some saw that boyhood heat is stronger and, therefore, grows more, their actions of appetite and digestion stronger and lasting, and the innate heat of the zygote is still available to them and strong. On the contrary, other physicians state that the young have stronger innate heat because their blood is stronger due to its plentifulness and strength, and this is the reason they get epistaxis (or a nosebleed [al-rou'af, الرُعاف]) more often and harder, and their temperament is closer to choleric, while boys are closer to phlegm. Youths have stronger actions; their movement is supported by their heat, and their appetite and digestion are stronger because of their heat. However, appetite is not formed by heat but rather by coldness, and this is the reason that bulimia (canine appetite [shehwa kelbiya, شهوه كلبيه]) takes place due to coldness. Youth are stronger because they are less afflicted by what causes nausea, vomiting, and indigestion in boyhood. Evidence that youth are closer to choleric temperament is that all their illnesses are hot, such as tertian fever [humma al-gheb, حمى الغب] and choleric vomit.

Most of boyhood diseases are wet and cold, phlegmatic fevers, and most of their vomit is phlegmatic. Boyhood growth is not from the strength of their heat, but rather from the excess of their hydration; additionally, their appetite indicates lack of heat. These are the two points of view of the two schools and their reasoning. However, Galen replies to both opinions. He sees that heat is initially equal in both ages, boyhood and youth, but the boyhood heat is more in quantity but poor in quality, while youth's heat is less in quantity but better in quality. To explain this, imagine the same quantity of heat spread through a wet object such as water, and through a hard object such as a stone; you will find that hot water has higher quantity and softer quality, and the stone has lesser quantity but sharper quality. According to this, evaluate the heat in boys and youths. Boys are a product of a zygote with excessive heat that has not been weakened, and with their continued growth there is no reason for the heat to diminish. However, youths have not attained any reason to increase or decrease their innate heat, and the heat is preserved by wetness of less quantity and quality until the age of decline. The decline in wetness affects heat preservation but not growth; wetness is initially sufficient for both [preserving heat and promoting growth], but in decline will not support either, therefore, it has to preserve one over the other. It is impossible to say that it will assist growth by abandoning innate heat. How will it support growth if it cannot maintain what is currently there? So, wetness in this case preserves innate heat but not growth. This is the age of youth.

The second opinion that the growth in boyhood is due to wetness without heat is invalid. This is because wetness is a substance for growth and it does not act and produce itself but rather through the action of an acting power on it; the acting power here is the breath ([نَفَس], or nature by the will of God), and its action is through an instrument: the innate heat. Additionally, their opinion [i.e., the second opinion] that boyhood appetite is due to cold temperament is invalid, because the corrupt appetite of a cold temperament does not induce nourishment and assimilation. Nutritional assimilation in boyhood is at its best all of the time, otherwise they would not intake nutrients more than what is used for growth. However, they may have bad assimilation due to their excessive eating of poor quality and moist food and additional inappropriate actions that result in the accumulation of toxins that require a lot of purifying. These affect their lungs and result in higher rate and faster pulse without greatness [the best state of pulse] for lack of complete power. This was the opinion of Galen on the temperament of boyhood and youth, and I expressed it here.

You should learn that after the period of youth heat starts to diminish due to the decline in moisture and in agreement with the internal innate heat and support of physical and psychological actions that are needed, therefore, in the absence of a natural reversal, all bodily functions reach their end. This was proven by physical science, that faculties' action cannot always be building up. If faculties were infinite and always building up, decomposition would remain constant, but it does not and constantly increases day after day, and decomposition consumes moisture; what would the situation be if they both are reducing and declining? If this is the situation, then the material should vanish and extinguish the heat, especially if it is assisted by the abnormal moisture that always takes place due to weak digestion, which participates in its extermination in two ways: the first, by suffocation and drowning [i.e., hypoxia], and the other, by an opposing quality, the cold phlegmatic moisture [i.e., due to incomplete assimilation]. This is the eventual death for every individual according to their first temperament's strength in preserving moisture.

"For each person a certain age and for each age a certain end,"* therefore, longevity varies in people according to their temperaments; these are the natural ages, but there are also premature deaths. The conclusion is that the bodies of boyhood and youth are moderately hot, and those of the middle age and elderly are cold. However, the bodies of boyhood are moister than moderate in order to promote growth, and this is evident from the softness of their bones and nerves—measuring this from their proximity to inception [zygote formation] and moist breath [womb environment]. The middle age and elderly are drier since they are colder, and this is evident from the hardness of their bones and dryness of their skin—gauging by their distance from their inception, blood, and moist breath. The fiery [temperament] is equal in boyhood and youth, while airy and watery is more in boyhood, and earthy more in middle and older age—and even more in the elderly. Youth is more of moderate temperament than boyhood, but drier than boyhood, and hot temperament in comparison to the middle aged and elderly. The middle age is drier than youth, and the elderly's original organ temperament is moister than both [youth and middle age] by the abnormal wetting moisture.

Gender temperaments differ. Females have colder temperament than males, which is the reason they are shorter than males in physique and less moist. For the coldness of their temperament they are more curious, and for their lack of exercise their flesh is soft. Although a man's flesh, from the composition point of view, is smoother due to what mixes with it, the cooling effect due to the penetrating vessels and nerve fibers makes it denser.

The inhabitants of the northern countries are more moist, and the opposite is true, and water workers are also more moist. Signs of temperaments will be listed in the total and partial signs.

----

*A Qur'ānic verse.

CHAPTER 5

The Humors
(Akhlāt [ʾḥlat], أَخْلَاط)

Fourth Lesson of the First Art: The Humors

- **First Section: The Definition of Humor and Its Types**
- **Second Section: How Humors Are Generated**

The concept of humors is very important and a fundamental basis of Unani medicine, as well as ayurvedic and Chinese medicines. The introduction mentions some of the issues associated with the interpretation of the humors, their history, and some of the viewpoints on this concept. However, this section is restricted to the Unani view of humors. Because of the importance of this section as a theoretical base of Unani medicine, and due to the many circulating misconceptions associated with humors, we present a literal translation in its entirety. This will also permit readers to reach their own conclusions on the meanings of humors and synthesize their own interpretations of these concepts.

The term *humor* is derived from the Greek word *chymos* and its equivalent in Latin, *humor,* which simply means "fluid," however, the Arabic terminology means "a mixture" (أَخْلَاط) (singular khālt, خَلْط ، أَخْلَاط). The Arabic term can be applied to liquids and nonliquids, which fits well with the concept of humors since not all humors are soluble, such as black bile, which encompasses solid substances. Avicenna defined humors as a "runny substance" that originates from food; they are carried throughout the body by the blood and used for nourishment and growth. However, humors are not the blood itself but only fractions of its composition. Therefore, one should distinguish, for example, between blood as the liquid circulating in the body and blood humor as a substance because blood humor refers to a fraction carried by the blood that represents good, available nutrients. The humors (the liquid ones) are neither the only liquids of the body nor the only cause of illness.

Retrospectively, there are clearly a few missing elements in Unani medicine that were beyond the knowledge of the time because the science of a thousand years ago could not have resolved them. One of the most obvious is the lack of a clear description of the chemical composition of humors. The exact molecular chemistry of our food was unknown; the major groups of our diet—carbohydrates, fats, proteins, and other macromolecules—were unresolved a thousand years ago. Albeit one may infer, from the descriptions of Avicenna in the *Canon*, the nature of these substances. When Avicenna referred to blood humor as being red in color and sweet, he was describing the characteristics of a proteinaceous and sugary substance; his descriptions are similar for the yellow bile as fatty; the phlegm as a heavy, thick, polymerized proteinaceous substance that required further processing to become available for the body; and black bile as biochemical compounds other than the three other categories and substances of various origins, such as broken cellular components from necrosis or apoptosis, or the byproducts of certain foods as uric and lactic acids, for example. Although Unani physicians had known that breath mixes with blood in the lungs before circulating to the heart, they had not speculated on the mechanism of breath attachment to the blood (that is, the binding of oxygen to hemoglobin in red blood cells) or its components. Nowhere in the *Canon* can one find a discussion of this point.

Also, there is a potentially confusing disconnect between the humors and their corresponding blood fractions as described by Avicenna. His description of yellow bile from blood as bright red in color does not fit well with the nature of the material as a foamy, fatty substance unless he was describing a blood-mixed fat; and also the black bile is not really black or sedimentary at all times. Our own interpretation of such confusion is that Avicenna tried to maintain allegiance to the original descriptions of Galen and Aristotle while introducing his own ideas, as is evident from the extremely respectful and frequent references to both throughout the *Canon*. However, if one takes his various descriptions as a general concept that he himself always viewed as a feasible framework to practice medicine, then his humors truly approximate our known four major groups of biological macromolecules that are essential for life.

Avicenna viewed the task of gathering and studying basic knowledge as well as proving various hypotheses to be restricted to scientists who were referred to during his days as physicists or natural philosophers. For Avicenna there were basic scientific facts that were axiomatic, such as the elements, the characteristics of the temperaments, and the humors. The body of knowledge on these scientific facts was handed down to physicians by the physicists, who had already worked out the verification of facts, and according to Avicenna, it was not the duty of the physician to prove any of the facts related to them but rather to use them as the theoretical and practical basis for understanding the disease and treating the patients. Avicenna's perspective as a physician was not to let theoretical "mechanisms of action" overcome clinical observations, and empirical evidence, regarding human physiology and therapeutics.

Although many references credit Hippocrates for the development of the humoral theory, the theory is even older, with roots in ancient Egypt and Mesopotamia (Iraq), and cannot be attributed to a single person or region. Avicenna accepted Hippocrates's and Galen's classifications of four primary humors and their subtypes and added the secondary humors of the tissue fluids (inter- and intracellular).

Unani recognizes four primary humors, the blood (dam [dām], الدم), phlegm (balgham [bālghām*], البلغم), yellow bile (safra' [ṣāfrā'],

---

*The accent marks included in the second spelling of balgham indicate proper pronunciation.

الصفراء), and black bile (sauda [sāudā'], السوداء), and secondary humors that include waste and nonwaste. Ancient Greek medicine differed from Egyptian medicine in that it used only three humors: blood, phlegm and bile. The addition of the fourth humor, black bile, to ancient Greek medicine was done by Thales (ca. 640 BCE–ca. 546 BCE), who had been educated in ancient Egypt, in order to bring Greek medical practice into alignment with that of Egypt. According to Unani tibb the four main humors exist in the bloodstream at different quantities and proportions to each other and are considered among the essential components of the body that exist in the vascular system. Good health is attributed to the balance of good humors; therefore, Unani treatment focuses on restoring humoral balance in sick individuals.

Each humor can exist in two states: normal and abnormal, with several subtypes of the latter. Additionally, a humor is described according to two natures, such as blood humor is hot and wet, phlegm is cold and humid (or wet), yellow bile is hot and dry, and black bile is cold and dry. As we have learned earlier in the chapter, these two natures are permanently associated with physical states. The temperament of the individual is the net result of the proportions of the four humors. The predominant humor determines the type of temperament that characterizes the individual: when blood humor predominates it is called sanguine (damawi, دموي), it is phlegmatic when phlegm humor predominates (balghami, بلغمي), bilious or choleric when yellow bile humor predominates (safrawi, صفراوي), and melancholic when black bile humor predominates (saudawi, سوداوي).

Every individual has a unique balance of the humors in their normal healthy state. Humoral balance is maintained by the faculties (quwa, قوى; described in detail later), which are the metabolic processes, functions of organs, and psychological strengths. Unani places significant emphasis on diet and digestion for the maintenance and restoration of humoral balance and health, as well as the restorative power of the faculties. Medicines are used only when diet and exercise need to be fortified.

FOURTH LESSON OF THE FIRST ART

The Humors
(2 Sections)

The Definition of Humor and Its Types

The humor is a moist, runny substance that originates from food first; it encompasses a beneficial type that becomes an essential component of the body either by itself or in combination with others. The transformed food resembles the humor in its independent form or when in combination. Overall, the newly transformed humor replaces the decomposed portion, and it also comprises waste products and a bad portion, which rarely becomes a good humor and should be sent out of the body.

We state that the body's fluids are primary and secondary. The primary ones are the four humors that we mention, and the secondary humors are the waste humors and nonwaste tissue humors [In *The General Principles of Avicenna's Canon of Medicine,* Shah translated the latter as "essential"]. We will mention the waste humors. The nonwaste tissue humors are transformed from their essential states and infiltrate the organs but have not become part of the single organs by complete transformation. These are of four types: (1) the liquid in the tiny blood vessels that are adjacent to the proper organs that supply them; (2) the liquid that keeps the organs moisturized (similar to dew), and this humor could turn into a nutritional source when supply is scarce and replenish the organ's moisture when lost due to violent movement or other effects; (3) a close-to-maturity humor that is similar to that of the organ in temperament and composition but not in complete texture; (4) the humor in the original organs that exists since inception, originating in the zygote, which originates from humors and keeps the parts of the organs in contact [*milieu interieur* is the extracellular fluid].

We state, also, that the beneficial and waste humoral fluids are restricted to four types: blood, phlegm, yellow bile, and black bile. **Blood** (dam, الدم), hot in nature and moist, is of two kinds: normal and abnormal. The normal blood is red colored, without a stench, and very sweet. Abnormal blood divides into two types: (1) changed from good blood humor without any admixing with other material but due to dystemperament such as development of cold or hot temperaments; (2) mixed with a bad humor that arises in two ways: (a) the bad humor is external, mixes with it, and corrupts it; or (b) the bad humor originates within it by putrefaction and transforms that layer to bitter yellow bile and dense, bitter black bile, and one or both remain in it. This latter type varies depending on the material with which it mixes, and its types are like those types of phlegm, black bile, or yellow bile, and watery; it becomes sometimes turbid, light, dark black, or white, and other times changes its smell and taste to bitter, salty, or acidic.

Phlegm (balgham, البلغم) also is normal and abnormal. The normal type could turn into blood at some time because phlegm is an immature blood (a type of sweet phlegm); it is not very cold in comparison with the whole body, but cold in comparison with the blood and yellow bile. Some of the sweet phlegm is abnormal: this is the tasteless phlegm that we shall mention if it gets mixed with normal blood as experienced in colds (inflammations) and menstruation. However, Galen stated that nature has not prepared a reservoir for the normal sweet phlegm like the two bitter humors [yellow and black biles] because phlegm is very similar to blood, all organs need it, and that is why it flows like the blood. And, we state that this occurs for two purposes: one is necessity and the other is beneficial. There are two reasons for the necessity; the first, to be close to the organs; when supplies to the organs from stomach and liver are scarce, it becomes blood. For such unusual circumstances, the organs' faculties use its innate heat to mature it, digest it, and use it as a nutrient. The innate heat ripens, digests, and turns it into blood, however, abnormal heat corrupts and ruins it. This process is not necessary for the two bitter humors since they are not similar to the phlegm in that the innate heat transforms it into blood, but they are similar to it in that the abnormal heat turns them into putrefaction. The second reason, for necessity, is that it mixes with blood to prepare it for nurturing the organs with phlegmatic temperament that require a certain amount of phlegm in their blood supply, such as the brain. This is also shared with the two bitter humors. The benefit comes from the wetting of joints and organs with excessive movement, so that they do not dry out because of the movement and friction. This is a benefit of extreme importance.

Abnormal phlegm [numbered 1–8] comprises the waste phlegm, such as (1) the **mucoidal** (al-mukhatee, المخاطي), which has a heterogeneous texture to the touch; (2) the **raw** (al-kham, الخام), which is homogenous to the touch; (3) the **watery** (al-ma'ee, المائي), which is light; (4) the **gypsoid** (al-jissee, الجصي), which is very dense and separates and precipitates into a layer in the joints and exits; it is the thickest of all; and (5) **salty** (al-maleeh, المالح), which is the hottest, hardest, and driest of the phlegm types. The cause of all saltiness that takes place is the balanced mixing of watery moisture, of little or no taste, with burned earthy parts of dry temperament and bitter taste; its excess increases bitterness. From this, salts are generated and water becomes salty. Salt can be made from ash, alkali, and lime, as well as other sources, by cooking them in water, filtering, and then boiling and reducing the water until crystallization occurs, or leaving it alone to dry and crystallize. **Yellow phlegm** develops by balanced mixing of **light phlegm** that is tasteless, or with little and weak taste, with burned bitter dry humor that turns it salty and hot. The respected physician Galen stated that this phlegm adds saltiness due to its putrefaction or admixing with watery humor; and we say that putrefaction makes it salty due to the burning effect followed by the mixing of ashiness (al-ramadyeh, الرمادية) with its moisture; watery phlegm does not by itself cause saltiness without the second reason [mixing of ashiness]. There is also (6) **acidic phlegm. Sweet phlegm** is of two kinds: (a) sweet by nature, and (b) sweet from mixing with strange matter.* So is the acidic phlegm, it can be of two kinds: one due to mixing with strange abnormal substances such as the acidic black bile (we will mention it later), and the other reason is from within,

---

*Sweet phlegm is normal phlegm that may become abnormal. Avicenna is trying to explain how the sweet phlegm may turn into abnormal forms such as acidic phlegm.

such as what happens to sweet phlegm (or on its way to be sweet) and other sweet humors of boiling, then acidity. Phlegm can be (7) **acrid** (aafss, عفص) due to mixing with acrid black bile or because of extreme cooling that converts its taste to acridity by increasing the rigidity of its water and its tendency to dryness, therefore, it did not mature because of the heat weakness and instead turned acidic. Some of the phlegm is (8) **glassy** (zujajee, زجاجي), thick and resembles the melted glass in its density. It can be acidic or insipid (tasteless). The dense insipid resembles the raw or can be converted to the raw; and this type of phlegm is watery and cold in the beginning, so it does not become corrupt or mix with others but stays confined until thickened and colder. Therefore, the types of abnormal phlegm according to taste are four: salty, acidic, acrid, and insipid (tasteless) (musseekh, مسيخ); and also four according to density: watery, glassy, mucoidal, and gypsoid. Also, the raw is counted as mucoidal.

Yellow bile (al-safra, الصفراء) also is normal and abnormal; the normal is the blood foam, which is bright red in color, lightweight, and hot in temperament. The warmer it is, the more red in color. When generated in the liver, one part of it goes with the blood and the other to the gallbladder. The portion that goes with the blood meets a necessity and confers a benefit. The necessity is supplying the organs that require yellow bile for their temperaments with a normal portion of yellow bile, and the right proportion as in the lung. The benefit is to ameliorate the blood and facilitate its entry into very small vessels. The filtered portion that goes into the gallbladder is necessary for the elimination of wastes and benefits the gallbladder by supplying it with nutrients. The benefit is also in that it rinses the intestines of the residues and viscous phlegm, and it stimulates the large intestine and sphincter to encourage excretion. Therefore, sometimes colic develops when the (biliary) tract from the gallbladder to the (small) intestine gets blocked.

The abnormal yellow bile occurs due to admixing with strange abnormal substances or by deviation from normal due to intrinsic abnormal change. Of the first type, the most well known is the one that mixes with phlegm, and it is generated in the liver most of the time and termed **bitter yellow bile** if it mixes with light phlegm or **bitter yolk** if it mixes with thick phlegm, and there is the less known type that mixes with black bile, which is called **burned yellow bile**. The latter may happen in two ways: first, when the yellow bile burns by itself and produces ashiness that makes it difficult to distinguish between its good part and its ashy part, and if the ashiness becomes trapped then it is bad; second, when the black bile arrives from a different location and mixes with it, which is better than the previous one. The color of the latter is reddish-yellow, not bright or radiant, but similar to blood, and its color could change.

The abnormal type that is caused by intrinsic deviation from normal is generated mostly in the liver, but is overproduced by the stomach. The one from the liver is of one type that is light and, if it burns, produces black bile. The one from the stomach is of two kinds: leek green (kerathee, كراثي) and verdigris (zenjaree, زنجاري). The green is produced by the burning of yolky, yellow bile when the blackness mixes with yellow and produces green color. The verdigris is generated from the green yellow bile by excessive burning that displaces all of its moisture, and its color tends to be whitish. Heat initially produces blackness in a moist body, and then blackness starts to disappear with the dissipation of moisture, and eventually bleaches it into white. Observe what takes place in a piece of (burning) wood; it first turns into charcoal because the heat turns the moist object black and a dried object white. Coldness turns a moist object white, and a dry one black. My description of the green and verdigris yellow biles is a hypothesis. The green is the hottest, worst, and most fatal type of the yellow biles.

Black bile (es-sawda, السوداء) is also normal and abnormal. In a fine blood, the normal black bile is sedimentary (rusubee, رسوبي), residual (thefel, ثفل), and causes its turbidity (aa'keer, عكر), and tastes between sweet and acrid. If it is generated in the liver it gets distributed to the blood and spleen. The part that mixes with the blood fulfills a necessity and confers a benefit. It is necessary in the blood supply to the organs, such as bones, that their temperament comprises a black bile. The benefit comes from its effect on the blood, where it strengthens, thickens, and prevents its disintegration. The part that goes to the spleen is a fraction that the blood gives away for a necessity and a benefit. The necessity is a cleansing of the whole body from dregs and nourishment of the spleen. As for the benefit, it occurs when the black bile breaks down at the stomach mouth; it binds, thickens, and strengthens it. Black bile also stimulates with acidity the stomach mouth and gives the feeling of hunger and appetite. Also note that the yellow bile effusing to the gallbladder is unwanted by the blood, and the yellow bile effusing out of the gallbladder is an excess. The same applies to the black bile effusing to the spleen; it is the excess in the blood, and what is released from the spleen is from the excess there. The latter yellow bile [coming out of the gallbladder] stimulates excretion from below while the latter black bile [at the stomach mouth] stimulates food intake from above.

The **abnormal black bile** differs from the normal one in that it is not sedimentary, but similar to the ashiness of charring. A substance of earthy temperament shows its earthiness in two ways: (1) by precipitating, and an example of this is black bile, or (2) by charring, where the light part disintegrates and leaves the thick part in the blood and humors; an example of this is the waste black bile that is called the **bitter black bile**. Precipitation is a blood characteristic, whereas phlegm is viscous [dissolving well] and does not cause any sediment [precipitation], and yellow bile is light, constantly in motion, lacks earthy temperament, and also does not separate from the blood in appreciable quantities. That which separates, putrefies, or is excreted loses its light [useful] fraction and its thick [waste] part becomes charred black bile and is not sedimentary.

Waste black bile may be the ash and charring of yellow bile, which is bitter. The difference between this and burned yellow bile is that the latter has this waste black bile mixed with it, and it also exists by itself. Waste black bile has lost its good fraction; some is the ash of phlegm charring. If the phlegm is very light and watery it gives salty ash, otherwise it tends to be acidic or acrid. Some waste black bile is the product of blood charring, and this tends to be salty to sweet. Black bile may give rise to abnormal types; the light black bile produces very acidic ash like vinegar boiling at the surface of the earth with acidic fumes that repel flies and alike. The thick black bile produces less acidic ash with some acridity and bitterness. There are **three types of bad black bile**: the charred yellow bile that lost its good fraction, and the other two types that follow [i.e., phlegmatic and blood black biles]. The phleg-matic black bile is slow in its harming effect and less dreadful. The burned four humors may be listed according to their vileness: black bile is the worst in form and effect, and yellow bile is the most susceptible to corruption but the easiest to treat. The other two are worse, depend-ing on their acidity—the more acidic the worse—but they accept the treatment the earliest it is applied. The third is less reactive with earthy substances, less attached to organs, and slow to become fatal, but more difficult to disintegrate and mature, as well as to accept the treatment. These are the natural humors and the waste ones.

Galen said, "It is incorrect what some state that the only normal humor is the blood and the other humors are useless waste"; this because if blood were the only humor that nourishes the organs, then all the organs would be similar in temperament and texture. And since bone is harder than flesh, then its blood is mixed with black bile, and since the brain is softer, then its blood is mixed with soft phlegm. The blood itself is mixed with the other humors and separates from them when placed in a container, according to touch, into a fraction that is a foam, which is the yellow bile, a fraction that resembles egg white, which is the phlegm, and turbid sediment that is the black bile. There is also a watery fraction that is waste and is released in urine; however, the watery part is not a humor because it does not nourish but is necessary to soften the food and infiltrate it. The humor originates from the nourishing food and drink, and by nourishment we mean that, by its power, it is similar to the body, which is the human body, that is, of mixed temperament, and not simple. Water is simple. It is not true what some people think that the strength of the body is due to excess of the blood, and its weakness due to its scar-city, but if the weakness is caused by it then fixing it will fix the weak-ness. Some people think that if the ratio of the humors to one another is maintained as the human body requires, then health is preserved, but this is not the case. Every humor should have its own constant quantity, not in comparison with other humors, and at the same time, a fixed ratio to the other humors. There are other issues about the humors, but their discussion is not suitable for physicians because it is not their specialty and should be left to the scientists; therefore, I kept it out.

SECOND SECTION

How Humors Are Generated

Note that the food is digested by mastication because the surface of the mouth is connected with the surface of the stomach as if the two are one, and it has a digestive capability; it changes the state of the masticated food via the innate heat* of the saliva. For this reason, masticated wheat by itself has an effect on the maturation of pimples and boils that is different from its water-soaked grains, or from cooked flour. Others have stated that the evidence that masticated food undergoes a little digestion is that it loses its original taste and odor. Then when it enters the stomach it gets fully digested not only by the heat of the stomach, but by the additional heat that comes from the liver on the right side, and from the left side by the heat that is generated in the vasculature of the spleen, as well as by the heat dissipating from the frontal (abdominal) fat layer because of its capability to generate heat and its fatty supply to the stomach. As from the top, the heart heats the middle of the diaphragm. If the food gets digested it becomes (in many animals), together with the drink it mixes with, into chyle [from Greek *chylos*, juice], which is a whitish thick substance that resembles dissolved, dried yogurt paste and has the texture and color of barley water. After that, its good portion seeps from the stomach and the intestine through a network of veins that is connected with all of the intestines called mesentery. Through the mesentery it gets to the portal vein and gets distributed throughout the liver in a network with small, hairy branches that meet the openings of the roots of the vein leaving the liver at the *kyphosis* [hump]. Water, in excess of that needed by the body, assists in the movement of the chyle through the vessels, and it gets distributed through the whole liver and acts on it intensely and fast. When this takes place, the chyle is cooked, and like all cooking there is a foam and there is a sediment, and there may be some burning when cooking is prolonged or rawness [uncooked] when shortened. The foam is the yellow bile, the sediment is the black bile, and both are normal. The light

---

*Its capability to carry out action, which is digestion in this case.

portion of the burned substance is waste yellow bile, and the thick portion is bad black bile. The raw, uncooked portion is the phlegm. The remaining mature substance is the blood, which after passing through the liver is lighter than it should be due to the excessive water that was needed initially. When the blood leaves the liver, waste water separates from it, and this waste water goes through a vein to the kidneys, carrying with it some blood that is sufficient by quality and quantity to nourish the kidneys with fat and blood, and the rest goes to the urinary bladder and ureter. The rest of the good blood in the liver goes through the vein at the hump of the liver, then the branching veins, the creeks, the canals of the branching veins, the feeders of the canals, and then the fibrous hairy veins; it percolates from their mouths into the organs.

Blood humor is actively produced by moderate heat, and it is made from moderate food and good drinks, and its formative cause is good maturity, and its purpose is to nourish the body. Normal **yellow bile,** which is the blood foam, is generated by moderate heat, but the burned one is due to excessive burning heat, especially in the liver, and both types come from slightly hot and sweet, fatty food. Its formative cause is overcooking, and its purpose is necessity and benefit, as we mentioned before.

The **phlegm** is generated by undercooking [i.e., insufficient digestion], from heavy, moist, viscous, and cold foods. Its purpose, as mentioned earlier, is necessity and benefit. Normal **black bile** is produced by moderate heat, and burned black bile by heat that surpasses moderate from very heavy, dry foods, especially the hot ones. Its formative cause is the sediment that resists movement or decomposition, and its purpose is the mentioned necessity and benefit.

Black bile increases due to heat of the liver [overdrive or incomplete breakdown of toxins], the weakness of the spleen, excessive freezing cold, permanent congestion, or lasting chronic diseases that brought the humors to ash. If black bile increases, it settles between the stomach and the liver and reduces the generation of blood and other good humors and thus decreases blood.

You need to know that heat and cold are two causes, in addition to other causes, that generate the humors; however, moderate heat generates the blood humor, excessive generates yellow bile, very excessive produces black bile by charring, coldness produces phlegm, and the very cold produces black bile by freezing. However, you should take into consideration the active faculties, along with reactive faculties, and must not think that every temperament produces the biles that resemble it, and accidentally the opposite. If it is not exact, the temperament could excessively produce the opposite; the cold dry temperament produces the abnormal strange humidity due to weak digestion, and such a human being is usually thin with loose joints and fearful, their body cold and oily with narrow surface vessels. Older people are cold and dry with similar abnormal moisture.

In circulation, blood and the other humors undergo a third digestion. A fourth one takes place when the humors enter the tissues. The waste of the primary digestion of the stomach is excreted through the intestines. Most of the waste from the secondary digestion in the liver goes out in the urine, and a small fraction goes to the gallbladder and spleen. The waste of the third and fourth digestions is removed by unfelt decomposition, by sweating, by felt secretions of the nose and ear wax, by unfelt secretion like that of skin pores, or unusual discharges via boils and abscesses, as well as extra growth of hair and nails. Know that a person with thin humors gets weakened by their reduction and suffers weakness from the wide pores because decomposition is followed by weakness and thin humors are easier to decompose and eliminate. Elimination of thin humors weakens the vital force, thus further increasing their decomposition.

Know that, as there are reasons for the generation of humors, there are reasons for their movement. Movement and hot things induce the movement and strength of the blood and yellow bile and may move the black bile. However, rest strengthens phlegm and types of black bile. Mental activity moves humors, such as looking at a red object induces the movement of blood; this is the reason that a person with a nosebleed is told not to look at bright red objects. This is what we say about humors and their generation, and those who are in disagreement in the correctness of this should discuss it with philosophers [scientists] and not physicians.

TABLE 5.1. A SUMMARY OF THE PRIMARY AND SECONDARY HUMORS AND THEIR SUBTYPES

Primary Humors

1. Blood Humor (dam, الدم)

Normal Blood Humor:

Red colored and very sweet without any stench.

Actively produced by moderate heat.

Made from moderate food and good drinks through good maturity.

Its purpose is to nourish the body.

Abnormal Blood Humor:

1. Abnormal due to cooling or heating.

2. Abnormal due to admixing with other humors:

 a. Mixes with external bad humor.

 b. Bad humor originates within such as bitter yellow bile or dense bitter black bile. Form: turbid; light; color: dark black or white; and taste: bitter, salty, and acidic.

2. Phlegm Humor (balgham, البلغم)

Normal Phlegm Humor:

Resembles egg white. Sweet phlegm.

Generated by undercooking [i.e., insufficient heat], from heavy, moist, viscous, and cold foods.

Its purpose is necessity and benefit (see text).

Abnormal Phlegm Humor:

Tasteless sweet phlegm (when mixed with normal blood humor).

According to taste:

1. Salty (المالح).
2. Acidic (الحامض).
3. Acrid (العفص).
4. Insipid (التفه).

According to density:

1. Mucoidal (المخاطي).
2. Raw (الخام): counted under the mucoidal.
3. Watery (المائي).
4. Glassy or vitreous (الزجاجي).
5. Gypsoid (الجصي).

3. Yellow Bile Humor (الصفراء)

Normal Yellow Bile Humor:

Blood foam that is bright red in color, lightweight, and hot in temperament.

Generated from slightly hot and sweet fatty food through overcooking.

Its purpose is necessity and benefit (see text).

Abnormal Yellow Bile Humor:

A. By admixing with other humors:

1. Bitter yellow bile, mixes with light phlegm.
2. Bitter yolk, mixes with thick phlegm.
3. Burned yellow bile, mixes with black bile.

B. By deviating from normalcy:

1. Burned yellow bile, abnormality arises within the humor:

   a. Produced in the liver.

   b. Produced in the stomach.

     i. Leek-Green (كراثي): produced by the burning of yolky-yellow bile.

     ii. Verdigris (زنجاري): produced from the green by excessive burning.

4. Black Bile Humor (السوداء)

Normal Black Bile Humor:

It is the part of the blood that is sedimentary, residual, and causes its turbidity.

Produced by moderate heat from very heavy, dry foods, especially the hot ones.

Its formative cause is the sediment that resists movement or decomposition.

It serves a necessity and a benefit (see text).

Abnormal Black Bile Humor:

Produced by heat that surpasses moderate from very heavy dry foods, especially the hot ones.

Bitter black bile arises from the charring of yellow bile.

Salty to acidic or acrid black bile arises from the charring of phlegm.

Salty to sweet black bile arises from the charring of blood.

Very acidic substances (like vinegar, lactate, citrate, and so forth) arise from the charring of black bile.

Secondary Humors

Nonwaste Interstitial Humors:

Transformed from their essential states and infiltrate the organs but have not become part of the single organs by complete transformation.

a. The liquid in the tiny veins that are adjacent to the proper organs that supply them.

b. The liquid that keeps the organs moisturized (similar to dew), and this humor could turn into a nutritional source when supply is scarce and replenish the organ's moisture when lost due to violent movement or other effects.

c. A close-to-maturity humor that is similar to that of the organ in temperament and composition but not completely in texture.

d. The humor in the original organs that existed since inception that keeps the parts of the organs in contact [intracellular fluid = cytoplasm]; it originated in the zygote, which originates from humors.

Waste:

Such as urine, feces, and sweat

Implications of the Humoral Theory
on Diet and Food Preparation

The concept of humors, as outlined in the writings of Avicenna, extends beyond the body and enters into our diet and food sources and, importantly, methods of food preparation. Avicenna established the humors as the connection between the food we ingest and its effects on our body by defining them as the substances into which food is converted in the body. This is not surprising given that the vast majority of what we eat ends up as the building blocks of our body's tissues, drives our metabolism, provides energy, generates the waste we must excrete, and ultimately helps determine our state of health (or illness). An important point that should be reemphasized is that the humors are not the whole constituents of the blood fluids or solids, but rather the nutritional fraction of them that is available to the tissues for sustenance and growth. As such, the humors are important for the well-being of the individual, and their imbalance according to Unani medicine may have pathological effects that are signs of abnormal states of health.

Avicenna defined body humors as the materials into which the food we ingest is transformed (i.e., their source is the food we eat), and this has implications for the food we select and its methods of preparation. He further explained how the digestive processes are similar to the cooking process, which transforms the food into substances ready to be converted into humors. The food is digested through the first digestion in the stomach and intestine, the second digestion in the liver, the third digestion in the blood, and the fourth in the tissues to produce the humors. He also considered mastication as a form of digestion. More importantly, Avicenna considered the cooking process as a generator of humors; he stated, "Like all cooking there is a foam and there is a sediment; and there may be some burning when cooking is prolonged, or rawness when shortened. The foam is the yellow bile, the sediment is the black bile, and both are normal. The light portion of the burned substance is waste yellow bile, and the thick portion is bad black bile. The raw uncooked portion is the phlegm. The remaining mature substance is the blood." *It is unmistakably clear that Avicenna thought that the body's digestive processes for food are similar to the effect of cooking, with the end product of both being the humors.* Simply put, both processes break down food into its basic components, the humors. If conditions are within the optimal range, they produce the normal humors; otherwise, they give out abnormal humors depending on the severity of deviation from the normal range of "cooking."

Traditional Old World cooking within many cultures emphasizes well-prepared food that should be soft and easy to digest. It is usually a process where the end product does not resemble the raw starting materials in color, taste, or texture, and where the fusion of oils, spices, and other condiments presents tasty, healthful, and sustaining dishes. Probably, no microwave cooking can produce the same results! Within the humoral context, it is obvious that healthy living requires a proper method of food preparation and cooking; it also points out what to eat and what to reject. One should favor well-cooked food whose components have been cooked through, turned into light texture, and contain a minimal amount of burn (no black sediment), and reject food (or at least minimize its consumption) that is lightly cooked, dense, or overcooked with black sediment. Differences in cooking styles mean that the same food may have different effects and results within the body; two people may eat the same food prepared in two different ways, and each may experience different effects and benefits from it. Avicenna tells us that well-cooked food has more "blood humor" in it (the most beneficial type of humor) than the halfway cooked, which will have more "phlegm humor" that requires more of the body's energy and resources to digest later before it is converted to a fully useful form—usually the blood humor. Also, burned food contains the harmful types of the yellow and black humors. The latter statement may explain the harmful effect of burning foods produced by barbecuing and grilling, as well as severe microwaving.

The quality and quantity of humors are determined by several factors: the quality and types of food we start with, the cooking process that transforms the food into digestible and available substances, the quality of stomach digestion, and the processing or digestion in the blood and tissues. However, let us not forget that the body's humors may change into their abnormal types by the exposure of the body to environmental factors such as coldness or toxins.

Black Bile: Cause or Consequence of Diseases?

We know by now that the humoral theory is ancient, with historic roots in Egypt and Mesopotamia (Iraq). However, one of these humors stands out in the Unani literature as the most detrimental. Many adverse effects are attributed to black bile; for example, according to Hippocrates, tumors were caused by an imbalance of the four humors: blood, phlegm, yellow bile, and black bile, with black bile particularly having the worse effect. Galen adopted the black bile theory of Hippocrates and speculated that black bile caused severe, ulcerated, and incurable cancer, whereas thin bile was responsible for nonulcerated and curable cancer.* The reader may be confused here as to how bad black bile, a humor either ingested as such or produced from the other three humors, can be so powerful as to cause cancer in addition to other illnesses.

When trying to interpret the writings of ancient physicians, it is always central to keep in mind that Unani physicians were excellent observers of metabolic changes and they tried to explain their observation within the knowledge of their time. Our current knowledge tells us that black bile can be produced by a state of disease that was not necessarily originally caused by black bile. For example, some cancers are the result of exposure to harmful radiation that causes mutations within the genetic material, and these cancers, like all other cancers, produce "black bile" substances such as lactic acid (lactate), succinic acid (succinate), fumaric acid (fumarate), and oth-

---

*Hajdu, "Greco-Roman Thought about Cancer," 2048–51.

ers. These substances are normal when they are within their normal ranges and when their corresponding metabolic enzymes are normal and functional. Hence they can represent normal black bile; however, when their production is out of control they become the harmful, abnormal black bile. An example of black bile produced from blood humor is uric acid, which is a metabolic product from purines, a component of DNA; certain foods such as meat, some fish, and dried beans will increase uric acid concentrations in the blood and lead to painful joints (gouty arthritis).

Our current biology predicts that black bile substances in the body are produced when something goes wrong with metabolic processes at the cellular level such as a mutation in an enzyme gene that affects a metabolic reaction, ingestion of a toxin (or its accumulation over time) that disrupts a metabolic reaction, or an infection with a virus that affects nuclear or mitochondrial functions. The products of a metabolic disorder are usually harmless substances under normal conditions where they are broken down or excreted; however, their accumulation above the upper normal limit will eventually overload the organs and lead to sickness in the individual. Furthermore, these abnormally high accumulations of some substances trigger alternative metabolic pathways (e.g., hypoxia pathway) that may permanently alter the metabolic fate of the cell and thus its phenotype.

We conclude from this discussion that black bile as a cause or a result of diseases can have two sources of accumulation in the body: the first by its ingestion, either as black bile or as other humors that are then transformed into black bile, and the second by its production from abnormal metabolic processes. While the first will produce humoral imbalance and sickness, the latter is a result of cellular metabolic disruptions that may eventually cause disease.

CHAPTER 6

The Organs according to Avicenna

Fifth Lesson of the First Art:
The Organs according to Avicenna

• Authors' commentary

Avicenna attributed the origin of organs (a'dha', الإعضاء) to the "benevolent humors of the zygote, which are generated by the first elemental temperament" and defined the essential organs as the ones needed for the preservation of the body and species. He classified the organs into simple and compound, with the simple organs having parts that are similar to each other like the flesh, bone, and nerve, and the compound organs having dissimilar parts such as the face and the hand. He then described the simple organs from the inside out, starting with the bone, "the first of organs with similar parts: it is hard because it's the foundation of the body and supportive of movement." Then he went on to describe the simple organs and their functions, such as joints, nerves, ligaments, arteries, veins, flesh, brain, and liver, and classified them according to their acceptance and sharing of breath and heat, and their faculties. For example, he stated that there is a consensus that the brain and the liver accept nutrients, heat, and breath ("spirit") from the heart, and each of them has a faculty that affects other organs, so both are receivers and donors. However, the skin for example is a receiver and not a donor. Avicenna concurred with his predecessors that the heart is the universal donor to all other organs that require nourishment, perception, and movement. Avicenna cited Galen as saying, "Some of the organs have only action, some others have only benefit, and others possess both action and benefit. The first like the heart, the second like the lungs, and third like the liver."

Most of the remainder of this section, however, is anatomical descriptions that do not represent, in retrospect, a unique strength of the *Canon,* and we will leave it out for the sake of brevity and in order to focus on more important topics.

CHAPTER 7

A General View of the Faculties and Actions

·············

(Quwa and Af'al,

(القوى و الافعال)

Sixth Lesson of the First Art:
A General View of the Faculties and Actions

- Authors' commentary
- Chart of the faculties and their relationship to each other

---

A faculty is a sense, capability, or functionality that is based on the biological system of an organ; therefore, faculties and actions are characteristics of the organs. Galen thought that each faculty belongs to a certain organ that represents it and carries out its actions. Unani medicine recognizes three types of faculties: the psychological, the natural (physical), and the vital (animalistic).

The psychic faculties (quwa nafseyeh, القوى النفسيه) represent the conscious and unconscious mind; they reside in the brain, which is the source of their actions: behavioral, voluntary movement, and sensation.

The natural faculties (quwa tab'yyah, القوى الطبيعيه) have two types; one is concerned with the preservation of the individual, such as nutrition, it resides in the liver, and the second type governs the reproductive biology and resides in the gonads. Because they fall into those that serve other faculties and those that are served by others, they have a hierarchical relationship (see chart on page 90). For example, the growth faculty is served by three others: assimilative, adherent, and receptive. These three supporting faculties serve the growth faculties' receiving, keeping, and synthesizing. The growth faculty serves the forming faculty, which in turn serves the generative faculty.

The animalistic faculties (quwa hayawaniyyeh, القوى الحيوانيه) are the source of the motive faculty or life force (referred to by classical Greeks as *thymos* [θυμός]); they manage the issues of breath that underlie perception and movement. According to Avicenna, the source of this faculty is the heart. However, Avicenna stated that Aristotle attributed to the heart the origin of all faculties and to the other organs the actions; however, other physicians attributed perception to the brain and to each faculty an organ that carries its action. Avicenna concurred with Aristotle, but stated that knowing the exact facts on this issue is the job of the philosopher and the naturalist and not the physician, who need only know the actions of these organs.

We explain the faculties and their relationship to each other by a flow chart on page 90 to simplify the diversity that Avicenna presented in the 1st Book.

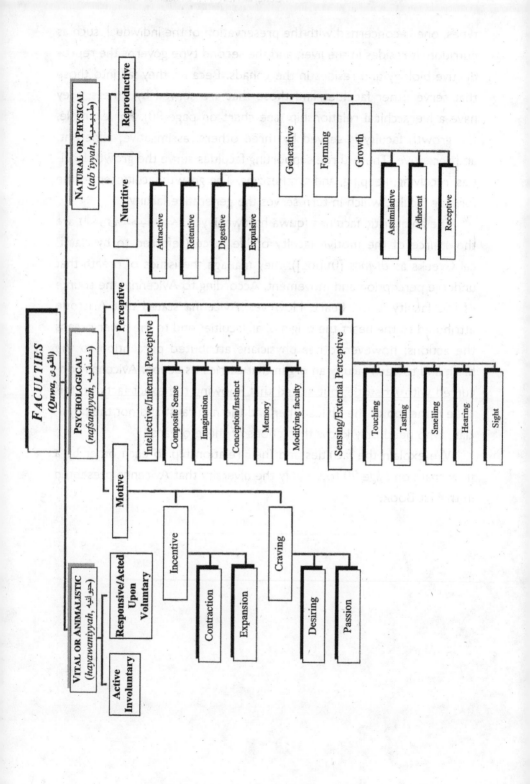

DISEASE, CAUSES, AND GENERAL SYMPTOMS

3 Lessons

In general, diseases are of three types: diseases of dystemperament, structural diseases, and diseases of discontinuity.

AVICENNA

DISEASE CONCEPT

A unique characteristic of Unani is the concept of disease, which differs from that of the WMS. It may be surprising for many that there are different ways of defining what constitutes a disease. The disease concept of a medical paradigm is a foundation of the system's practice. It defines what composes a disease, circumscribes the role of the physician, and sets parameters of treatment, prognosis, and therapeutic expectation. The differences among various disease concepts are not trivial since each concept is based on (or emphasizes) different aspects of the disease process (symptoms vs. cause, or a set of abnormal parameters). Thus medical systems differ in their disease etiology, their assessment of symptoms, and their implications, treatment regimen, and definition of a complete recovery.

Unani has a well-defined disease concept and thus differs from the more loosely defined concept currently followed in Western medicine. Therefore, it is important to explore the Unani concept of disease in order to understand its framework and its application in practice. In several places of this book, including the translations below, there is a central emphasis on the causes of the pathological condition as they relate to *temperaments* and *humors* rather than symptoms. It is also reflected in the disease classification system that Avicenna had outlined.

In the current WMS, and aside from genetic disorders and infectious diseases, there is really no clearly defined concept of disease similar to the Unani concept. Traditionally, the WMS defines a disease by a number of symptoms that are then traced back (or not) to the corresponding pathophysiological factors that link each effect to its cause; the causes are then attributed to the abnormal parameters in diagnostic test results. Diagnosis and treatment in the WMS are based on the simple correlation of clinical syndromes and a reductionist pathological analysis; this approach limits our knowledge about the disease processes over time and limits our knowledge on when to intervene and to what degree.* In the WMS, none of the causes are attributed to dystemperament or a class of "molecules" such as a humor. In the reductionist scheme of the WMS, it is usually one biochemical compound that is the culprit (e.g., prostate-specific antigen, C-reactive protein, creatinine, serum glutamic oxaloacetic transaminase, and others). The disease then gets attributed to one abnormal reading, and the treatment usually targets this one molecule.

Take for example the extreme overemphasis on LDL and its associated cholesterol. Without understanding the cause behind the rise in LDL and cholesterol, the WMS physicians prescribe statins to lower cholesterol, incidentally creating the latest generation of "blockbuster" drugs for the pharmaceutical industry. Many do not even give you the option to try to adjust your LDL and cholesterol by following a healthy diet and attaining a healthy weight, which is the real reason behind the problem most of the time. By examining the temperaments in the patient, Unani assesses more parameters; for example, important parameters are the tissue's energy and hydration measured as temperaments. In the WMS, there is no measure of energy production or hydration of

---

*Roukos, "Networks Medicine," 695–98.

the body or its organs; therefore, it does not have any concept equivalent to dystemperament.

The same is true for humoral imbalance as a causal factor in Unani; the WMS does not attribute the cause of disease to a class of molecules but rather to one or a few molecules, as if one metabolic pathway works totally independently from other pathways. As a matter of fact the WMS still struggles to define what causes a disease at the cellular and molecular levels, and on a more serious note remains unsure of what is the normal range for some parameters. Cholesterol's upper range has been adjusted and readjusted several times without any consideration to gender, race differences, and geographical location. Unani medicine has a well-defined chronological notion of disease phases and progression, and most diseases have four phases: incipience, increment, acme (peak), and decline (see the 7th Section in this Lesson). The duration for each of these phases is specific to the resulting disease. The disease phases are significant in Unani because each is a chronological phase with its specific treatment. The phases concept is almost absent in the clinical practice of the WMS since its reductionist framework continues to define disease and diagnosis as the relationship of symptoms to single blood chemicals and imaging technologies, which in fact do not exist in complex, dynamic physiological and pathophysiological processes.

Over the last fifty years, tens of billions of taxpayer and investor dollars have been spent in the United States alone on reductionist biomedical research to find out the "key" gene expressions, proteins, and other metabolic changes that are presumed to be associated with disease initiation and expansion, yet without producing any meaningful results. Despite the impressive body of knowledge that has accumulated over the past half century, biomedical research within the WMS has been conducted without a well-defined molecular framework of disease concept. For example, despite the large number of cancer researchers working on all types of cancers, whether to find a cure or to understand its particulars, we are still in the dark as to when a cell becomes cancerous (i.e., the molecular events that transform a cell to a cancerous phenotype). The WMS has not provided us with any meaningful or effective early detection method for the majority of diseases. Recent studies have shown that even some of the biomarkers that have been in use as "reliable" indicators of pathology such as prostate specific antigen (PSA) and cancer antigen 125 (CA-125) are actually of questionable value for early detection.*

By contrast, within the Unani paradigm, Avicenna had long ago given us an accurate general understanding of cancer's biochemistry that is compatible with our recent findings about cancer and, in a step far ahead of its time, prescribed a suitable diet for individuals with cancer that is consistent with the ketogenic diet (calorie-restricted diet with high-fat and high-protein content) that is now emerging as the most suitable diet for cancer patients. This last point tells us that one may find some remedies in Unani medicine for certain ailments that the WMS does not offer.

Unani medicine also differs from the WMS in its view on infectious diseases. While the WMS views the invasion

---

*Abu-Asab et al. "Biomarkers," 105–12.

and establishment of a pathogen as the beginning of the disease, Unani attributes the success of the pathogen to the individual's susceptibility to infection (host factors) due to dystemperament or humoral imbalance. Supporters of the Unani view observe that in an epidemic (even of catastrophic proportions) not everyone gets infected despite the ubiquity of the infectious agent, just as most people with streptococcus in their respiratory tract do not develop strep throat infection.

CLASSIFICATION OF DISEASES ACCORDING TO AVICENNA

Avicenna defines illness as an abnormal state that leads to dysfunction. While he classifies dysfunction into two types (dystemperament or structural abnormality), illness is classified into three types (disease of dystemperament, structural diseases, and disease of discontinuity); any illness should belong to one of these types and attributed to it. As Avicenna explains in the section on temperaments, on page 50, there are sixteen dystemperamental conditions that produce sixteen diseases of temperaments; eight of these are pure temperamental problems while the other eight are associated with humoral imbalances. Humors, as we have learned earlier, are the main natural classes of biological substances that exist in the body (proteins, fats, organic acids, etc.), they are obtained from food, and through digestions form the nourishing material that sustains and builds the tissues. They are carried in circulation by the blood, but they are not by themselves the whole blood itself.

Diseases are also categorized in Unani as single or compound. The single diseases encompass one type of dystemperament or one type of structural disease, while the compound diseases have two types that work simultaneously to produce an illness. Therefore, in Unani disease is a symptomatic dysfunction that may be caused by dystemperament, a combination of dystemperament and humoral imbalance, structure (acquired or inherited), or discontinuity; all these causes may also act in various combinations.

One may wonder how this classification of disease encompasses infectious and genetic diseases, which are caused by infectious agents (bacteria, fungi, viruses) and various types of genetic problems, respectively. Ancient Unani physicians were aware of the nature of infectious and contagious diseases and suspected "malicious bodies" in causing them. For Unani physicians the effects of these invisible microorganisms, or "germs," were visible as dystemperaments and humoral imbalances, and therefore, they addressed the latter two as the targets of the treatment.

HOW DOES UNANI MEDICINE DEAL WITH GENETIC DISEASES?

Although the genetics and molecular knowledge of today were unknown to Unani physicians of that time, we find that they explained what we call today genetic diseases within the paradigm of humors, or body constitution. They incorporated genetic disorders into the Unani disease concept without the knowledge of the underlying gene defect, which is the "cause" of the disease. They did so by empirically describing the effect of these genetic defects on the humors; one may say that they confused the effects for the cause. However, a positive aspect is that, by attempting to ameliorate the effect, they did the best that could be done in such situations.

A combination of dystemperament and humoral imbalance is the hallmark of many diseases, such as degenerative diseases, genetic disorders, and cancer. The genetic abnormalities (such as single nucleotide mutation, translocation, copy number variation [duplications], etc.) that underlie disease were unknown to physicians before the second half of the twentieth century, so like most traditional physicians, Unani physicians described mostly the metabolic effects of these diseases and attributed the disease manifestations to the obvious dystemperament and humoral imbalance, and at the same time they sought to minimize the adverse effects of the symptoms on humans by treating with diet and drugs that brought relief but not cure. This notion is clearly stated in the *Canon* where Avicenna professed that "not every tumor has an obvious reason," however, he went on to describe the physical events that lead to the increase in the size of the tumor.

Additionally, by attributing the disease to a humoral imbalance, Unani physicians have effectively pointed us in the right direction in order to associate a disease with its gene. For example, a metabolic disease that is caused by a genetic mutation in the DNA and thus encodes a defective enzyme will lead to the excessive accumulation of a metabolic compound (an abnormal humor in Unani terminology) that will produce the sickness. Therefore, knowing the humor type narrows the search to a particular class of compounds. In Unani, relief for patients comes from reducing the intake of that class of humor that feeds the accumulation of the metabolic compound. In practice, this could be very beneficial today in diseases where the etiology of the disease is unknown to the medical community. A good example of applying the Unani disease concept is the case of methylmalonic acidemia where the accumulation of organic acids (abnormal black bile humor in Unani terminology) due to a defective enzyme (methylmalonyl-CoA mutase) is treated with dietary management.*

DYNAMIC NATURE OF DISEASE IN UNANI MEDICINE

In Unani the disease is not a static condition but rather a dynamic, changing state with phases that reflect the changes over the course of the illness. Most diseases have four phases: incipience, increment, acme, and decline. These phases are not meant to describe the severity of the disease but rather to determine the most suitable treatment for that phase; each phase has its own treatment regimen and expected outcome. This contrasts with the one-drug-fits-all paradigm of allopathic pharmacology of the WMS.

Diseases are also described according to their reaction to treatment; the disease may be responsive or resistant to treatment due to a contraindication. Also, diseases may transform to other diseases, and the new disease may be a

---

*Hauser, "Variable Dietary Management."

cure from the old, or it may make the situation worse (see examples in the 8th Section).

In Unani, with its simpler methods of patient examination, the caregiver does not have to rely on calibrated machines and delayed test results to treat an illness. It offers a cost-effective, real-time evaluation of the patient's status relative to any known method. Therefore, the patient benefits from real-time assessment and receives the proper treatment that is suitable for their phase of the disease.

AVICENNA'S VIEWPOINT ON SWELLINGS AND TUMORS

Avicenna places all swellings and tumors, both benign and malignant, under the category of compound diseases. He reasons that the swellings or tumors recapitulate all the types of diseases according to Unani classification; they have a diseased dystemperament, humoral imbalance, discontinuity of structure and form (since every tumor produces problems with form and quantity [volume, number] and maybe location), and a shared disease of discontinuity; every swelling or tumor produces discontinuity where waste products fill in the area between tissues. Within the humoral framework, Avicenna explains that swelling or tumor manifestations are due to harmful humors that are left behind after normal humors are evacuated. Harmful humors are pushed out to the skin (in the case of infection, as a draining abscess) and form swellings. The swellings separate from tissues by various ways according to their cause; these causes are the substances that form them (the four humors as well as aqueous and gaseous materials).

Avicenna classified swellings and tumors according to their temperaments into hot and cold tumors (see Table 8.1, page 111). The hot ones are produced by the abnormal humors of blood and yellow bile or a combination of the two. The cold swellings or tumors are of four types produced by abnormal black bile, phlegm, and watery and gaseous humors. Malignant tumors (cancerous) are produced by abnormal black bile (see also the section on abnormal black bile in the **chapter on humors**). However, as we now know, genetic mutations precede (are the cause of) abnormal black bile accumulation in tumors; abnormal levels of black bile (or catabolic compounds) in cells can cause hypoxia and lead to the activation of oncogenes (genes that promote a cancerous phenotype).* Abnormal levels of succinic acid due to mutation in the enzyme succinate dehydrogenase are an example of abnormal black bile leading to a tumorigenic cell type.

---

*Chandel, "Cellular Oxygen," 1880–89.

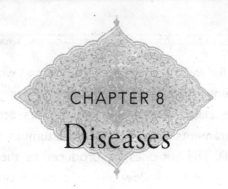

CHAPTER 8

Diseases

First Lesson of the Second Art: Diseases

- First Section: Cause, Disease, and Symptoms
- Second Section: States of the Body and Types of Disease
- Third Section: Structural Diseases
- Fourth Section: Diseases of Discontinuity
- Fifth Section: Compound Diseases
- Sixth Section: Topics Included Under Diseases
- Seventh Section: Phases of Disease
- Eighth Section: Concluding Remarks on Diseases

The following is a translation of the *Canon's* 1st Lesson of the chapter on disease. It is comprised of eight sections encompassing (1) cause, disease, and symptoms; (2) body states and disease types; (3) structural diseases; (4) diseases of discontinuity; (5) compound diseases; (6) topics included under diseases; (7) phases of disease; and (8) concluding remarks on diseases.

FIRST LESSON OF THE SECOND ART

Diseases

(8 Sections)

FIRST SECTION

Cause, Disease, and Symptoms

In medicine, there is first the cause; it produces a condition in the human body that may persist. Disease is an abnormal state that produces a problem in the function of the human body as either a dystemperament or an abnormal structure.

The symptom reflects the state of disease, and it is abnormal whether it is opposite to normal as in the pain accompanying biliary colic or not opposite such as the redness of cheek in pneumonia due to putrefaction. An example of disease is fever, and its symptom such as thirst and headache. An example of cause is the blockage of lower vessels of the eye. Another example of disease is the blockage of the iris, which is mechanical-structural disease. An example of a symptom is loss of vision, and an example of cause is catarrh. An example of disease is ulceration of the lung, the symptom is redness of both cheeks and curving of nails. The symptom is called such for what it presents, by itself or in relation to the situation, and is also called a sign because the physician uses it to diagnose the disease. Sometimes, one disease becomes the cause of another, such as biliary colic may turn into fainting, palsy, or epilepsy. The symptom could become the cause of the disease, such as severe pain may become a reason for swelling due to the convergence of material to the effected location. The symptom itself may become the disease such as the headache due to fever; it may persist until it becomes the disease. One thing, in relation to itself, to something before it or after it, can be a disease, a symptom, and a cause, such as pneumonic fever; it is a symptom of lung ulceration, a disease by itself, and a cause for the weakness of the stomach. And, headache caused by a fever, if it persists, then it is a symptom of fever and by itself a disease and it may bring phrenitis,* and thus becomes the cause of the two diseases.

SECOND SECTION

States of the Body and Types of Disease

The states of the body according to Galen are three: (1) healthy, a state where the human body in its temperament, structure, and actions are all correct; (2) diseased, which is the opposite; and (3) a state where it is not healthy or diseased, or incomplete health or diseased like the bodies of old people, recovering from disease, and as in children. The third state is also produced due to a combination of the first two states in two organs, or one organ but in two distant types such as proper temperament by structural dysfunction. Or, one organ in two similar types such as proper structure but improper in quantity and form, proper in the two reactive temperaments but not the active temperaments, or due to the succession of the two issues at different times such as in the individual who is healthy in the winter and sick in the summer.

Diseases are single and compound. The single is one type of dystemperament or one type of structural diseases that we will mention later. The compound diseases have two types that unite to produce a disease. The single diseases are of three types. First, diseases afflicting homogeneous organs are dystemperament diseases. They are symptomatic of homogeneous organs and cannot be thought of in the compound organs. Second, diseases of mechanical organs are the structural diseases within the homogenous mechanical organs. Third, the shared diseases of homogeneous organs also afflict mechanical organs without similarity in symptoms to the homogeneous organs. These are also termed diseases of discontinuity and disintegration. Discontinuity becomes symptomatic of the dislocated part without any symptoms for the

---

*Phrenitis is an old term that refers to the acute inflammation of the brain; it is known in Arabic as sirsam or birsam (السرسام الحار) and is equivalent to meningitis. It is also referred to erroneously as qranitis ("قرانيطس," which should read phrenitis فرانيطس).

homogeneous parts that make up the organ. These symptoms appear only for nerve, bone, and vessels. In general, diseases are of three types: diseases of dystemperament, structural diseases, and diseases of discontinuity. Every disease belongs to one of these types, originates from the type, and is attributed to it. Dystemperament diseases number sixteen, and we have mentioned them in the 1st Section, 3rd Lesson, 1st Art.

THIRD SECTION

Structural Diseases (amradh al-tarakeeb, امراض التراكيب)

Structural diseases are restricted to four types:

1. Diseases of form or shape (amradh al-khelkeh, أمراض الخلقه). These fall into four subtypes:
   a. Diseases of appearance (amradh es-shekl, أمراض الشكل). These involve a change in the normal form that results in abnormal function. For example, flexion of penis, straightening of the curved, squaring of the round such as in megalocephaly if it produces harm, extreme rounding of stomach, and lack of curvature in eye pupil.
   b. Diseases of ducts, canals, and tracts (amradh al-majaree, أمراض المجاري). These fall into three conditions:
      i. Dilatation: as in the dilation of pupil (الثقبه العنبيه), widening of blood vessels of eye, and in varicose veins.
      ii. Constriction: as in pupil, bronchial tube, and esophagus.
      iii. Blockage: such as the obstruction of eye pupil, liver vessels, and other structures.
   c. Diseases of vasculature and cavities (amradh al-awe'eyeh wa et'tajaweef, أمراض الاوعيه والتجاويف). These fall into four conditions:
      i. Enlargement: as in the swelling of testicles.
      ii. Reduction: as in the shrinkage of stomach or the ventricles of the brain in epilepsy.
      iii. Obstruction or fullness: as in the blockage of vessels

lining brain ventricles after a stroke that leads to apoplexy.

    iv. Emptiness: as in the emptying of the blood from heart cavities in extreme states of excitement or ecstasy that leads to death [or "high output" heart failure].

  d. Diseases of organs' surfaces (amradh safayeh al-aa'dah, أمراض صفائح الأعضاء). These describe the smoothness of a normally rough surface such as the lining of the stomach and intestines or the roughness of a normally smooth lining such as the trachea.

2. Diseases of quantity or size (amradh al-mikdar, أمراض المقدار). These fall into two conditions:

  a. Increase in size: as in elephantitis or enlargement of penis, which is a disease termed *priapsim.**

  b. Decrease in size: as in shrinkage of tongue or iris, and emaciation.

3. Diseases of number (amradh al-a'dad, أمراض العدد). These fall into two forms:

  a. Increase in number: normal, like an extra tooth or finger, or abnormal, like a tumor or a stone.

  b. Decrease in number: natural, like a missing finger since birth, or unnatural, such as losing finger in an accident.

4 Diseases of position or location (amradh al-wadhe'e, أمراض الوضع). According to Galen, these may require a location or sharing.

  a. Position diseases fall into four conditions:

    i. Separation of an organ from its position.

    ii. Dislocation without separation as in hernia.

    iii. Abnormal and involuntary movement such as tremors.

    iv. Immobility of organ as in the fossilization of joint in gout.

  b. Shared diseases involve the change in position in relation to another organ. They fall into two conditions:

*The original term that Avicenna used is phrysimyos (فريسميوس), probably a modified Greek word that refers to priapsim, which is derived from the name of a Greek god, Priapos, who is depicted with a large penis.

i. Inability to move closer as when a finger cannot move closer to another (adduction).

ii. Inability to move away as with eyelid paresis, laxity of joints in palsy, and not opening the palm.

FOURTH SECTION

Diseases of Discontinuity (or Separation); (amradh tafarouk al-eetessal, امراض تفرق الاتصال)

Diseases of discontinuity may happen in the skin, called a scratch (khadsh, خدش) or an abrasion (sahj, سحج), or take place in the flesh and around it; one without pus is called a wound (jurh, جرح) and one with pus (keeh, قيح) is called a sore or ulcer (Kurha, قرحه). The pus accumulates in the latter because of its weakness and inability to use nourishment, which turns into waste, and also because it acts as a sink for waste. This process also takes place in the bone when it breaks into two or more parts, large or very small, or is broken longitudinally. The same process may take place in cartilage or nerve. If it is crosswise in direction it is termed a cut (batr, بتر), lengthwise but shallow is a slit (shak, شق), but deep lengthwise is a split (shadkh, شدخ). In the muscle, a severance near the insertion (ligament or tendon) is a tear (or rip), (hetk, هتك), in the middle of the muscle is a cut (jez, جز), lengthwise with a few deep cuts is called open slits (fadgh or fadr, فدغ), however, the one with many deep cuts is termed a tear or rip (faskh, فسخ). All these terms are used interchangeably for all issues inside the muscle. In the vessels (arteries and veins), where a discontinuity is usually termed a rupture (infijar, انفجار), crosswise is a cut, lengthwise is a rift (sada', صدع), and a small opening is called a perforation (thokb, ثقب). A leak from an artery that forms a blood sac that can be squeezed back into the artery is called an aneurysm (oum ed-dam, أم الدم), which is a term given by some to all arterial ruptures.

Note that not all organs can tolerate cuts; heart cuts lead to death. Ruptures in membranes and septa are called hernias (fetk, فتق). When two parts of a compound organ separate without affecting the homogenous parts, it is called separation or dislocation. A movement of a nerve from its place is called displacement (fak, فك). Discontinuity may take place in ducts and tracts and dilate them or create canals where they did not exist. An organ with good temperament may recover quickly from discontinuity, but this may take longer in an organ with dystempera-ment, especially in the bodies of those with edema (dropsy) (estiska', استسقاء), anemia (*cacochymia**) (sou' al-kenyeh, سوء القنيه), or lep-rosy. Also note that the prolonging of summer sores may lead to gan-grene (al-akleh, الآكله). You will find later more explanation in detailed books on the disease of discontinuity.

FIFTH SECTION

Compound Diseases (al-amradh al-murakabeh, (الامراض المركبه

By compound diseases we do not mean a group of diseases taking place simultaneously, but rather one disease that encompasses a group of dis-eases [conditions as classified above] such as a swelling and/or tumor (waram, ورم). Pustules (pimples, boils) (buthur, بثور) are a small swell-ing type, whereas swellings are large pustules. The swelling and/or tumor captures all the types of diseases; it has a dystemperament accompanied by a [humor] substance, disease of structure and form since every swell-ing and/or tumor produces problems with form and quantity and maybe position, and a shared disease of discontinuity; every swelling/tumor pro-duces discontinuity where waste products fill in between.

Swellings and/or tumors occur in soft organs, and a similar process to swelling and/or tumor takes place in the bones, where they enlarge and increase edema. The latter is not strange since the organ, which takes up food for growth, will allow a swelling and/or tumor to take hold if it hap-pens. *Every swelling and/or tumor does not have an obvious reason;* however, its physical cause is the movement of a substance from an organ by gravity in a process termed catarrh (nazleh, نزله). The physical reason that prob-ably gives rise to swellings and/or tumors and boils is obscured by unharm-

---

*The term *cacochymia* referred to a depraved habit of the body, replete with ill humors, from various causes.

ful normal humors. When these normal humors are evacuated (naturally, as in the case of lactating puerperia, or abnormally, as in a bleeding wound), the harmful humors are left behind and cause irritation, thus are pushed out to the skin and form swellings and boils. The swellings separate from tissues by various waste substances such as those that cause them in the first place, and these are the substances that form the swellings.

The origins of swellings are six, the four humors as well as aqueous (ma'yeh, ما ئيه) and gaseous (reehia, ريـحـيـه). Hot swellings originate from a sanguine and choleric humor or other hot-natured substance, become hot by putrefaction, and are named after their humors. These types are subtyped according to their qualitative composition. The purely sanguine tumors are called phlegmon (phalghamonia, فلغا مونيا), the choleric carbuncle (jamra, جـمـره), and the combination of the two is abscess (kharaj, خـراج). The last type, when it occurs in soft tissues, such as under the axilla and behind ears, is termed plague (ta'oon, طـاعـون) [indicative of an infection by *Yersinia pestis,* creating bubos, or swelling of lymph nodes due to infection with bubonic plague, the "black death" of history].

The beginning of a **hot swelling** is marked by the accumulation of humor and appearance of size, then it increases in size until it reaches its fullness; afterward, it starts to decline by maturing, which is disintegration, pus formation, or other. It sometimes becomes solid. There are four origins for **cold swellings:** melancholic, phlegmatic, aqueous, and gaseous. There are three types of melancholic tumors: solid, cancerous (most biting), and glandular, such as scrofula (lymphadenitis of the cervical lymph nodes associated with tuberculosis; khanazeer, خـنـازيـر) and lipoma (sal', سلـع). The glandular differs in that they are contained within the tissue where they originate, like in glands (ghudad mahdeh, غدد مـحـضـه), or superficially attached to it, like in scrofula, while the other two are "mixed with" (infiltrating) the normal tissue of their origin. The difference between the cancerous tumor and solid swelling is that the later is a continuous, painless growth, while cancer is mobile, continuously growing, with primary roots in organs, and will not silence the sensation unless it continues to grow, thus eventually destroying sensation and the organ itself. It is not far-fetched that the distinction between the two is by their symptoms and not their forms.

Melancholic solid swellings start as solid, or could become solid as in sanguineous or phlegmatic ones. They differ from glandular, lipomas, and alike, such as the knotting of nerves (ganglia, which are confined to the nerve and feel as such); they reappear after manual manipulation but disappear completely with a strong medication. Most ganglia develop from fatigue, and they may be treated by manual pressure or placing a piece of heavy lead (الأسرب) or something similar on them.

Phlegmatic swellings are of two types: soft diffused tumors (rakhu, رخو) that are mixed and indistinct and the soft encapsulated lipomas (sal' layen, سلع لين). Most of the winter swellings [of the upper respiratory tract] are phlegmatic; even the hot ones with white color [pus]. Their phlegm varies in density, fluidity, and softness; sometimes it is similar to the melancholic or gaseous ones. More often the light phlegm moves down in catarrh due to a problem in the nerve fiber until it reaches the lower part of the larynx and maybe beyond, into the lungs.

Aqueous swellings develop due to the accumulation of liquids in cysts such as pustules (بثور), or within the tissues such as edema (الأستسقاء), hydrocele* (القيله المائيه), and hydrocephalus (ورم القحف المائي) and the like. Pustules are as many as the causes of swellings (i.e., six.) There are sanguineous pustules like smallpox (الجدري); purely choleric as in urticaria (yellow rash, الشري الصفراوي) and miliaria (الجاورسيه); and mixed as in measles (الحصبه), herpes (النمله), clavi [corns] (المسامير), scabies (الجرب), warts (الثآليل), and others. They may also be aqueous in origin such as blisters (النفاطات) or gaseous such as bullae of emphysema (النفاخات).

Gaseous swellings result from gas accumulation in the organ's cavity or within the organ's tissue and are of two types: puffiness (التهيج) and distension (النفخه). The two differ in form and localization; whereas puffiness infiltrates the soft, pressured tissues, the distension is confined to one area with extensive pressure (see Table 8.1). You will find more detail on tumors and pustules in the 4th Book of the *Canon*, which is more suitable for this topic.

---

*A hydrocele denotes a pathological accumulation of serous fluid in a body cavity.

TABLE 8.1. AVICENNA'S CLASSIFICATION
OF SWELLINGS AND TUMORS

Swellings and Tumors According to the Material that Causes Them

1. Blood humor
2. Phlegm humor
3. Yellow bile humor
4. Black bile humor
5. Aqueous substance
6. Gaseous substance

Types of Tumors

1. Hot Tumors
   a. Phlegmon
   b. Choleric
   c. Mix of a and b: pus
2. Cold Tumors
   a. Melancholic
      i. Solid
      ii. Cancer
      iv. Glandular
   b. Phlegmatic
      i. Soft
      ii. Lipoma
   c. Aqueous
      i. Edema
      ii. Pustules
         1. Sanguinous: e.g., smallpox
         2. Choleric: e.g., urticaria, miliaria
         3. Mix of 1 and 2: e.g., measles, herpes, corns, scabies, warts
         4. Aqueous: boils
         5. Gaseous: bullae of emphysema
      iii. Hydrocele
      iv. Hydrocephalus
   d. Gaseous
      i. Puffiness
      ii. Distension

SIXTH SECTION

Topics Included under Diseases

There are issues that are not generated by disease but are included under diseases. They concern appearance; they are about hair, color, odor, and physique. Hair problems may include: falling (تناثر), alopecia or glabrousness (تمرط), stuntedness (قصر), splitting (شقاق), lightness (دقه), thickness (غلظ), excessive curliness (جعوده), excessive straightness (سبوطه), grayness (شيب), and any other color change. Problems of color are of four types: first, change of color due to bad humor such as in jaundice (يرقان) or another substance of single humor as in measles (حصبه); second, change due to obvious reasons such as exposure to sun, cold, or wind; third, the spreading of abnormal color such as vitiligo nigra (البهق الاسود) and its persistent effect afterward such as moles (خيلان) and freckles (نمش); fourth, marks and effects left after healing from a disease of discontinuity such as pockmarks and deformations of skin left from smallpox and sores. Problems of odor are such as "lamb" odor [comes out from sweating in wool clothes] and other bad odors of the body. Physique problems include excessive weight loss or gain.

SEVENTH SECTION

Phases of Disease

Most diseases have four phases: incipience, increment, acme, and decline. Health is assumed to be restored after these phases. It is not meant that the incipience and decline are phases when disease is not taking hold, but rather that each is a timely phase with its specific treatment. Incipience is the time of appearance of disease; it could remain steady without feeling any advancement. Increment is the phase where its manifestation increases with time. Acme is the steady phase of the disease. Decline starts with subsiding and continues with time. The durations of these phases are specific to the disease occurring and are called general phases (أوقات كليه), and may take place within episodes (paroxysms) of the disease; in such a case they are called partial phases (أوقات جزئيه).

EIGHTH SECTION

Concluding Remarks on Diseases

Diseases are named in various ways. Sometimes (1) according to the organs they afflict, like pleurisy (side disease, ذات الـجـنـب) and pneumonia (lung disease, ذات الرئـه); by (2) their symptoms, like epilepsy (الصـرع), (3) according to the causes, like our saying "melancholic disease," (4) by analogy (lionitis [lion's disease, داء الاسد], elephant disease); (5) named after the person who first described the disease, or eponymous, as in Telephic ulcer, named after a man called Tyleanus; (5) named after a town where the disease is endemic, as in Balakh sores; (7) after the person who was most successful in treating it, like Cirotinia ulcer; or (8) according to the nature of the disease, such as fever or tumor.

Galen said that some diseases are obvious and can be felt; others are internal and can be figured out, like the pain of stomach and lung; some are difficult to figure out, like diseases of liver and lung vessels, or can only be guessed, like problems with urinary tracts. Some diseases are specific for an organ or shared, such as two organs sharing the disease of the other either because (1) they are connected by instruments like the nerve between the brain and the stomach; (2) through blood vessels, like the uterus and the breasts; (3) one organ is the path to the other, as the groin (الأربيتين) to leg swelling; (4) they share because one is next to the other, like the lungs and brain [the brain abnormal humors drain into the trachea and can cause problems with the lungs], especially if one of them is hot and weak so it accepts from the other its products, like the axilla to the heart; (5) because the first's action is needed for the other to function, like the diaphragm to the lungs in breathing; (6) because one serves the other, like the nerve to the brain; or (7) because the two are sharing (dependant on) a third organ, like the brain and kidneys share the liver.

Such dependency may be harmful; for example if the brain does not involve the stomach, the digestion will get weaker and produce low-quality nourishment and pain in the brain increases. Sharing problems take place according to periodicity and sequence that also characterize primary diseases [see the section on the phases of disease on page 112].

States of health and disease are six according to our description: body in perfect health, less than perfect, in-between intermediary (neither healthy nor diseased), recovering and capable of quickly becoming healthy, slightly diseased, and fully diseased. Every disease is either compliant (responsive) or resistant. A compliant disease is the one that presents no problem to proper treatment, and the resistant is associated with a hindrance that prevents its treatment, such as the headache associated with catarrh.

Also learn that a disease that is compatible with the temperament, age, and season is less dangerous than the incompatible one. Incompatible diseases occur due to a serious cause. The disease of one season should disappear in its opposite season. Diseases get transformed to other diseases and the original disappears, which is better since the new disease is a cure to the old one; for example, quartan fever (حمى الربع) [or malaria (reminiscent of the old "malaria cure" for syphilis)] often cures epilepsy, gout, varicose vein, arthritis, scabies, itching, furunculosis, and spasm. Likewise, sprue* (ذرب) cures conjunctivitis, lienteric diarrhea, pleurisy, and bleeding anus [hemorrhoids], and benefits every melancholic disease (e.g., coxalgia [وجع الورك] and pains of kidney and uterus). The situation could get worse if a disease transforms into another, such as the change from pleurisy to pneumonia, or phrenitis (السرسام الحار) to lethargia (السرسام البارد).

Some diseases are contagious, such as leprosy, scabies, smallpox, epidemic fevers, and infected sores, especially if dwellings are tightly enclosed; also factors are: living in the direction of wind coming from an infected area, such as with conjunctivitis; looking closely at an infected person; and tooth ache may start if you think of something sour; [also contagious are] pannus (vascular keratitis, سبل) and leprosy. Some diseases are inherited, such as baldness, leukoderma (برص), gout, pannus, and leprosy.† Some of the sexually transmitted diseases are specific to a tribe or an area where they are endemic. Remember that the weakness of organs is attributed to dystemperament and decomposition of structure.

---

*Sprue is a tropical disease of unknown origin involving deficient absorption of nutrients from the intestine and marked by persistent diarrhea, weight loss, and anemia.

†Avicenna's grouping of leprosy with heritable diseases is a reflection of his time, when it was thought that certain families were afflicted with a particular disease. It is now known that leprosy is not heritable.

CHAPTER 9

Causes

Second Lesson of the Second Art: Causes

- **First Statement: Causes from General Factors (19 sections)**
- **Second Statement: Listing of Causes of Each Bodily Symptom (29 sections)**

Bodies may vary in their reaction to causes; the same cause may produce different diseases in different bodies, different disease at different times, and its effect varies among the strong and the weak as well as among the sensitive and the very sensitive.

AVICENNA

Diseases have causes, and in Unani there are three sets of causes: (1) bodily predisposition (also termed *prior causes*) that are humoral, temperamental, or structural; (2) external causes that are mostly environmental; and (3) bodily connecting causes essential to inducing change that result from the interaction of the first two sets. Avicenna classified the causes that affect the body, and that preserve it, into (1) essential and (2) unessential. The essential causes are those that are necessary for life to continue; they are six: the air, food and drink,

bodily movement and stillness, psychological activity, sleep and wakefulness, and eating and emptying.

Avicenna describes disease inception as mostly an interplay among
the state of the body, the environment, and the changes that induce illness. For this reason, he goes into a detailed account of the effects on
health of the seasons, climate and weather temperaments, direction of
wind, and geographic location. He also includes in the 1st Statement a
discussion on the effects of movement and rest, sleep and wakefulness,
and psychological states.

THE ROLE OF AIR AND AERATION IN HEALTH

Of the necessary causes for life, air is the first on the list. Avicenna
emphasizes in several places in the 1st Book of the *Canon* the primary
importance of fresh, clean air for life and health preservation. The 1st
Statement (2nd Lesson of the 2nd Art) contains detailed descriptions of
the characteristics of good air and of the various types of air in relation
to the four seasons, wind direction, precipitation patterns, topography,
location, and habitat, as well as housing location and design. He presents each of these factors in relation to its effects on health.

In the 2nd Section of the 1st Statement on the effect of air, Avicenna
provides a very refined explanation that almost borders on molecular
description of the function of air in the body. Although Avicenna did
not know this in his own time, he was in fact describing the function of
oxygen, which was not yet discovered,* in the body. He distinguished
between (1) air as a structural component of the body and (2) its role
as an active, interacting element responsible for the well-being of the
body, while its corruption causes illness. He states that air is essential
in the body and necessary for its functions, however, it does its function not only as structural element but also as an active participant in
bodily interactions.

In addition to its function in the respiratory process and the

---

*Oxygen was independently discovered by Carl Wilhelm Scheele in 1773 and Joseph
Priestley in 1774. The name *oxygen* was given in 1777 by Antoine Lavoisier.

generation of innate heat, Avicenna ascribes other beneficial functions to air that he calls aeration and cleansing. First, because the air is usually cooler than the body's temperature, it reduces the heat generated from respiration's innate heat and restores the temperament balance to its normal state, especially in the case of hypoxia. Second, air is responsible for the cleansing act of carrying out from the lungs the "smoky vapor" (i.e., carbon dioxide).

In discussing the effect of air on the human body, Avicenna was ahead of his time in broadly describing this process in terms that have been proven true at the molecular level.

His description of hypoxia, carbon dioxide release, and the respiratory quotient (the ratio of carbon dioxide released as a measure of respiration) predicted what we know today at the cellular level. Further, you will find Avicenna's description of what he considers good air in the 5th Section.

HYDRATION IN RELATION TO HEALTH AND AGING

Tissue and body hydration is a main theme in Unani, and it considers lack of body moisture as a sign of senescence in older people and as a portent of illness in younger people. Here Avicenna presents a connection between aeration (oxygenation and respiration in today's terminology) and hydration. He affirms the role of air in moisturizing the tissues (remember that the cellular respiratory cycle in the mitochondria produces water, thus being an important process for hydration of the cells, as well as providing energy to the cells). Avicenna stressed the importance of this factor in health and the preservation of life throughout the book.

By pointing to the amount of water in the cells and tissues (i.e., metabolic hydration) as directly related to their proper functions, physicians of Unani medicine devised a practical method for measuring the metabolic health of an individual. As we have known since the last century, water in the tissues, other than from drinking water, comes from the respiratory processes—glycolysis and the Krebs cycle. The higher the respiration rate, more water is produced within the cells and more energy is produced as chemical bonding (ATP*) and as heat. Similar methods that are also related to measuring other byproducts of the respiratory process have just recently started to appear in the modern scientific literature. Among these is the measuring of lactic acid content in the blood. The increase of lactic acid in the body signifies the dimensioning efficiency of the respiration phase in the mitochondria and could be indicative of disease in the young or senescence in the old.

In the section on the conditions of water (16th Section, 1st Statement), Avicenna details the qualities of good water for the body. He describes the water's function in the body as well as its part in food conditioning. He also gives a lengthy account of water sources and the quality of their waters, as well as the effect of boiling on water and its purification.

ACTIONS OF FOOD, DRINK, AND DRUGS

Avicenna classifies the reactions of the human body to consumed food, drink, or drugs into three forms. The immediate reaction is to the temperament of the ingested substance, with the body gaining or losing heat before the substance's constituents become available to be assimilated within the body; he calls this **reaction to quality.** The second reaction is to the individual elements of the ingested substance, for example, amino acids, fatty acids, and sugars; these elements are the building blocks of the substance that are similar to those of the body, and they become part of its organs. The second reaction brings about the substance's **neutralization of temperament.** The third reaction emanates from the substance's specific chemical components that give the substance its specific nature. This reaction is substance-specific, depending on its unique chemical composition. Avicenna calls it the **action of essence**, and completion of the action is called total essence.

---

*Adenosine triphosphate (ATP) is the cellular currency of energy. It transfers the chemical energy within cells for metabolism.

These three reactions may take place sequentially or, as in some strong poisons, at a reduced reaction of the first two.

Unani classifies food (including medicinal food), drink, and drugs according to their reactions on the body into two main categories, hot and cold, where each category has a different mechanism of action. The terms *hot* and *cold* here mean the effect on the innate heat and not the sensation they produce upon touch (i.e., not the feel). The severity of their effect (also termed potency or degree) is classified on a scale of one to four (i.e., there are four degrees for each). The first degree is the lightest and the fourth is the strongest, which includes most of the poisons. A detailed explanation of the scale is in the 15th Section of the 1st Statement.

Avicenna also discusses the nutritional value of food and how the food's quality and quantity affect the body. Tables 9.1 and 9.2 summarize two food classifications, one according to the food's texture and its nutritional value and the second according to the type of chyme* produced by the food and its nutritional value.

TABLE 9.1. TYPES OF FOOD ACCORDING TO TEXTURE AND NUTRITIONAL CONTENT

Light food	Very nutritious	Wine, meat juice, warm egg yolks, or half-boiled eggs
	Slightly nutritious	Julab (or *jallab*) legumes with moderate texture and quality, and fruits such as apples, pomegranates, and the like
Dense Food	Very nutritious	Boiled eggs and beef meat
	Slightly nutritious	Cheese, dried meat, eggplants, and the like

*Chyme (from the Greek χυμός, *khymos*, meaning "juice") is the semifluid mass of partly digested food expelled by the stomach into the duodenum.

TABLE 9.2. TYPES OF FOOD ACCORDING TO THEIR PRODUCED CHYME

Good chyme	Light, slightly nutritious	Lettuce, apples, and pomegranates
	Dense, slightly nutritious	Egg yolks, drinks, and meat juice
	Dense, very nutritious	Boiled eggs and meat of one-year-old lambs
Bad chyme	Light, slightly nutritious	Radishes, mustard, and most legumes
	Light, very nutritious	Lung and the meat of young birds
	Dense, very nutritious	Beef, duck, and horse meat
	Dense, slightly nutritious	Dried meat

THE CONTENTS OF THE SECOND STATEMENT

In this part of the *Canon,* Avicenna summarizes the effects of warmers, coolers, moisturizers, and dryers; causes of deformity; causes of obstruction, constriction, and dilation of ducts; causes of coarseness and smoothness; causes of dislocation, displacement, and ill proximity; causes of abnormal movement, size, and number; causes of discontinuity, ulceration, and swelling; causes and types of pain, as well as its cessation and effect; causes of pleasure; mechanisms of movement pain; mechanisms of humor pain; causes of retention and evacuation; causes of indigestion; and causes of organ weakness.

Causes from General Factors

(19 Sections)

FIRST SECTION

General Description of Causes

Causes of the previously mentioned states of the body (health, disease, and in-between) are three: predisposition (السـابقـه), external (البـاديـه), and connecting (الـواصـلـه). The predisposition and connecting are similar in that they are bodily issues; I mean they are humoral, temperamental, or structural. The external causes are issues that are external to the body [environmental], such as trauma, hot weather, and ingested hot or cold food, or psychological (since psychology is different than the physical body), such as anger, fear, and alike.

The predisposing and external causes may share an agent in order to affect the states of health. And, the external and connecting causes may not share an agent to affect the state of the body. However, the predisposing causes are different from the connecting causes in that the first are not followed by a change of a state, but rather there are other causes that are more directly linked to the change. The predisposing causes differ from the external in that they are bodily and require an instrument to cause the change in the state, while the external causes lack these characteristics. The connecting causes do not need an agent to induce the change of state of health.

The predisposing causes are bodily, meaning that they are humoral, temperamental, and structural, and not essential to induce a change of state and require an instrument to do that. The connecting causes are bodily causes that are essential to inducing a change in the health status without any agent. The external causes are not bodily causes and are essential or unessential to inducing a change in health status.

Examples of predisposing causes are stomach indigestion (fullness) for fever and edema of eye vessels. Examples of connecting causes are putrefaction for fever, excess moisture during menstruation for obstruction, and scybala for fever. Examples of external causes are sun's heat, excessive heat, depression, insomnia, or eating hot food such as garlic; all these for fever or a trauma for dilation of pupil and edema of the eye [glaucoma].

A cause could act directly by itself, such as pepper heats up and opium cools down, or secondarily, such as cold water causes heating by shrinkage or causes congestion when heated, hot water causes a cooling effect by evaporation, and scammony [*Convolvulus scammonia*] causes cold by the evacuation of a hot humor [hot fecal matter]. The effect of cause does not take place unless three conditions are met: (1) the cause has sufficient power, (2) predisposition of the body, and (3) interaction of the two for a duration that permits the effect to take place. Bodies may vary in their reaction to causes; the same cause may produce different diseases in different bodies, different diseases at different times, and its effect may vary among the strong and the weak, as well as among the sensitive and the very sensitive.

Causes vary in the duration of their effects. Some causes are long lasting, even after they are gone, while others have no effect after they depart the body. We say that the causes that affect the body and preserve it are either essential in that life cannot continue without them or unessential.

The essentials are six types: the kind of surrounding air, the kind of food and drink, the kind of bodily movement and stillness, the kind of psychological activity, the kind of sleep and wakefulness, and the kind of eating and emptying.

SECOND SECTION

The Effect of Surrounding Air

The air is an element within our bodies and their functions, and although it is an element, its effect reaches our breath to keep us healthy, not as an *element, but as an active actor.* We have explained earlier what we meant by respiration or breath (روح); we do not mean what philosophers call it, "a being" (نَفْس). The air acts on our breaths in two ways: aeration (ترويح) and cleansing (تنقيه). Aeration modulates the hot temperament of the internal breath* during times of congestion† and changes it—I mean the additional modification to restore balance. This modification benefits from the aeration of the lung as well as the pores adjoining the arteries. The air surrounding our bodies is cold in comparison with the temperament of innate heat or the dystemperament due to air deprivation [hypoxia], so aeration prevents overheating (fiery condition, ناريه) and prevents air deprivation that produces dystemperament, thus eliminating psychological resistance to accepting the cause of life and preventing the disintegration of its vaporous moist nature.

The cleansing that air performs takes place during exhaling by carrying out the smoky vapor‡ (given to the air by the discerning faculty); the ratio of the smoky vapor in the breath is equivalent to the ratio of the superfluous humor (خلط فضلي) in the body. Modification by air happens when inhaling and the mixing of air and respiration, and cleansing by exhaling. The inhaled air is beneficial when it first enters the body as cold, and later warms up and loses its beneficial effect, and the body sends it out. By exhaling, the body needs fresh air to replace the outgoing air and to send out the excesses of respiration. Moderate clean air that is free of impurities that antagonize respiration is supportive of good health and preserving of it. Air is modulated by normal and abnormal changes that are unnatural and antagonistic to its nature. Natural changes are the seasonal changes in temperament that occur at each season.

---

*Here, "internal breath" refers to the heat generated by the mitochondria due to the lack of oxygen as an electron acceptor.

†Here "congestion" refers to oxygen deprivation, anaerobic condition.

‡Ancient authors associated a "smoky" nature with nitrogen-containing ammonia, and we interpret it sometimes as referring to protein made of nitrogen-containing amino acids; however, in this section it refers to carbon dioxide.

THIRD SECTION

Characteristics of Seasons

Learn that seasons according to physicians are different from those according to astronomers. Astronomers define seasons as the solar movements in quarters from the tropics starting with the vernal point; however, physicians consider the spring when the countries of moderate temperature do not require heating to protect their people from the cold or fanning to lower heat, and it signifies the growing of trees. It starts between the vernal equinox (a little before it or a little after it) when the sun is in the middle of Taurus zodiac [April 20–May 20]. Autumn is cross-wise of spring in our land; in other countries, the spring may advance and the autumn may delay. The summer is all the hot times, and winter is all the cold times. According to physicians, the spring and autumn times are shorter than those of the summer and winter. Winter is cross-wise of summer, longer or shorter depending on the country.

Spring is the time of flowering and the beginning of fruiting, and autumn is the time of leaves changing and the beginning of their fall; the summer and winter are the other times. We say that the temperament of the spring is the moderate temperament and, as some think, that it is the hot and moist. The verification of this is through the physical philosophy, which says spring is moderate and summer is hot because the sun is closer to the top of the heads and the excessive reflection of its rays, either in acute angles or straight back in its original angle of incidence, amplifies its strength. The real explanation is that the incidence of the sun's rays is more similar to a cone than to a cylinder, and the cone seems to originate from the center of the sun and spreads to its vicinity. Some of the rays are direct, circumferential, or close to circumferential, and the strength is highest at the center because it is fortified from all sides, and anything beyond the sides is weaker; therefore, we are exposed in the summer to the center, or close to it, for a time in the northern latitudes. In the winter, we are at the periphery of the cone. The light during the summer is brighter although the distance between us and the sun's closest surface is farthest. This issue of closeness and distance is elucidated by mathematical astronomy of (natural) philosophy; however, the evidence for the increase of heat due to an increase of light intensity is verified by physical philosophy.

Summer is hot and dry because of the evaporation of moisture from high heat and the lightness of air and its acquisition of "fieriness," as well as the rarity of dews and rains. The winter is cold and moist for the opposite reasons. In autumn, the heat is reduced but the cold has not settled in yet, as if we are in the middle, between the center and edge [of the solar radiation cone], so it is close to moderation in heat and cold but immoderate in moisture and dryness because the sun has dried the air and there are not yet any wetting factors to oppose the drying ones. The situation in cooling is different from moistening because it is easier to cool but more difficult to moisturize. Also, it is not the same to moisturize by coolness and to dry by heat since drying with heat is easy with minimal heat, but minimal coolness does not moisturize. Perhaps minimal heat is more moisturizing if the substance is available than is minimal coolness because minimal heat does not induce evaporation of dissolution. Minimal coolness does not induce condensation, confinement, and aggregation. For this reason, the spring's preservation of the winter's moisture is not similar to the autumn's preservation of the summer's dryness since the spring's moisture is moderated by the heat at some time, but the dryness of the autumn is not moderated by the coolness; the moisturizing and dryness here are similar to possessing or not, and do not occur by the action of two opposites, since drying here is only the loss of moisture.

Moisturizing is not the loss of the essence of dryness but the acquisition of the essence of moisture. We do not say in this situation that an air is moist or dry in order to indicate its form or temperament (maybe slightly), but we mean by moist air that a moisture has mixed with the air or that by condensation it became moist; we say dry air to mean that it has lost its water vapor or expanded by heat, thus becoming lighter, and also by its mixing with earthy vapors that are similar to earth in their dryness.

The spring loses its winter moisture by the slightest of heat when the sun reaches its zenith,* and the autumn does not become moist with the slightest of cold. If you would like to know then watch if the dry objects accumulate dew in cold weather like the drying of moist objects in warm weather by keeping the cold in its coldness as the hot in its warmth [equal amount of coldness and warmth]. If you examine them, you will find that the two issues are different for another important reason; moisture does not persist in a cold or warm weather without continued supply. Dryness does not need any supply. Moisture in exposed bodies or air does not persist without a continued supply. It is said that air is cold in comparison with our bodies (it does not reach it coldness until it carries some moisture from the land before us on its way into us); in all cases air takes up moisture [by drying objects] because it acquires energy from the sun and other planets. The lack of supply encourages uncoupling and dryness.

In the spring, there is more uncoupling than evaporation because evaporation takes place for two reasons: heat and little moisture in the air as well as strong heat in the Earth that affects light objects close to the Earth's surface. Even during winter, the Earth's interior stays very warm, as indicated by original natural sciences, and the air's heat is low; therefore, two reasons converge for moisturizing: evaporation and condensation, and coldness induces condensation and clouds in the air.

In the spring, the air's uncoupling is stronger than its evaporation effect, and the Earth's internal latent heat decreases sharply, pushing some of it to the surface, thus leading to evaporation; this is met with an increase in the air's heat that aids evaporation. This takes place according to the consensus of reasons or their single actions without the presence of other contradictory reasons other than what we have mentioned. During spring, there is not excess of moisture to evaporate and temper, thus spring is moderate in wetness and dryness, as well as

---

*The word zenith (azimuth) derives from the inaccurate translation of the Arabic term سمت الرأس (samt ar-ra's), which means "direction of the head" or "path above the head," by medieval Latin translators (during the fourteenth century), probably through Old Spanish. It was incorrectly reduced to samt (direction) and imprecisely written as senit or cenit by those scribes. Through Old French cenith and Middle English senith, zenith finally first appeared in the seventeenth century.

in warmth and coolness. Early spring is moist, and its time away from moderation is not as far as the autumn's dry temperament from moderation. Those who judge the autumn as far from moderation in heat and cold are not far from the truth since its early days are "summery" due to the dryness of autumn's air, which accepts heat easily and acquires fieriness; therefore, its nights and middays are cold where the sun is distant from its zenith and the expanded air accepts coolness.

Spring is closer to moderation in both temperaments because its weather does not accept what makes the autumn's weather warm or cool; therefore, its night is not much different from its day. Someone may ask why the autumn's night is colder than the spring's and its air should be warmer because of its lightness! We reply by saying that the well-expanded air more readily and/or quickly accepts the heat or cold, and that also holds true for expanded water; therefore, if you heat up some water and then freeze it, it would freeze faster than cold water due to the faster effect of freezing on expanded water. Bodies do not feel from the coldness of the spring what they feel from the coldness of the autumn because the bodies in the spring are transitioning from cold to warm and habituated to coldness, but it is the opposite in the autumn, when the autumn is heading into winter while the spring is moving away from it. *Know that the transitioning between seasons in every region induces a set of diseases that the physician should be aware of and prepared for in order to preempt them.* A daily (diurnal) cycle also may resemble some seasons; a day may be wintery, summery, or springy, warming and cooling, all in the same day.

FOURTH SECTION

Seasonal Rules and Their Meanings

For every season the individual exhibits a temperament that is most suitable to it, and the season antagonizes the person who has a temperament that is unsuitable to that particular season; however, if the season departs from moderation, then it antagonizes both the suitable and unsuitable temperaments and weakens their individuals. *Also, every*

season is compatible with a temperament that is opposite to its tempera-
ment [for example, a person with hot and dry temperaments is healthier
in a cold and moist winter]. If two successive seasons departed from
their moderation in opposite ways without excess, such as when the
winter is southern and the spring is northern, then the second is compatible with and moderates the bodies because the spring modulates
the harshness of the winter. If the winter was very dry and the spring
moist, then the spring moderates the dryness of winter as long as its
moisture is not excessive and does not last a long time to enter into
harmful moisturizing.

Multiple weather changes in one season are less conducive to epidemics than many changes over several seasons, and this is not similar
to water expansion, as we have mentioned above. The first seasonal temperament to induce putrefaction is the hot and moist air temperament,
and it is most harmful in the areas of variable topography and lower
valleys and least harmful in plains and high areas.

Seasons ought to be within their normal ranges, thus the summer
should be hot and the winter cold; however, a departure from these ranges
will encourage illnesses. A year with similar seasons as when the whole
year is moist or dry, and hot or cold, is harmful since it will be compatible with diseases that are similar to its temperament, with a prolonged
duration of the disease. If a season can precipitate the disease with which
it is compatible, then what about a whole year? For example, in a cold
season, a phlegmatic body is vulnerable to epilepsy, palsy, apoplexy, spasm,
and alike, and in a choleric body, a hot season may induce insanity, acute
fevers, and hot tumors; imagine if the entire year continues in a similar
fashion to the one season. When the winter sets in early its diseases also
appear early, and the same is true for the summer, and the diseases will
change accordingly. A prolonged season will prolong its diseases, especially the summer and the autumn. Know that the sudden change of a
season affects the temperament and induces immense change, even if the
weather change lasts for only a day from hot to cold, due to the changes
it induces in the body. The most healthy of times is when the autumn is
rainy, the winter moderate with some coldness but without excess to the
region, the spring rainy, and the summer with some rain.

The Good Air

A good quality air is without contamination by strange vapors or smokes, open to the outside, and not confined to rooms, except during a general contamination when the inside air is better; otherwise the outside air is better. The good air is clean and pure without vapors of lagoons, marshes, ditches, bamboo fields, farm vegetables (especially those of cabbages and arugula), trees of bad nature (such as walnuts and figs), not mixed with smelly wind, mixed with good wind from high lands and plains, unconfined, warms up at sunrise and cools down at sunset, not confined to tanks or alike that have not completely dried, and easy to breath without pressure on the throat.

Air changes could be normal, abnormal and harmful, or abnormal but not harmful. Abnormal air changes, whether harmful or not, are periodic or irregular, and the healthiest are regular in temperament, otherwise they are conducive to illnesses.

SIXTH SECTION

Air Temperaments and Effects of Seasons

Hot air disperses and softens; when moderate, it brings blood to the surface and reddens the skin; when excessive, it produces yellowness by disintegrating what it brings to the surface. It increases sweating, reduces urine, weakens digestion, and induces thirst. Cold air firms up and strengthens digestion, increases urine since it retains moistures, and reduces sweating and alike. It reduces evacuation due to the contraction of the anal sphincter and the rectum, thus increases retention of feces, and their water is diverted to urine. Moist air softens the skin and moistens the body, and dry air thins the body and dries the skin. Turbid air reduces breathing and stirs humors. Turbid air differs from thick air; the latter is uniform in its density while the turbid is mixed with coarse objects. Distinguishing between the two can be done by looking at the stars; turbid air will mask small stars and extinguish the brightness of fixed planets like Antares (المرتعش) because of excessive vapors and smokes and lack of good winds.

The spring in its proper temperament is the best season and the most suitable for temperaments of respiration and blood. As a moderate season it is close to gentle, airy heat and normal humidity. It reddens the skin because it brings the blood to the surface [of the skin] in moderation without breaking it down like in the summer. The spring triggers chronic diseases because it moves settled humors and makes them runny. For this reason it sets off melancholy in melancholic individuals; also those with excess humor in the winter from overeating and inactivity should be ready in the spring for the diseases associated with these substances because the spring will disintegrate them. The prolonging of a moderate spring will reduce summer's diseases. Spring diseases include hemorrhagic diarrhea (إختلاف الدم), nosebleed, activation of melancholy of the bitter black bile, swellings, furuncles (boils), fatal suffocating afflictions, and all forms of abscesses. Also, it increases the incidents of ruptured vessels (إنصداع العروق), hemoptysis (نفث الدم) [spitting of blood or blood-stained sputum], and cough, especially in a wintery spring, which also worsens tuberculosis, and for stirring phlegm materials in phlegmatic individuals it precipitates apoplexy [sudden death], palsy, and joint pain. Excessive physical and mental activities as well as hot dishes promote the aforementioned illnesses because they fortify the temperament of the air. The best treatment of spring diseases are venesection, elimination, reducing food consumption, increasing drinking, and mixing of alcoholic drinks with water. Spring is agreeable with children and others of close age.

Winter is best for digestion because the cold confines the warmth,* thus strengthening it and preventing its decomposition; also, due to people's reduced consumption of fruits [fruits induce coldness] and eating a light diet, as well as reduced movement when full and staying warm around fires. Its coldness, short days, and long nights make it the highest in black bile. It has the maximum in retention of substances and

---

*The coldness of winter constricts the surface blood vessels and thus the best circulation is occurring deep in the body, and, hence, better digestion.

requires the help of digestives and soothers. Winter's diseases are mostly phlegmatic. Phlegm is excessive in that most of the vomit is phlegm, and the color of swellings is white most of the time. Cold [nasal catarrh] is rampant in winter; cold starts with change in air temperament from the autumn, followed by pleurisy, pneumonia, voice hoarseness, and throat pains, then followed by pain in the waist and back, nerve problems and chronic headache, and possibly sudden death and epilepsy. All this is due to the accumulation of phlegmatic material. Winter is harmful to the elderly and alike, beneficial for the young. There is more sediment in the urine, more than that of the summer, and urine quantity is larger.

Summer breaks down humors and weakens strength and natural functions due to its excessive disintegration. It reduces blood and phlegm and increases the bitter yellow bile, then at its tail end, black bile increases because it disintegrates the light fraction of it and retains and condensates the thick part. It strengthens the elderly. It turns the skin color yellow because it disintegrates the blood it brings to the [skin] surface. It shortens the time of illness because its air temperament strengthens the body to mature the disease humor and push it out; however, if the body is weak then the air temperament will weaken it further by relaxation, which increases sickness and favors death. A hot dry summer cuts short the illness, while a hot humid summer lengthens it; therefore, most ulcers turn into gangrene, and edema, lienteric diarrhea (زلق الامعاء), and softness of the bowels (تلين الطبع) are induced—all facilitated by the movement of humidity from top to bottom, especially from the head. Hot diseases include tertian fever, incessant fever [typhoid fever], burning fever [hyperpyrexia], and shrinkage of the body. Summer pains include earaches, ophthalmia (conjunctivitis, رمد), erysipelas (becomes frequent especially if air movement is lacking), and pustules (pimples, بثور) of suitable nature.

If the summer is springlike, then fevers are mild and gentle without dryness; it also induces sweatiness (this is expected in sailors because of heat and humidity) because heat loosens and the humidity softens and widens the skin pores. A southerly summer increases epidemics as well as smallpox and measles. A northerly summer increases the frequency of squeezing diseases (أمراض العصر); these occur by cold liquefaction and squeezing of hot humors, either deep or superficial. These diseases are like catarrh and those associated with it. However, if a northerly summer is dry, it benefits phlegmatics and women and causes ophthalmia and hot chronic fevers for cholerics as well as converting burned, yellow bile to black bile.

The autumn is full of illnesses because people are exposed to hot sun and then coldness, excess of fruits that corrupt humors, and weakness of strength in the summer. Autumn corrupts the humors due to substandard diet as well as the disintegration of light [humor] and the retention of thick [humor] and their charring. Additionally, every time nature erupts, trying to disintegrate and push a humor out, the coldness retains it. Blood humor is decreased in autumn, which is opposite in its temperament to blood humor and does not support its generation; this is in addition to the summer's degeneration of blood and the lowering of its quantity. The autumn increases the bitter yellow bile (some of it was generated in the summer) and black bile due to the charring of humors in the summer. The black bile increases during autumn because the summer causes charring and the autumn cools down. The beginning of autumn is somewhat agreeable with the elderly; however, the tail end of it is extremely harmful to them.

Autumn's diseases include excoriating scabies and/or eczema (جرب متقشر), ringworm (قوبا، قوابي), cancers, joint pains, irregular fevers (حميات مختلطه), quartan fever (for excess black bile), enlargement of the spleen, strangury (تقطير البول)* due to the bladder's temperamental fluctuation between hot and cold, also difficulty in urination (عسر البول), lienteric diarrhea by cold pushing light humor deep into the body, sciatica (عرق النسا), and bitter bilious angina (ذبحه) that is phlegmatic in spring since the beginning of each starts in the preceding season. There is also the frequency of dry ileus,† apoplexy and its diseases, lung diseases, backaches, and pains in the thighs due to

---

*Strangury is a painful, frequent urination of small volumes that are expelled slowly only by straining and despite a severe sense of urgency, usually with the residual feeling of incomplete emptying.

†Dry ileus is an intestinal obstruction that is either partial or complete blockage of the bowel that results in the failure of the intestinal contents to pass through.

the movement of morbid humor during the summer and then congestion during autumn. Intestinal worms are frequent due to weak digestion and expulsion. A dry autumn encourages smallpox, especially if
preceded by a hot summer. Insanity is also common in autumn because
of abnormal bilious humors and mixing with black bile. Autumn is very
harmful to people with lung ulcers and tuberculosis (it uncovers the
problem if it is asymptomatic) and single hectic fever due to its drying
effect. Autumn is suitable for the summer diseases that did not appear
then. The best autumn is wet and rainy, worse is a dry one.

SEVENTH SECTION

Rules of the Year's Structure

When a northerly spring follows a southerly winter and provides a long
summer with water, the fall in this case will witness many deaths among
children, abrasion and ulceration of the intestine, and long impure tertian fever (الـغـب). If the winter is very humid it aborts pregnant women
who are expecting in the spring for the weakest of reasons, or they will
deliver babies that will be weak, dead, or sick. It will increase conjunctivitis, hemorrhagic diarrhea, and catarrh, especially in the elderly (and
could cause in them sudden death when it afflicts nerves and blocks the
respiratory passages).

If a wet southerly spring follows a northerly winter, then its summer
will induce excess of hot fevers, conjunctivitis, bowels looseness, hemorrhagic diarrhea, and a lot more of catarrh. Additionally, this situation
will cause the movement of phlegm by warmth to internal cavities, especially for people with wet temperament like women, and the increase
of putrefaction and its fevers. However, the rise of the dog star (Sirius,
الـشـعـري) accompanied by rain and northerly wind ameliorates these illnesses and improves the outlook. This type of a season is most harmful to women and children; those who survive it could develop quartan
fever (حـمـى الربـع) due to the charring and ashiness of humors, as well
as edema after the quartan, spleen pain, and weakness of the liver. Its
harm is less on the elderly and those that should avoid coldness.

If a dry northerly summer is followed by a rainy southerly autumn, then in the winter the bodies will be ready for headache, cough, scratchy throat (hoarseness), and tuberculosis because they will tend to get catarrh. If a dry southerly summer is followed by a rainy northerly autumn, the winter will also see [some of] the same illnesses: headache, catarrh, cough, and hoarseness. If a northerly autumn follows a southerly summer, squeezing diseases and congestion become prevalent. When the summer and autumn are both southerly and wet, they tend to increase wet humors, and the winter will induce squeezing diseases. Accumulation of bad humors will encourage illnesses of putrefaction during winter.

If winter is both northerly and dry, it will benefit those with excessive wetness and sciatica, dry conjunctivitis, chronic catarrh, hot fevers, and melancholy. Know that a rainy cold winter induces urethritis (حرقه البول).

An excessively hot dry summer produces fatal and nonfatal, as well as explosive and nonexplosive, suffocating afflictions (خوانيق) [may be interpreted as inflammation of the throat]. The explosive ones are internal and external [they rupture internally or externally]. It also produces dysuria, measles, chicken pox (جدري الماء), synonyms are العنكز, العنقز, الحمقاء), benign smallpox (جدري سليمات), conjunctivitis, blood putrefaction, anxiety, amenorrhea, and hemoptysis.

A dry winter followed by a dry spring is bad; plants get infected, thus animal feed becomes degraded and animals become contaminated, which adversely affects the humans who eat them.

EIGHTH SECTION

Effects of Weather Changes That Are Not Very Opposite to the Normal

We need to complete the discussion of all abnormal weather changes and the changes that oppose temperaments that occur due to celestial and terrestrial causes. We have mentioned many of these in the discussion of seasons. Celestial effects occur due to the influence of planets. The aggregation of many bright planets in a region, or near the sun, increases temperature substantially, especially when these planets are at their zenith or close to it. The planets are sometimes far from their zenith and thus heat is reduced. The zenith effect is influenced by its duration; however, it is not the same effect as proximity. Terrestrial effects are due to latitudes, altitude, presence of mountains and seas, wind, and some because of the soil. Latitudes closer to the Tropic of Cancer in the north and the Tropic of Capricorn in the south are warmer during their summers than are locations closer to the equator or away from the two tropics. It must be believed that the spot that is located within an equitable day is the closet to equitability because the only factor responsible for it is the presence of the sun at its zenith most of the time. This explains why the afternoon is warmer than midday. For this, the heat is more intense at the end of Cancer [July 22] and the beginning of Leo [July 23], when the sun is at its maximum declination. When the sun moves down slightly from the zenith of Cancer, it is hotter than if it had reached the Tropic of Cancer and remained at the same degree of declination. The sun remains at the orbital nodes of the equator (العقدتين) [during equinox] only for a few days because the increase in declination there is more than at the two tropics [Cancer and Capricorn] (المنقلبين). The sun remains at the two tropics for three to four days; therefore, countries that are at the tropics are the warmest, and next are the countries that are 15 degrees toward the poles on both sides of the tropics. Heat at the equator is not as excessive as when the sun's zenith is at the maximum of the Tropic of Cancer; however, these countries to the north of the tropic are much colder. This explains the similarity in conditions across one latitude.

Regarding the location of the country in a high or low land, the ones that are in a valley are always warmer, and those on high locations are always colder. The air closer to the Earth gets warmer because of the warming effect of the sun closer to the Earth's surface, and the farther it is the colder it gets. The explanation in physical philosophy is that the deeper the valley the more it retains the sun's heat and becomes warmer. The effect of the mountain depends if the location is on top of the mountain or next to it. We have explained the first and now will explain the second. The mountain affects the weather in two ways: one, by reflecting the rays on the location or shielding the location from the sun, and the other is its protection from wind. A mountain located north of a location will warm it up by the reflection of the sun's rays on the mountain; similarly if the mountains are on the western side and the eastern side is exposed to the sun. If the mountains are on the eastern side, then there is less exposure to the sun every hour because the sun keeps moving away from the location, which is the opposite if the mountains are to the west. As for preventing wind, a mountain can protect a location from northerly cold wind or expose it to warm southerly wind. The location between two mountainsides is exposed to wind with higher intensity than in an exposed desert because the wind is pulled into a narrow pathway and continues; the same occurs with water, which is known in natural sciences. *The most moderate location regarding exposure and protection is that exposed from the east and north and shielded from the west and south.*

Seas increase the humidity in the vicinity. If the sea is to the north, then it will have a cooling effect due to the air's gentle passage over the water surface that is naturally cold. If the sea is to the south, it increases the thickness [humidity] of the air, especially if a mountain traps the wind. An eastern sea humidifies better than a western sea because the sun increases evaporation more than a western sea. In general, a seaside location has higher humidity and is healthier if the wind moves freely without mountains to block its movement. However, wind scarcity induces infections and humoral putrefaction. In this regard, the healthiest of winds is the northerly, followed by the easterly and westerly, and most harmful is the southerly.

There are two sides to the effects of the wind, one general and the other specific to each location. In general, southerly winds in most countries are hot and humid; their heat is carried from the warm areas, and they are humid because most of the seas are to the south of us. The sun acts on the southerly wind by reducing its vapors and thus making it lighter. Northerly winds are cold because they move over cold mountains and lands with lots of snow, and dry because they lack vapor where less evaporation takes place in northern lands and no bodies of liquid saline water are present, but rather, winds cross frozen waters and prairies. The easterly wind is moderate in warmth and humidity, but drier than the westerly since the northeast is less humid than the northwest. We are in the north where, without a doubt, the westerly wind is more humid because it passes over seas and moves in the opposite direction to the sun's movement, thus it is not loosened by the sun as is the easterly wind, especially since most of the blowing of the easterly wind takes place at the start of the day. Most of the westerly wind blows at the end of the day. Therefore, the westerly wind is less warm than the easterly and tends to be cold, while the easterly is warm, and both are moderate in comparison with the southerly and northerly winds.

The effect of the wind may be different in some countries due to other reasons. In some countries the southerly wind is colder because it passes over snowy southern mountains, and the northerly wind warmer than the southerly one because it passes over warm prairies. Breezes are winds that pass over very hot prairies or smoke that has the horrific effect of fire; the heavy type of them causes inflammation by drying light humor and releasing the heavy humor that causes inflammation and fieriness (ناريه).

All strong winds, according to ancient scientists, start in the upper atmosphere, even if their initiating material comes from below; however, their initial movement, direction, and speed are determined in the above atmosphere. This can be a general rule, or takes place in the majority of cases, but its proof rests with physical philosophy. We will have a section on housing. As to soil differences, there is pure clay, calcareous, sandy, muddy (marshy), and black, and some is mostly affected by usage; all of this affects the air and water.

NINTH SECTION

Bad Weather Changes That Are Opposite to the Normal

These changes in air are either in its composition or qualities. The change in composition happens when one of its components becomes excessive or rare, and this induces epidemics due to the putrefaction in the air that is similar to that occurring in a pond or stagnant water. Air here is not the pure air since this is not what surrounds us. Every simple component of the air does not rot but changes in quality; it may change to another component like the water becomes vapor. Air is a substance that is spread in the atmosphere, that is, a mixture of true air, watery vapors, earthy smoke and dust, and fiery components [the energy associated with the components]. Similarly, despite its mixing with air, earth, and fire, we still refer to the water of the sea and ponds as water. Air with high humidity is conducive to epidemics and putrefaction. Additionally, stagnant waters also become moldy. Most of the adverse changes of water such as putrefaction and rotting take place at the end of the summer and autumn. We will explain the symptoms of epidemics in a different place.

Qualitative change is an extreme hot or cold that cannot be tolerated and causes the devastation of plants and animals. The change may be of the same quality, such as excess of heat, or of opposing qualities, like extreme cold in the summer. A change in the air is reflected in the body; a corruption of the air leads to the corruption of the humors, and it reaches the heart first because it is the closest to it. If it becomes excessively hot it loosens the joints, evaporates the humidity and induces thirst, and weakens respiration, thus it deteriorates the faculties and digestion by reducing the innate heat that is nature's machine, changes the color to yellow by decomposing blood humor, brings yellow bile to dominance, liquefies and putrefies humors, and sends them into the cavities and weak organs, which is not healthful for intact bodies but helpful to edematous and palsy sufferers, as well as people with cold tetanus (كزاز), cold catarrh, wet spasms, and wet facial paralysis (اللقوه).

Cold air confines innate heat in the body unless it is excessive and has deeper effect, and then it is deadly. Moderate cold air prevents the humors from becoming runny and holds them in place; however, it induces catarrh, weakens nerves, and damages the trachea (قصبه الريه); it may also strengthen digestion and all other internal functions as well as appetite (شهوه). In general cold air is more agreeable with healthy people than is excessively hot air. Its hurts neural functions, closes pores, constricts viscera, and loosens the bones.

Humid air is congruent with most temperaments, improves skin and its color, softens it, and keeps pores open, however, it encourages putrefaction.

TENTH SECTION

Effects of Winds

We have mentioned the characteristics of winds in the part on the changes of weather; however, here we provide general description in a different organization, starting with the north.

Northerly wind strengthens, tightens, prevents superficial secretions, clogs skin pores, strengthens digestion, produces constipation, is a diuretic, and corrects the putrefactive and epidemic air. When the sequence of a northerly, a southerly, and then a northerly wind takes place, the southerly liquefies humors, and the northerly pushes them to the abdomen, which may lead to an outside bulging and rupture; this is the reason for the increase of movement of liquids from the head [catarrh fluids moving down], chest illnesses, northerly diseases, and nerve pain, as well as diseases of the bladder, uterus, dysuria, cough, shivering, and pains of ribs, waist, and chest.

Southerly wind weakens the faculties, opens skin pores, excites and moves humors to the outside; dulls senses; putrefies wounds; relapses disease; weakens; produces ulcers, gout, itching, and headache; induces sleep; and induces putrefied fevers but not sore throat (تخشّن الـحـلـق).

Easterly wind blowing at the end of the night and early in the day originates from air that has been ameliorated and lightened by the sun, and its humidity has been reduced so it is dryer and gentler. If the wind moves in at the end of the day and early night then the situation is the opposite. In general, the easterly is better than the westerly.

Westerly wind blowing at the end of the night and early in the day originates from air that has not been modified by the sun; therefore, it is denser and heavier, and it is of opposite quality when it blows at the end of the day and early night.

ELEVENTH SECTION

Effects of Locations and/or Habitat

We have mentioned under the topic of weather changes the characteristics of locations and/or habitats, however, here we provide general description, in a different organization, and it does not matter if we repeat some of that we have mentioned earlier.

You have learned that location affects the body due to altitude, surrounding topography such as mountains, soil (whether clay, damp, muddy, metallic, wetness), and the presence of woods, metals, graves,* and such. You have known how to figure out the temperaments of air from its latitudes, soil, the presence of adjacent seas and mountains, and the winds. In general, air cools rapidly when the sun sets, and warms up, and becomes gentle, when it rises; and the opposite is true. Bad air congests the heart and suffocates.

Hot areas darken the skin, curl the hair, and weaken digestion. The increase in evaporation and the lowering of body humidity accelerate aging; for example, Ethiopians look old at the age of thirty years due to weakness of the heart and respiration. People of hot areas have softer bodies.

People of **cold areas** are stronger, braver, and have better digestion. When a cold area is also humid, its people are fleshy and fatty, with sunken vessels and joints, and healthy skin.

People of **humid areas** are good-looking, soft-skinned, and quickly fatigued by exercise. Their summer is not excessively hot, and their winter is not excessively cold. They have chronic fevers, diarrhea, menorrhagia,† and hemorrhoids. Also common among them are ulcers, putrefaction, thrush,‡ and epilepsy.

People of **dry areas** tend to have dry temperaments, dry cracked skin, and dry brain. Their summer is hot and winter is cold.

People of **high areas** are healthy, strong, and enduring, and live long lives. People of **low areas** are always depressed and sad. Their areas

---

*Here Avicenna is referring to cemetaries.
†Menorrhagia is unusually heavy or prolonged bleeding during menstruation.
‡Thrush is a yeast infection (candidiasis) of the mucus membrane lining of the mouth and tongue.

have warm, stagnant, muddy, or salty waters, and because of their low air quality the waters are also the same.

Unexposed **stony areas** have very hot weather in the summer and cold in the winter, and their people have solid compact bodies with thick hair, strong joints, and mostly dry temperament. They stay up late, have ill manners, and are arrogant and totalitarian, strong fighters, clever craftsmen, and possess acuity.

People of **snowy mountainous areas** have the same characteristics as other cold areas. These areas are windy. During the snow season the winds of these areas are pleasant, however, after the snow melts, they become muggy, especially if mountains block the wind.

Coastal areas have moderate weather due to the stabilizing effect of their humidity, which is prevalent in these areas. If the area is located in the north, then the coastal and valley locations are the best; however, in the south it is the opposite.

Comment on Northern Areas

These areas fall within the characteristics of cold locations and seasons, where diseases of congestion, squeezing, and internal aggregation of humors prevail. Also, people of these areas are known for good digestion, longevity, nosebleed due to fullness, and low evaporation that leads to the rupture of vessels. Epilepsy is rare because of their good health and strong innate heat; however, if it takes place it is usually severe because it appears due to a strong problem. Ulcers heal quickly because of the people's bodily strength and the good quality of their blood, and also for the lack of external causes that loosen and soften the ulcers. Due to the excessive innate heat of their hearts, they display wild manners. *Their women do not fully bleed and cleanse during menses due to the constriction of vessels and lack of liquefaction and softness; therefore, the incomplete discharge of menses induces sterility.* This is opposite to what we see in Turkey, and I say that the strong innate heat opposes the lack of external inducers of liquefaction and softness. It is said that women of cold areas rarely abort, and that is evidence that the wombs of these women are contracted and constricted, but miscarriage mostly happens due to cold. Their milk is reduced and thickened by cold that prevents liquefaction and movement. In these areas, tetanus and tuberculosis may occur in weak individuals such as women, and especially in post-partum women. Severe tetanus may complicate childbirth, thus ruptur-ing vessels in the chest or nerve fibers and causing tuberculosis in the first [rupture of vessels] and tetanus in the second [rupture of nerve]. It may also lead to the rupture of the hypochondrium [solar plexus, the upper part of the anterior abdomen caudal to the lowest ribs of the tho-rax] due to severe difficulty in childbirth. Newborn boys may develop a hydrocele that disappears later. Young women may develop ascites and hydrouterus that disappear with age. They rarely develop ophthalmia, but it is usually severe when it occurs.

Comment on Southern Areas

These areas fall within the same characteristics of warm locations and seasons. Their water contains salt and sulfur. The heads of their inhab-itants are full of moist humors because the south does that. Their bow-els are instable due to the continued leakage of catarrh liquids from their heads to the stomach. They have organs that are lax and weak, dull senses, and weak appetite. They are heavy drunks because of their weak heads and stomachs. Their ulcers are soft and difficult to heal. Frequently, their women have menorrhagia, difficulty getting pregnant, and miscarriages due to their many illnesses. Their people past the fifti-eth year of age are susceptible to palsy as a consequence of their catarrh. Others develop hemorrhagic diarrhea due to head congestion, asthma, distension, and epilepsy, and are afflicted with fevers that combine heat and cold and long nightly winter fevers with less of hot fevers due to their frequent diarrhea that causes loss of light humors.

Comment on Eastern Areas

The city that is open to the east is healthful with good air. The sun rises on it early in the day and purifies the air, which moves on with even higher purity; also, the sun sends it gentle wind that is followed by the sun and affected by its movement.

Comment on Western Areas

The city that is exposed to the west and shielded from the east does not receive the sun until later, and as soon as the sun gets closest, it starts moving away, therefore, the sun does not moderate the air or dry it but rather leaves it moist and thick. When the sun sends wind it is westerly and nightly, thus these areas are similar to those with humid temperament and moderate but dense temperature. If it was not for the humidity, it would have been similar to spring. However, it is less in quality than the eastern areas, and one should not pay attention to the saying that it has the same absolute effects as the spring, but in comparison with other countries it is very good. One disliked aspect of this area is the late and sudden exposure to the sun's heat after the night's coldness, thus the humid temperament of the weather and its effects on voice hoarseness, especially in the winter due to catarrh.

On the Selection of Areas for Residency and Features of Buildings

One who selects a residence should know the soil, altitude, exposure, water supply and its quality, type of wind (whether it is the cold healthful), close water bodies, plains, mountains, and minerals, as well as the prevailing and usual illnesses of its population, the strength of their digestion, their type of food, and the source of their water (from widely open sources or small constricted outlets). The windows and doors should be northeastern, and supporting columns should permit the eastern wind to enter the building and the rays of the sun to reach every spot inside, since it improves the air. The residence should be close to deep, clean, fresh running water that cools down in winter and warms up in summer (unlike well water), which is beneficial.

We have discussed the weather and locations, and now we should talk about what comes after them as causes that we count with them.

TWELFTH SECTION

Effects of Movement and Rest

Movement affects the human body by its severity and duration, as well as interspersed rest. According to philosophers, this is a section by itself that also includes the substances consumed. Vigorous movement, whether for long or short duration, mixed with rest excites the body's heat; however, vigorous but short differs from long and mild, and the long interspersed with rest warms a lot and induces little sweating.

The long movement induces sweating gently due to warming; however, each of the two factors [movement and heat] will cool down the body because they exhaust the body's resources and disperse its moisture. The consumption of a substance may affect the outcome; for example, the bleacher benefits from his profession by getting cooling and moisture, and the iron smith get heat and dryness. Rest is always cooling for the lack of refreshing of the innate heat, congestion, and moistening because it stops the loss of moisture in wastes.

THIRTEENTH SECTION

Effects of Sleep and Wakefulness

Sleep is very similar to rest, and wakefulness is very similar to movement, but they have some specifics that we should consider; therefore, we say that sleep strengthens the natural faculties because it retains and saves the innate heat and relaxes the psychological faculty by moisturizing its components, thus making breath available and reducing evaporation. Sleep removes the causes of fatigue and restrains excessive evacuations because movement increases liquefaction, except for skin wastes that are pushed out during sleep because they aid in heat retention to the interior. Sleep distributes food in the body, pushes whatever is close to skin, and retains it everywhere else; however, wakefulness is more effective in this because it includes acquiring the substance and not only its slow gentle decomposition.

Whoever sweats profusely during their sleep, without other known causes, has excess of food that the body cannot tolerate. During sleep, the food that is ready for digestion and maturing gets converted into blood humor, warmed, and sent throughout the body, thus increasing the innate heat; however, existing bitter hot humors will give the body an abnormal type of heat. Sleep will produce coldness if there is no substance to work on or if there is an indigestible humor. Wakefulness does exactly the opposite, and its excessive action corrupts the brain's temperament to dryness, thus weakens it, induces confusion, chars humors, and produces severe illnesses.

Excessive sleep causes dullness of psychological faculty, heaviness of brain, and cold diseases by preventing evaporation. Wakefulness at night increases appetite, induces hunger by decomposition of substance, and reduces digestion by lowering faculties; decomposition between wakefulness and sleep is bad in all situations. During sleep, heat is internal and cold appears externally; this is the reason for the need for bed covers for the whole body that are not needed during wakefulness. You will find more details on the effect of sleep, its indication, and its conditions in future books.

FOURTEENTH SECTION

Effects of Psychological Movements

All psychological syndromes are followed or accompanied by breath movement to the outside or inside, all at once or little by little; outside movement results in internal cooling, and an excess of it weakens exhalation, thus resulting in internal and external cooling followed by loss of consciousness or death. Inhaling results in external cooling and internal warming, and when congested it cools down both the internal and external, resulting in coma or death. Exhaling is either all at once as when angry, or slowly as during ecstasy or moderate happiness. Inhaling is also either all at once as during fright or slowly as in sadness or choking.

Gradual reduction in respiration [including innate heat] happens slowly, bit by bit. Reactive breathing may take place in two directions if the situation requires, that is, in anxiety or grief that includes anger and sadness; also shyness induces inhalation, then the mind relaxes the contraction and exhales, thus causing blushing.

The body may react due to psychological situations other than what we have mentioned. For example, the imagination may induce physical effects, as when a woman delivers a baby who looks similar to what she imagined during intercourse and the baby's skin complexion is similar to what the father imagined at ejaculation. These are situations that some reject in disgust because they are not aware of these mysterious situations of existence; however, people who are aware of such knowledge do not deny their existence. Similarly, a person may increase blood circulation by staring at a red object, develop toothache when watching someone eating sour food, experience pain induction in an organ by looking at another person with pain in the same organ, and experience the alteration of temperament by imagining a happy or sad matter.

FIFTEENTH SECTION

Effects of Food and Drink Consumption

The human body reacts to three aspects of food and drink: the reaction to its **quality** [i.e., temperament], the reaction to its **elements** [i.e., monomers, building blocks], and the reaction to the **essence of its substance** [i.e., chemical constituents]. The linguistic meanings of these terms or concepts are close; however, we will explain their meanings. The active, by its quality, may gain or lose heat from the human body, thus producing either warmth or coolness without becoming part of the body. The **active, by its elements**, loses its own characteristics and transforms to that of an organ; initially its elements retain their own nature until becoming part of an organ. Some of its qualities are stronger than that of human temperament and are retained long after digestion and integration within the human body, for example, the lettuce has cold temperament that is colder than that of humans and cools down the blood, while garlic has an opposite effect [i.e., warms up the blood].

The active, by its essence, describes the actions of its specific composition [chemistry], not its quality [temperament], which results from its distribution within the body without any homologous similarity to the body. By quality I mean one of the four temperaments.

The **active by quality** does not involve its matter into the action [no chemical bonding]. The active by element releases its elements [monomers such as amino acids] from its essence and strengthens the body by replenishing its nutrients, increases the innate heat by enriching the blood humor, or acts by its remaining temperament [the portion that was not incorporated into humors].

The **active by essence** [specific action] is the one that acts by its new form after the temperamental change has taken place and after it has spread in the body and produced a new form and quality that is different from that of its initial element and temperament. It is an endpoint [resting point] that happens to the element [substance] according to its temperament, like the attractive power of the magnet and the nature of every species of animal and plant that benefits from what comes after the temperamental reaction by preparing the temperament, and it is not as the simple temperament or the temperament itself since it is not simple or mixed, warmth, coolness, moisture, or dryness, but similar to color, odor, breath, or another form that is not felt by the senses. This form, produced after the temperamental reaction, may become complete by the action of other substances if this form is reactive or by its action on others if the form is active. If it is active on others it may act within the human body or not. An active substance within the body may produce a suitable or unsuitable action. The complete action is called total essences because it is not based on the temperament but on the substance's specific effect after the temperamental balancing has taken place, by its kind not quality (i.e., without the four temperaments or their combinations). A suitable substance is like the peony (*Paeonia* sp., فاوانيا) for curing epilepsy, or unsuitable like aconite (*Aconitum napellus*, البيش), which corrupts the essence of the body.

Now, we are back to say, if we describe something that is ingested or spread [ointment, oil] as hot or cold, we mean the effect and not the feel. We mean by hot effect or cold effect on the body that the effect is on the body's innate heat after the substance has reacted with the heat of the body. We may also mean another thing, and that is the general quality of the substance such as when we say the sulfur is hot. We say in short that the substance is hot or cold in its temperament without attention to its effect on the body. We may say that this drug is such, meaning the characteristic possessed by the drug, like our saying that a person possesses the skill to write or that aconite is poisonous. The difference between the first and the second meanings is that the first means that the body has to interact with the substance to produce an action, while the second appears immediately, like a snake's poison, or by little change in its quality, like the aconite. There is an intermediate effect between the two, similar to poisonous drugs.

The degrees [grades, potencies] of medication are four. The first-degree drugs are those that have unfelt effect of heating and cooling; it is only felt if repeated and increased in dosage. The second degree has a higher effect than the first and does not harm the body functions in an obvious manner or change its normal functions except as side effects or when repeated and increased in dosage. Third-degree drugs cause obvious harm but do not lead to death or disease. Fourth-degree drugs induce death and disease, which is the characteristic of poisonous medications; the fatal medications are poison.

We say from the top that all that goes into the body and interacts with it (through action and reaction) is either (1) changed by the body but does not change the body, (2) changed by the body and changes the body, or (3) unchanged by the body and changes the body. The one changed itself, but not affecting the body, or slightly affecting it, is either similar to the body or not. The one similar to the body is food, and the dissimilar is balanced drugs [i.e., nonassimilable].

Drugs that are changed by the body and change the body may affect the body the same way they are affected by the body, or the changes in the drugs may take place after a while from ingestion and be neutralized by others or eventually corrupt the body. The first type when similar to the body is **medicinal foods**, and when dissimilar is **absolute medicine**, while the second type is **poisonous medicines**.

The drugs that do not change themselves but change the body

are the **absolute poisons**. We do not mean that, because it does not change, it is not warmed up by the innate heat of the body, most of the poisons do, but rather we mean that its natural form is not altered and it continues to act on the body in a fixed strength and form until it corrupts it. The poison's hot temperament [in the body] assists its specific essence [chemical effect] in the destruction of respiration, such as snake venom* and aconite. While poisons of cold temperaments assist their specific effects by weakening and extinguishing respiration, such as scorpion venom† and hemlock (الشوكران), and all induce coldness in the body.

Heating is a normal body change that is induced by all nutrients, and when nutrients are converted to blood humor they increase heat; even lettuce and pumpkin [considered as cold food] produce this heat. However, by change we do not mean this kind of heat but rather that which is produced by the drug's quality and specific action at the end [after temperamental reaction and digestion]. The body changes the specific action of medicinal foods as well as their quality [temperament], however, it first changes its quality. Some of the foods show, first, their heating effect, such as garlic, and some their cooling effect, such as lettuce. When the change in quality is complete then most of the effect is heating by increasing the blood humor; how could it not heat when it has turned hot after it has released it coldness? Additionally, the change in the specific action may be accompanied with a leftover of the original quality, so there will be some cooling in the blood humor from lettuce, and some warming from garlic.

Some medicinal foods are more medicinal and others are more nutritive, and some are closer in their characteristics to blood humor, like wine, egg yolk, and meat juice, while others are somewhat less, like bread and meat, and some exceedingly less, like medicinal foods. We say that food changes the body by its quality and quantity (you have known

---

*Snake venoms hydrolyze protein bonds and nucleic acid (DNA).

†Scorpion toxins affect sodium (Na⁺) and probably potassium (K⁺) channels in nerves attached to muscles, thus causing loss of function and control of skeletal muscle through involuntary tremor.

that [as described previously]), where excess of quantity leads to indigestion, obstruction, and putrefaction while deficiency in food weakens. Excess of food produces coolness unless it putrefies, then it gives heat because it is generated by abnormal heat and produces abnormal heat.

We say that there are the **light** food, the **dense**, and the **moderate**. The light produces light blood humor, and the dense produces heavy blood humor. In these three food types, the food may be very nutritious or lightly nutritious. Examples of light very nutritious food are wine, meat juice, warm egg yolk, or half-boiled egg. It is very nutritious because most of its essence gets converted to nutrients. Examples of dense and slightly nutritious foods are cheese, dried meat, eggplant, and the like; only a small portion is converted to nutrients. Examples of dense and very nutritious are boiled eggs and beef meat. Examples of light and slightly nutritious foods are *julab,* or *jallab* [an Old World drink made from diluted honey or molasses with dates, rose water, pomegranates, and floating pine nuts—usually a summer drink], legumes with moderate texture and quality, and fruits such as apples, pomegranates, and the like. These types produce either good or bad **chyme** (*chymos*). Examples of dense, rich food with good chyme are egg yolk, drinks, and meat juice; light, slightly nutritious with good chyme are lettuce, apples, and pomegranates; light, slightly nutritious with bad chyme are radishes, mustard, and most legumes; light, very nutritious and bad chyme are lung and the meat of young birds; dense, very nutritious with good chyme are boiled eggs and meat of one-year-old lambs; dense, very nutritious with bad chyme are beef, duck, and horse meats; and dense, slightly nutritious with bad chyme are dried meat. And, it is up to you to find in all of this the moderate.

SIXTEENTH SECTION

Conditions of Water

Water is one of the elements, and it is specified in the description of the elements that water is the only element that is part of all that is ingested, not because it is nutritional, but rather because it carries through the foods and improves their texture. We said that the water is not nutritional because such a substance becomes part of the blood humor and further becomes part of an organ. A simple element does not change into the form of blood humor or that of a human organ unless it becomes part of a compound. Water assists in the liquefaction of food, making it lighter, and in its transport through vessels in both ways; this is very essential for the completion of the nutritional functions. Waters differ not in the essence of water but in what mixes with them and their dominant qualities. The best waters are those from springs, not all springs but those in a land free from contamination or stony soil without any soil putrefaction, however, the waters from free clay are better than that from stony soils. Spring water has to be running water that is exposed to the sun and wind to be good water since stagnant water may become of less quality by exposure, which would not occur if it stays below the surface.

Water running over clay soil is better than one running over stones since clay filters out contaminants while stones do not. However, the clay should be free and not putrid, marshy, or other than that. The best water is deep and fast running (in which impurities do not change its nature), running toward the sun (especially in the summer), running far from its source, and then turning north. The one running west or south is of low quality especially when wind blows from the south. Water falling from a height is better if it also combines the other good characteristics.

Water with good characteristics should taste good and sweet and should not be mixed with alcohol in excess. It is light, heats up and cools down quickly due to is looseness, and is cold in the winter and warm in the summer, without taste or odor, goes down quickly through the epigastrium (الشراسيف), and is easy to cook food with because it cooks through with ease.

Know that weighing is one of the successful methods of testing water condition. Lighter in most cases is better, and its weight can be measured by weighing. This can be figured out by wetting two pieces of cloth with two waters, or two cottons of equal weight, and then drying them completely; the one with lighter cotton is better. Water quality can be improved by boiling and distillation or by cooking it, since scientists have testified that this way causes less distension and/or bloating and the water goes down faster. Ignorant physicians think that cooked water loses its light part and retains its dense part and thus there is no benefit in cooking since it becomes thicker; however, you should know that water in its natural ranges is similar in lightness and density because it is simple and not compound. Furthermore, water density increases by severe coldness or by admixing with very small earthy particles that stay suspended and do not settle because they cannot break through the water due to its lightness and water forces them to stay suspended. Cooking of water removes the condensation caused by coldness first, and then loosens it to become lighter in density, and the earthy particles precipitate through its density. The rest of the water is pure water that is close to the simple, and its vapor is similar and not far from it; this is because when water has no impurities it becomes similar in all of its parts and the vapor is not far from the rest. Therefore, cooking water removes cold condensation and precipitates impurities. The evidence for this is that if you leave dense water for a long time nothing significant precipitates, but after cooking a lot precipitates and the density is lighter; the reason for precipitation is the looseness that resulted from cooking. Do you not see that the waters of the large valleys like River Jayhon (also Gihon),* especially those far from their sources, are turbid at their sources, but the water becomes clear in a short while, and if you try to purify it, only insignificant precipitate comes out? There are people who praise very much the water of the Nile River and list four of its advantages: distant source, passing through good soil, going from south to north, and its depth, which is a characteristic shared by others.

Purifying contaminated water by decanting from one container to another every day shows some sediment; the sedimentation takes place slowly, however, it will not purify the water completely because the earthy contaminants separate easily from thin water that lacks

---

*Nineteenth-century, modern, and Arabic scholars have identified Jayhon with Amu Darya. Amu Darya was known to the medieval Islamic writers as Jayhun or Ceyhun in Turkish. This was a derivative of Jihon, or Zhihon as it is still known in Farsi.

thickness, viscosity, and oiliness, but not easily from thick water. Cooking increases the thinness of water, especially after cooking with agitation (churning, المـخـض).

Rainwater is good water, especially during the summer from thundering clouds. Water from stormy clouds becomes contaminated since the water vapor and their clouds are impure. Rainwater is thin and, therefore, becomes easily contaminated with earthy and windy impurities, and its putrefaction can cause humoral putrefaction and hurt chest and voice. Some have said that this is because it is generated from various moistures, however, if this was true then rainwater would have been disliked, but this is not the case. It is because of its lightness and its density's readiness to accept others; however, its corruption can be interrupted by boiling it to make it less acceptable to putrefaction. To prevent the harmful effect of rainwater susceptible to putrefaction, some acidity should be added to it [vinegar, lemon juice].

The water of **wells** and **canals** in comparison to **spring** water is bad, and this is because it is stored and exposed to earth material for a long time and thus may not be free from some putrefaction. It is collected by excessive force and not by its own tendency but rather by trickery and craft that eased its way to storage. Its worst type is that transported in lead pipes, thus picking up some of its nature and causing stomach ulcers.

Percolating water (مـاء الـنـز) is worse than well water because the latter is renewed by usage, and thus continues to get renewed without sitting in storage or underground passages for a long time. On the other hand, water of percolation remains for a considerable time in contaminated underground passages before moving out to the surface; its movement is slow because it is generated by its abundance, not by forceful pressure, and it mostly exists in unclean land.

Icy and **glacier** waters are thick. Stagnant **water of woody low land** (wetland, أجـمـه) is dense and of low quality; it cools down in the winter because of snow, thus generating phlegm, and warms up in the summer by the sun and putrefaction, thus generating gallbladder problems; and due to its thickness, earthy contaminants, and evaporation of its light part, it causes enlargement of the spleen, thinning of the abdominal wall, hardness of internal organs, and weakness of arms, legs, and neck; it enhances appetite and thirst, causes constipation and difficulty in inducing vomiting, and may produce edema because of water retention, pneumonia, diarrhea, and inflammation of the spleen. Furthermore, it is responsible for shrinkage of legs, weakness and shrinkage of the liver due to spleen problems, insanity, hemorrhoids, varicose veins, and soft loose swellings, especially in winter. Also, it causes difficulty in conception, labor, and delivery in women, the delivery of edematous fetuses, and frequent pseudocyesis (false pregnancy). Hydrocele appears in children, and sciatica and leg ulcers in adults (the ulcer being difficult to heal), increase of appetite, and difficulty in inducing evacuation, which takes place with harm and ulceration. They have frequent quatrain fever, and the elderly develop hyperpyrexia due to their dry temperament and constipation.

All **stagnant** water is always not good for the stomach. Drinking from a spring is similar to the stagnant, and the stagnant is preferred if it does not stay for long in its location; however, if it does not move, then without a doubt it has some contaminants and causes constipation. Such water warms up in the stomach, therefore, it is not recommended for people with fevers or with gallbladder issues, however, it is fine in cases where constipation or maturation are needed. Waters contaminated with minerals or alike, or infested with leeches, are worse; however, some have benefit, such as iron in water strengthens internal organs, stops diarrhea, and stimulates sexual desire. We will describe later the characteristics of these waters and similar ones.

Ice and snow if pure without contaminants are useful, whether melted into water or used to cool down water from the outside or added to water. Their different types do not differ much from water. They are denser than all other waters, hurt the individual with nerve pain, and heating removes the effect. If the ice was from low-quality water or the snow gained contaminants where it fell, then it should be used from the outside to cool water.

Cold water in moderate amount is more agreeable to healthy people although it may hurt the nerves and people with internal swellings; it increases appetite and strengthens the stomach. By contrast, **hot water**

corrupts digestion and neutralizes food, does not extinguish thirst, and may lead to edema, hectic fever, and wilting. Lukewarm water causes nausea, and warmer than that, if taken on empty stomach, washes the stomach and softens the stool; however, excess of it is bad and weakens the stomach. Very hot water reduces colic and disintegrates flatus. Hot water benefits people with epilepsy, melancholy, cold headache, and conjunctivitis, those with pustules in the throat and gums and pimples behind the ears, as well as people with catarrh, ulcers of the diaphragm, and weakness of the heart in the chest; it also acts as an emmenagogue, diuretic, and pain reliever.

Salty water reduces weight, dries, and is diarrheic; first by the cleansing it creates, then by drying; that is of its nature. It impairs blood, thus causes itching and scabies. **Turbid water** causes calculi (kidney stones) and obstruction, and a diuretic should be used. A person suffering from diarrhea benefits from all thick and heavy waters because of their retention in the stomach and slow release. Proper treatments of constipation caused by turbid water are fats and sweets.

Ammonia water induces the release of waste, whether as drink, bath, or enema. **Alum*** water is beneficial for menorrhagia, hemoptysis, and bleeding hemorrhoids. However, it induces fevers in bodies ready to accept them. **Iron water** reduces spleen enlargement and enhances sexual desire. **Copper water** improves temperament. When good and bad waters mix together, the strongest one will dominate. We explained the management of bad water in the section on travelers' precautions. The rest of water conditions and their characteristics and effects are in the section on water in the single drugs, so look under that.

SEVENTEENTH SECTION

Effects of Retention and Evacuation

Holding in that which should be expelled occurs because of weakness in expulsion, strong holding, weakness in digestion that keeps the food

---

*The specific compound is hydrated potassium aluminum sulfate (potassium alum), with the formula $KAl(SO_4)_2 \cdot 12H_2O$.

longer to complete its digestion, narrow passage and obstruction dense and viscous in form, its excessive quantity, loss of sensation to expel as in the case of biliary colic (القولنج اليرقاني), or when the body's resources are preoccupied with another crisis (بحارين) and produce strong isch- uria or constipation since evacuation crisis (الاستفراغ البحراني) hap- pens in other direction.

Retention without evacuation will produce illnesses. These may be from the structural type, such as obstruction, distention, humid spasm, and such; from the dystemperament type, such as putrefac- tion, the alteration of innate heat to fiery, the extinguishing of innate heat due to long duration of congestion or its strength that is followed by a cold, and the domination of moisture; from secondary diseases, such as rupture of vessels and bleeding and indigestion, which is a worse cause of disease, especially if it occurs after a long period of scarcity, such as overindulgence during the fertile season after hunger in the dry season; or from compound diseases, such as swellings and pustules.

Evacuation of what should be retained occurs because of strong expulsion, weakness of retention, or the harmful effect of the mate- rial's residues (dregs), such as excess, distention from resulting gas, and excessive acidity, hotness, or thinness. Thinness causes runniness, espe- cially if the ducts are wide, as in the oozing out of semen, or the slit- ting of ducts longitudinally or transversely, or the dilation of orifices, as in nosebleed. Evacuation of needed material that supplies the innate heat causes cold dystemperament; it may cause warm temperament if the expelled is cold, like phlegm, or excessive biliary heat if it is close to equitable, like blood humor, which results in dryness. The expelled material may cause moisture depending on the amount of heat, such as when the expelled is dry humor or indigested food, it increases phlegm; however, this type of humor is not normal. Such expulsion is ultimately followed by coldness and dryness of organs, even if it was initially fol- lowed by abnormal heat and useless moisture. Excessive expulsion in people with obstruction may be followed by dryness of vessels and their obstruction. Moderate retention and elimination that take place when needed are beneficial to maintaining good health.

We have discussed the important types of causes, although not all may be important, so let us take up other causes.

EIGHTEENTH SECTION

Commentary on Unnecessary and Harmless Causes That Are Compatible with the Body

Let us talk now about the unnecessary and harmless causes that are not by their nature in the temperament or against it. These are the things that touch the body other than air, such as **baths, massages,** and others.

We start with a general description of these causes by saying that factors acting on the human body by touching from the outside act in two ways: first by percolating through the skin pores by their own penetrating power, by pulling from the inside, or by both; second through a quality that affects the body like cooling or warming ointments and hot pads that warm. This is because their hot temperament acts through its power while the innate heat excites the active force into action or through its specific action.

There are substances that are affected by touch and inactive when ingested, like onion, which in external application causes ulcer and none of it internally; others are the opposite, like white lead, that has great effect when taken internally but is safe externally; and some are active in both situations. The reasons in the first type are six:

First, a thing like an onion when inside the body is digested and its temperament altered, therefore, it does not have the time to act and induce ulcers.

Second, most of the time it is ingested with other things.

Third, it gets mixed with mixtures that render it harmless.

Fourth, externally it is placed in one location while it is mobile internally.

Fifth, it is firmly fixed on the outside and barely touching on the inside.

Sixth, internally it is ameliorated by the body actions, its waste expelled, and its good parts are converted to blood humors.

However, it is different in the case of white lead, which has large parts, and thus does not pass through the [skin] pore from the outside, and if it does penetrate, will not reach respiratory organs or others, but when taken internally the opposite happens; additionally, its poisonous nature is activated by our innate heat, which does not take place externally. Some of this will be repeated in the book on single drugs.

NINETEENTH SECTION

Effects of Bathing, Sun Exposure, Sand Bath and Rub, Bathing in Oils, and Water Sprinkling on the Face

I was told by some that claim authority that the best bathhouse is an aging, spacious building with fresh air and water. Another authority added that its fireplace should be adjustable to the need of the users. Learn that the natural effect of the bathhouse is to warm up by its air and moisturize by its water. The first room is for cooling and moisturizing, the second for warming and moisturizing, and the third for warming and drying. No attention should be given to the person who says, "Water does not moisturize the original organs by soaking or wrapping," because bathing, as we have described its effects and changes, can cause further changes, some directly and others indirectly. Bathhouse air cools down the excessive innate heat and reduces moisture in the organs of digestive functions and the abnormal moisture, when beneficial. If water is too hot, it produces gooseflesh (temporary rumpling of the skin into tiny bumps, also called goose bumps) and closes its pores; thus it prevents the water from entering the body and does not produce any action. Bathhouse water may warm or cool; if its heat is below lukewarm it cools and moisturizes. Cold water pushes the heat internally into the body. Immersion in water cools in two ways: water is cold and eventually cools down the body even if it initially warms up the body because warmth will dissipate and the natural effect of imbibed water will be cooling; water is moisturizing whether it is hot or cold, however, excessive moisture limits innate heat and thus cools down. Bathing may also warm up by breaking down undigested food and cold humors [converting them to blood humor].

Using dry heat in the bathhouse dries and benefits people with edema and flabbiness. When humid it moisturizes, and a prolonged sitting session in it dries by decomposition* [of undigested food and humors] and sweating; a short session is moisturizing by penetration before it induces sweat. Bathing early in the morning on an empty stomach dehydrates, reduces weight, and weakens; being close to fullness will increase weight by bringing nutrients to the surface; however, this may induce obstruction by incompletely digested foods that move from the stomach and liver, and it is beneficial and increases weight when used at the end of the first digestion [in the stomach] before evacuation.

Individuals using the bathhouse for moisturizing, such as patients with hectic fever, should soak in water as long as it does not weaken them, then cover their skin with fat [or oil] to increase moisturizing and trap the water that filtered into their skin. They should stay for a good amount of time and select a moderately warm location, sprinkle water on the floor to increase humidity in the air, move out of the steam room without excessive effort or be carried out on a stretcher, scented with cold perfumes, left in the dressing room until their normal breath returns, and given drinks of barley water and milk of donkey. A prolonged stay in the hot bath may induce unconsciousness by warming the heart.

Although bathing has many benefits, it also has some harm. It facilitates the movement of waste products to weak organs, relaxes the body, is harmful to nerves, weakens innate heat, diminishes appetite, and reduces sexual desire.

Bathing has beneficial effects from the contents of the water in the

---

*Digestion requires water; therefore, when heat induces digestion water is used.

bath. Waters containing **sulfurous natron,*** seawater, ash, salt (naturally or by cooking) or **mistletoe** and **laurel** (cooked in it), sulfur, and others breakdown [undigested material] ameliorate, remove flabbiness (الترهل) and soft swelling (التربل), prevent the sinking of material into sores [prevent discharge], and benefit in case of **dracunculiasis**[†] (العرق المديني). Waters containing **copper, iron,** and **salt** benefit in cold and moisture diseases, joint pain, gout, muscle weakness (إسترخاء), asthma, and kidney diseases, aid in healing of bone fractures, and benefit in pustules and sores. **Copper** in water is beneficial to the mouth and uvula (اللهاه), lazy eye,[‡] and moistures of the ear. **Iron**-containing water is good for the stomach and spleen. Water of **borax**[§] (بورقيه) salt benefits the head and chest in those predisposed to accepting matter [prone to disease], humid stomach, edema, and distention. **Alum** and **ferric sulfate** (زاجيه محلول الزاج) waters are beneficial for menorrhagia, anal bleeding (hematochezia, نزف المقعده), stomach sensitivity, idiopathic recurrent miscarriage, puffiness, and excessive sweating. Sulfur water treatment cleanses nerves; relieves distension and spasm pains; cleanses the skin from pustules, chronic bad sores, roughness (سمج), freckles (كلف), leukoderma (برص), and vitiligo (بهق); decom-

---

*Natron is a naturally occurring mixture of sodium carbonate decahydrate ($Na_2CO_3 \cdot 10H_2O$, a kind of soda ash) and about 17 percent sodium bicarbonate, or baking soda, $NaHCO_3$) along with small quantities of household salt (halite, sodium chloride) and sodium sulfate. Natron is white to colorless when pure, varying to gray or yellow with impurities. The English word *natron* is a French cognate derived from the Spanish *natrón* through the Greek νιτρων (nitron), which derived from the Ancient Egyptian word *netjeri*, meaning "natron." The ancient Egyptians found natron in the dry lakes of the desert and transported it to the banks of the Nile River to be used for mummification due to its dehydrating and preservative effects. The current scientific chemical symbol for sodium, Na, is an abbreviation of that element's New Latin name, *natrium*, which was derived from *natron*.

†Dracunculiasis, also called guinea worm disease, is a parasitic infection caused by *Dracunculus medinensis*, a long and very thin nematode (roundworm).

‡Amblyopia, otherwise known as lazy eye, is a vision disorder characterized by poor or indistinct vision in an eye that is otherwise physically normal. It affects 1–5 percent of the population.

§Borax (sodium borate, sodium tetraborate, or disodium tetraborate) is an important boron compound, a mineral, and a salt of boric acid.

poses the wastes in the joints, spleen, and liver; and reduces hardness of the uterus; however, it weakens the stomach and appetite. Bathing in desert water or arid land water (مياه قفريه) congests the head, therefore, the head should be kept out of the water; it heats up the uterus, bladder, and colon, and it is bad for women.

Bathing in bathhouses should be approached in calmness, quietness, and gradually. There is more on the topic of bathing that should be added in the section of preserving health as well as on the uses of cold water (see 3rd Art, 2nd Lesson, 5th Section).

Sunbathing, especially with excessive movement like fast walking and jogging, strongly decomposes waste, moistens flatulence, breaks down soft swelling and edema, benefits asthma and orthopnea* (shortness of breath), resolves cold chronic headache, and strengthens cold brain; it also beneficial when remaining dry for hip pain, cauterization, leprosy pain, vascular blood congestion, and cleanses uterus. Exposure to the sun makes the skin denser, poorer, and warmer; it also burns (like cauterization) the pores' openings and prevents decomposition. Staying in the same location under the sun burns the skin more than moving around and severely prevents decomposition.

The best **sand** for drying the body moistures is sea sand. One may sit on it while hot, be buried in it, or sprinkle it on skin, little by little, to resolve pains and illness mentioned under sunbathing. In general, sand severely dries the skin.

An oil bath could be beneficial to individuals with fatigue, chronic cold fevers, and those with fevers accompanied with joint and nerve pains, spasm, tetanus, and urine retention. Oil should be warm and brought in from outside of the bathhouse. Oil with a fox or hyena cooked in it, diluted to half, is the best treatment for joint pain and gout.

Sprinkling of water on the face rejuvenates laxity after a fright, high fever, and unconsciousness, especially if mixed with rose water and vinegar. It may rejuvenate and excite appetite. However, it harms individuals with catarrh and headache.

---

*Orthopnea is shortness of breath (dyspnea). It is the opposite of platypnea.

Listing of Causes
of Each Bodily Symptom

(29 Sections)

FIRST SECTION

Warmers

There are a few types of warmers: moderate quantity of food; moderate movement, including sports; moderate massage; moderate pétrissage;* cupping without slitting the skin (since slitting cools down by evacuation); vigorous and plentiful movement without excess; hot food, hot medication, moderately hot bath warming by its hot air; hot profession; moderate touching of hot applications such as air and wraps; moderate late nights, moderate amount of sleep; moderate anger and worry (excessive worry cools down); moderate joyfulness; and putrefaction, which produces abnormal heat in the body that is an absolute heat, which is different than burning (الإحراق).

Heating without burning takes place often and does not cause putrefaction, and may happen before putrefaction since putrefaction stays after the dissipation of the factor that caused the initial heat; putrefaction acts on the moist humors by altering their moisture content and their normal functional temperament without converting them to any of the normal qualitative temperaments. Normal warming may prepare and change the wet heat from a qualitative temperament to another, which is called digestion and not putrefaction. However, burning is the separation of the wet material by dispersion from the dry one by precipitation. Simple warming (التسخين الساذج) is the increase in the

---

*Pétrissage consists of movements with applied deep pressure and compression of the underlying muscles. Movements include kneading, wringing, skin rolling, and pick-up-and-squeeze.

temperature of the wet material without changing its temperament to another. The condensation on the surface of the skin warms up because it pushes the water vapor inside, and more heat makes the vapor penetrate deeper.

Galen used to limit all warmers to five types: moderate movement, moderate contact with hot object, ingested hot matter, condensation, and putrefaction.

SECOND SECTION

Coolers

Coolers also have types: excessive movement (dissipates innate heat); excessive stillness (congests innate heat); excess or scarcity of food and drink; cold food; cold medication; excess of hot air, wraps, or bath; excessive looseness of the body (drives out innate heat); long contact with a warming body such as long stay in the bath; excessive condensation that congests innate heat; contact with a cooling matter acting by action or its specific power (even if it is initially warming); excess of retention (إحتباس) that congests innate heat; excessive vomiting that ties heat material by wetting of breath (إستنقاع الروح) and obstruction by waste; long period of organ tension that cools down by blocking heat; excessive worry, fright, and pleasure; cold profession; deep pit (الهوة); and raw humors upon putrefaction.

Galen used to limit all coolers to six types: excessive movement, excessive stillness, contact with cold matter or hot matter that eventually induces decomposition, cold food, considerably reduced food intake, and excessive eating.

THIRD SECTION

Moisturizers

There are several reasons for an increase in moisture, among them are stillness, sleep, holding what needs to be eliminated, elimination of dry humor, excess of food, excess of moist food, moisturizing medication, contact with moisturizers, especially the bath on a full stomach, contact with cooling matter that congests moisture, contact with a gently warming matter that liquefies moisture, and moderate pleasure.

FOURTH SECTION

Dryers

Causes of drying are also many, such as movement, sleeplessness, excessive evacuation, intercourse, fasting, dry food, dry medications, excessive alterations and succession of psychological moods, contact with a drying substance such as dehydrating water [salty], freezing cold with contraction that prevents nutrients from reaching the organ and causes obstruction, and excessive heat that causes excess perspiration, like repeated bathing.

FIFTH SECTION

Causes of Deformity

Among the causes of deformity are those that take place at inception, thus alter the forming power (قوه مصوره), or those in the gametes that prevent the zygote from completing its action [congenital causes]; causes that take place during birth; causes at infancy; external causes from accidents; causes at childhood, such as attempting to move before full development of organs; illnesses such as leprosy, pneumonia, spasms, weakness, and distention; obesity; wasting; swellings; diseases of position; improper healing of sores, and others.

SIXTH SECTION

Causes of Obstruction and Constriction of Ducts

Obstruction occurs by material in the duct; this material may be abnormal, such as a stone, or excessive in quantity, such as a superfluous substance, and different in quality, such as density (thick, runny, or solidified like a solid leech). These are the types of obstructive material. Some of these may be stuck in place in the duct, others moving within the duct space, or with the fusion of the duct during the healing of a sore or growth of a wart, or the collapse of the duct due to an adjacent growing, swelling, and/or tumor, or excessive cold, or dryness by astringents (مقبضات), excessive retentive power (قوه ماسکه), application of a very tight bandage, or a winter season that induces a lot of obstruction due to congestion and spasms from excessive cold.

SEVENTH SECTION

Causes of Dilatation of Ducts

Ducts get dilated because of the weakness of the retentive power or a strong movement by the expulsive power (قوہدافعه). In this category are holding breath, medications for decongestion, and warm and humid relaxing medications. Ducts constrict and clog for the opposite of these causes.

EIGHTH SECTION

Causes of Coarseness

Coarseness occurs by material that cleanses very well by its separating action, such as vinegar; acidic wastes; breakdown action like sea foam and sharp wastes; astringent that causes roughness by its acidity; cold substance that roughens by shrinkage; or the settlement of earthy particles on the organ, such as dust.

NINTH SECTION

Causes of Smoothness

Smoothness can be due to a substance with low viscosity or a substance causing an increase in liquefaction or evaporation of condensation from the surface of the organ.

TENTH SECTION

Causes of Dislocation and Displacement

Dislocation may take place by pulling an organ until it comes out of its place; violent movement over a supporting position that snaps the organ out of its place, such as the overturning of a leg; relaxing and moistening, as it happens in a hydrocele (قيله); or disintegration or infection of the integrity of the ligament, as in leprosy and sciatica.

ELEVENTH SECTION

Causes of Ill Proximity That Prevent Normal Closeness

The causes that prevent proper movement and proximity may be thickening, scarring, spasm, weakness, dryness and calcification of a joint, or congenital.

TWELFTH SECTION

Causes of Ill Proximity That Prevent Normal Separation

The causes that present normal separation are thickening, fusion, scarring, spasm, or congenital.

THIRTEENTH SECTION

Causes of Abnormal Movement

Abnormal movement is caused by weakening dehydration that is the source of dry tremor; dry spasm (such as dry hiccup [فواق]); spasmodic dregs; obstructive material; dregs that are harmful by their cooling effect, as in shivering (نافض), or their biting, such as in goose skin; and distance from and scarcity of innate heat that will show dregs as cold and induce wind that should be released, as in trembling (إختلاج). We say that this harmful substance is either simple vapor that causes stretching (تمطي) or, if stronger and immobile, causes fatigue sickness; when even stronger, causes goose skin; and the strongest of all causes shivering. If wind is mobile it causes other types of fatigue that we will mention. When the wind is confined within the muscle it induces trembling.

Causes of Increase in Size and Number

Increases in size and number are caused by wealth of material [humors], potency of attractive powers, increased potency of attraction by massage, and hot wraps such as tar wraps, which affect the size rather than the number.

Causes of Decrease in Size and Number

Causes of decrease in size and number may be congenital due to lack of material; a problem and weakness in the transformative power; external factors such as cuts, trauma, or harmful cold; others are internal, such as decomposition and infections.

Causes of Discontinuity (Separation)

These encompass internal and external causes. Internal may be due to harmful humors: corrosive, burning, moistening and relaxing, drying and tearing, filling and expanding wind, or piercing wind. Also, expanding, contracting, or piercing by the action of the humor, as a strong movement or penetration. All of these causes are due to violent movement or excess in quantity in an abnormal condition, such as movement on fullness [full stomach], fierce screaming, and rupture of swellings.

External causes include pulling the body like a rope or weight, cutting with a sword, burning with fire, beating with a stone (may produce a break if a space is present or rupture if the vessels are full), piercing by an arrow, or biting, as when a dog attacks another dog and the snake bites a human.

SEVENTEENTH SECTION

Causes of Ulceration

These are either from the rupture of swellings, infection of surgery, or pustules spreading into the tissue.

EIGHTEENTH SECTION

Causes of Swelling

Some of these causes are from substance [humors] and others from the organ structure. As for substance, it is the fullness by the mentioned six things [the four humors, as well as aqueous and gaseous substances]. As for the organs' structure, swelling may be caused by the organ's expulsive power; weakness of the receptive organ and its readiness to accept waste products either due to its nature, like skin, or for its simplicity, like loose flesh in the "three curvatures" (behind the ear from the neck, axilla, and nose tip); enlargement of vessels leading to it in comparison with those leading out; lower position [acting as a sink for other organs]; smaller size that fills up with nutrients; weakness in assimilating nutrients due to a problem; a trauma that leads to congestion; loss of its ability to decompose that which decomposes by exercise; or excessive heat that attracts [humors], and this heat is either normal, as in fever, or acquired, as from pain, violent movement, or some warmers. Fracture causes swelling due to some of the causes mentioned, as contusion (bruise), organ compression, or gripping of the fractured bone to fix it. A tooth may swell; because it grows from food and accepts moisture and putrefaction, it also accepts swelling.

NINETEENTH SECTION

Absolute Causes of Pain

Because pain is an abnormal condition that affects the animal body, then let us discuss its total causes. *We say that pain is feeling the opposite of normal.* All of its causes fall into two types: one type produces dystemperament, and the other introduces discontinuity. By dystemperament I mean that organs at first have good temperament, then are exposed to abnormal and opposite temperament, such as warmer or colder than their temperament, and the new opposite is felt as a pain. Therefore, the pain is feeling of the opposite effect as an opposite. A regular dystemperament does not produce pain and is not felt, such as when a dystemperament replaces the original temperament and becomes the new norm; then this is not painful because it is not felt. The affected should react with the effecter, however, it does not react to a gripping condition that does not change its nature. It reacts to the incoming opposite that changes its nature to a new. For this reason, a person with hectic fever does not feel as bad as a person with ephemeral fever, or tertian fever, although the hectic fever produces much higher temperature than tertian, because the hectic fever has a stronger grip on the organs while the fever of the tertian is caused by a seeping humor to the proximity of organs with normal temperament; therefore, the organs return to their normal temperament by the removal of the humor, and the fever goes away unless it is transformed to hectic.

Regular dystemperament takes hold of an organ gradually, and there is an example that brings this closer to understanding. If, during winter, a person was suddenly bathed in warm or lukewarm water they would initially feel unpleasant and may be hurt because the quality of their body is far from it and opposite to it; however, later they will start enjoying it and gradually feel warmer, especially after sitting for an hour. Now if this person is surprised by pouring on them the same type of water, they will feel that it is cold. If you learned this, then we say although dystemperament is one of the two causes of pain, not every dystemperament is bad enough to produce pain; the hot *per se* and the cold *per se* produce pain directly, while dryness does so indirectly, and wetness does not hurt at all; the first two are active, and the last two are reactive, not by the exerted effect of an object but by both objects affecting each other [one gains and the other loses]. Dryness hurts indirectly because it may be followed by a cause from the second type, discontinuity, because dryness induces shrinkage that could cause discontinuity and nothing else.

However, Galen attributes pain to a specific cause, and that is discontinuity and nothing else. That heat causes pain because it causes discontinuity, and cold also causes pain because it must produce discontinuity. Because of its strong condensation and shrinkage, cold brings in the parts where the condensation is taking place and separates them from the other end. Galen has exaggerated in this regard and made it sound, in some of his books, like all harmful things function this way. For example, staring at black objects hurts due to the attractive power of black; white due to its dispersive power; bitterness, saltiness, and acidity because of their dispersive effect; and astringents by their excessive contraction, thus, without a doubt, followed by discontinuity. Likewise, smells and loud noise produce pain by the violent movement of the air when it meets the ear canal (external auditory meatus, صِمَاخ). The truth in this regard is to make dystemperament a type of cause that produces pain even if it is accompanied by discontinuity. The evidence is not in medicine but in the natural philosophy; however, I will point to a small part of this evidence by saying that a painful organ is similar in all of its parts, but not so the one with discontinuity; therefore, the presence of pain in the parts that do not have discontinuity is due to dystemperament. Cold causes pain where it contracts and brings parts together and generally cools down. Discontinuity from cold occurs not at the exact spot where it cools but at its periphery. Additionally, pain is, without a doubt, the feeling of a sudden opposing effect as reflected in its severity, and every felt opposing effect is a pain. Do you see: if a dystemperamental cold is felt as dystemperament without causing discontinuity, is it a feeling of an opposite? Is it pain? Sometimes after pain disappears there is a remnant that is not a true pain and will disappear on its own, and the ignorant will work on it and make it worse.

TWENTIETH SECTION

Causes of Different Pain Types

The types of pain that have names are fifteen types:

1. Itching (hakak, حكاك), caused by a bitter or salty humor.
2. Rough (khashin, خشن), by rough humor.
3. Stabbing (nakhes, ناخس), by a humor extending the muscle membrane and separating it. It may be even or uneven in its action. The uneven may be due to the heterogeneity of the parts that the membrane touches between soft and solid, such as the clavicle (collarbone, ترقوه), to the membrane that covers the ribs if the swelling in pleurisy is pulling to the top, or heterogeneity in the movement of its parts, such as the diaphragm (الحجاب) in relation to the pleura. This pain can be due to unequal sensitivity within the organ or pathological problems with some of its parts.
4. Flattening and/or extending (moumaded, ممدد), by a humor or gas pulling the nerve or muscle from two opposite ends.
5. Pressing (daghet, ضاغط), by a substance or gas engulfing the organ and pressing on it.
6. Splitting (moufasekh, مفسخ), by a substance seeping out of the muscle or its membrane and separating the two.
7. Breaking (moukaser, مكسر), by a substance, gas, or coldness in between the bone and its membrane, or cold that forcefully contracts the membrane.
8. Softening (rakhou, رخو), by a substance that extends only the muscle without its tendon. It is called softening because the muscle is more extended than its nerve, tendon, or membrane.
9. Boring (thaqeb, ثاقب), by the trapping of a dense substance or gas between the tissues of a hard organ, such as the colon, and is felt as if a gimlet is going through.
10. Piercing (masalee, مسلي), as the boring pain but with the substance trapped during the piercing.
11. Dull (khader, خدر), by a very cold temperament or obstruction of blood supply by a nerve or filling.

12. Throbbing (dharabani, ضـربانـي), caused by warm swelling next to an organ. Solid or soft cold swelling does not cause pain unless it turns into a warm swelling. This type of pain is caused by a hot swelling when the neighboring organ is sensitive and with pulsing arteries next to it. The pain is not felt when the organ is healthy, but the swelling makes the pulse painful.

13. Heavy (thaqeel, ثـقيـل), a sense of heaviness in an insensitive organ such as lung, kidney, or spleen due to inflammation or tumor, or when the tumor disables the pain sensation, such as cancer in the mouth of the stomach [the opening of the stomach, the cardia], which only hurts because it kills sensation.

14. Tiring (a'ya'i, إعـيـانـي), could be due to fatigue, or by an extending humor and termed *tiring extension,* a gas, termed *tiring bloating,* or ulcerative humor, termed *tiring ulcer.* There are combinations of these that we will discuss in their specific areas; one of these compound pains is known as boraceous (بـورقيـه), which combines the extending and ulcerative.

15. Biting and/or incisive (lathe', لاذع), caused by a sour humor.

TWENTY-FIRST SECTION

Causes of Pain Cessation

Pain stops if its cause is stopped, such as draining the humor with a poultice of linseed [*Linum usitatissimum*] or dill [*Anethum graveolens*] or by applying wet sedatives, such as alcohols, or cold anesthetics, such as all narcotics. The true analgesic is the first [i.e., stopping the cause].

TWENTY-SECOND SECTION

Effect of Pain

Pain weakens, prevents the organs from carrying out their functions, and prevents proper breathing or disturbs its function or makes it irregular (متقطـع), frequent (متـواتـر), and abnormal in general. Pain initially warms the organ then cools it by decomposition and by the weakening of spirit and life [respiration and other metabolic processes].

Causes of Pleasure

These fall within two types: one that changes the normal temperament by expulsion to induce feeling, the other by returning to normal continuity by expulsion. All that takes place without expulsion is not felt and does not produce pleasure. *Pleasure is a feeling of compatibility,* and every feeling is perceived by the sensitive faculty and is felt by its reaction to whatever is suitable or opposing and whether it is pleasurable or painful according to what is affected. Since touch is the most sensitive of all senses and retains the memory of opposing or suitable feelings, it generates extreme pleasure in people with heightened senses of touch when they experience suitable feeling. Its opposing feeling is more painful than other faculties.

How Movement Hurts

Movement is painful when it generates extensions, contusions, or rips.

How Bad Humors Hurt

Bad humors hurt either by their quality, as they sting (burn), by their quantity, as in distention, or by a combination of the two effects together.

TWENTY-SIXTH SECTION

How Gases Hurt

Wind hurts by distention. Expanding gas occurs either in the cavities of organs, in bellies as bloating in the stomach, or in tissue layers and fibers of organs, as in flatulent colic;* in the muscle layers; beneath membranes; above bones; around muscles and among them, skin, and flesh; and embedded in the organ as it spreads through the thoracic muscle. Its speed of expansion and duration depends on its abundance and density, as well as the organ's thickness and density [looseness or tightness].

TWENTY-SEVENTH SECTION

Causes of Retention and Evacuation

Retention and evacuation are easy to understand if you look up what we said about them.

TWENTY-EIGHTH SECTION

Causes of Dyspepsia (Indigestion) and Fullness

These are either (1) external causes, such as heavy moisturizing that provides moisture to hydrate food and drink, thus combining the two produces excess of matter in the body that corrupts the normal function; examples are excessive bathing, especially after a meal, and inhibitors of digestion like repose, cessation of exercise, evacuation, extravagant eating, and bad diet; or (2) internal, such as weakness of digestive power that does not digest, weakness of expulsive faculty that leads to the accumulation and retention of humors, or constriction of ducts.

---

*Flatulent colic is also termed *tympanites* or *wind colic*.

TWENTY-NINTH SECTION

Causes of Organs' Weakness

Weakness of the organ may be due to a cause within the organ, the spirit carrying the functioning power in the organ [i.e., supply of oxygen and respiration], or the power itself [i.e., metabolic health]. The cause within the organ may be a chronic dystemperament, especially a cold one; however, the hot may weaken the numbing action of the cold that corrupts the spirit's temperament. This also happens with prolonged bathing and in those who faint. Dry dystemperament prevents faculties from functioning, and wet dystemperament, by inducing looseness and obstruction.

Weakness may be caused by a structural disease that is particularly asymptomatic—without pain or sickness, where pain is a weak spasm in the organ's nerve while all the normal and voluntary functions are carried out by the fibers and their functions. Digestion may also lack good grip and form because of fiber [problems].

The weakness where the cause concerns spirit is either a dystemperament or dispersion by evacuation of the organ or following the evacuation of other organs. Weakening actions of power are excessive functions and excessive repetition that may also be accompanied by weakening of spirit as a reason upon reason [one cause induces another].

If we approach these causes of weakness from a different direction and bring in the distant causes (الاسباب البعيده) that are the causes of the proximate causes (الاسباب الملاصقه), then dystemperaments take place. Among these distant causes are corruption of air, water, and food. Some of these may weaken the spirit [breath], such as foul smell, rancid water, and diffusion of toxic effects in air or body.

Among the general causes of weakness are those related to loss by depletion (إستفراغ), such as blood bleeding and diarrhea of light humors, excessive and sudden drainage of edema, excessive drainage of pus from a large number of cold abscesses at once or when they burst on their own, excessive sweating, excessive exercise, and when pains break up the spirit and cause dystemperament. Among these pains that have substantial effects are the distending or burning pains of the cardiac opening of the stomach (فم المـعـده) or a part of an organ and all the pains in the heart region. Fevers weaken by dissolution and depletion of body and spirit and induce dystemperament. Widening of pores promotes weakness by transpiration [a form of dispersion], and starvation is similar.

Weakness of the whole body may be induced by the weakness of an organ. An example is body weakness and dissolution of its powers due to an injury of the cardiac opening of the stomach. When the person's heart and mind react intensely to small injuries, this person is susceptible to quick breakdown and anxiety (ضجر) from the tiniest cause. The cause of weakness may be a prolonged torment by illnesses. Some organs are weaker than each other since birth [of the same organ type, e.g., one kidney weaker than the other] or than another organ, such as the lung and brain, and these weaker organs accept what the stronger organs excrete and export; if the brain was not placed higher, it would have been afflicted with more than it can handle of these, and it would have lost its power. Be aware of all of this.

CHAPTER 10

Symptoms and Signs

Third Lesson of the Second Art: Symptoms and Signs

- Introduction (11 sections)
- First Statement: Pulse (19 sections)
- Second Statement: Urine and Feces (13 sections)

When the organ function becomes abnormal then there is a problem with its energy, and a problem with an organ's energy causes a disease in the organ.

AVICENNA

AUTHORS' INTRODUCTION

The 3rd Lesson of the 2nd Art is a rich part of the *Canon* addressing the main symptoms of pulse and of urine and feces. In the introduction of this Lesson, Avicenna covers the symptoms and signs of health and disease; the six laws to diagnosing internal diseases; indicators of temperaments; differences between single and shared diseases; signs of normal, equitable, and abnormal temperaments; signs of fullness; signs of a humor dominance; and signs of poor constitution, blockage, gases, swellings and tumors, and discontinuity.

The 1st Statement addresses the detailed description of the pulse; its characteristics; irregularity and its types; causes and indicators of irregularity; pulse of genders, ages, temperaments, seasons, and geographic locations; effects of food and drink, sleep and wakefulness, exercise, bathing, pain, swellings, and psychological conditions on the pulse; and the pulse of pregnant women.

The 2nd Statement covers urine and feces. It includes indicators of urine characteristics, such as those of its color, texture, turbidity, odor, foam, sediment, quantity, maturity, age groups, gender, animals, and liquids that resemble urine. Additionally, the Statement includes indicators of feces characteristics, such as quantity, texture, color, turnaround time, and accompanying sound.

In this Lesson, Avicenna states, for the first time and in very clear terms, his theory of disease at the most basic level of body organization; in it he ties the disease process to the lack of available energy within the organ's tissue. He writes that when there is an organ dysfunction, there is a problem with the organ's innate heat (i.e., the respiratory processes), and that whenever there is a problem with innate heat, disease arises. Avicenna's explanation offers us a direct pointer to the molecular explanation of the disease initiation.

In modern medical science, the innate heat of the cells, tissues, and organs is provided by the tiny organelles within the cells called mitochondria; these are the powerhouses within the cells that produce free energy heat (referred to as delta G in physical sciences) and most of the chemical energy in the form of ATP (the cell's energy currency). The free energy heat can be likened to Avicenna's *temperament* of the tissue and organ, while the energy of ATP is used to initiate the biochemical reactions within the cell. ATP is used by enzymes and structural proteins in many cellular processes, including biosynthetic reactions, motility, and cell division. When the ATP energy is used in a reaction, it breaks down into adenosine diphosphate (ADP) and a phosphate group.

For the cells to carry out respiration and produce energy, they need to start with a high-energy chemical compound. The main chemical compound used by the cells for energy is glucose, which has a significant amount of energy in its bonds. The energy in glucose gets there when a plant traps light energy and uses it to synthesize glucose from simpler compounds. Other high-energy compounds such as fats (lipids) and proteins can be used for cellular respiration as well.

Not surprisingly, Avicenna also ties in the health of the pulse to the state of respiration in addition to the blood vessels' condition of softness or hardness (6th Section, 1st Statement). We have discussed in our introduction to the 2nd Lesson the relationship between the innate heat and/or respiration and moisture, which is a central theme in Unani medical theory and to which Avicenna attributes aging and death as well. In the modern interpretation of Avicenna, he can be understood as stating that cellular respiration fortifies the innate moistures and prevents the formation of abnormal heat and that the latter usually arises due to hypoxic conditions. If cellular respiration is strong it will enable the body to complete its actions of digestion, maturation, and preservation of health; therefore, metabolism acts properly and does not produce abnormal heat or putrefaction. However, if cellular respiration is weak, the body cannot carry out its metabolic functions due to the weakness; thus the moistures (of the cytoplasm, interstitium, and blood) are overtaken by abnormal activity that produces putrefaction (anaerobic environment and incomplete digestion and maturation). Avicenna further asserts that respiration "is an instrument for all faculties."

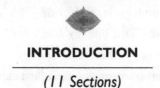

INTRODUCTION

(I I Sections)

FIRST SECTION

General Statement about Symptoms and Signs

Symptoms and signs that characterize one of the aforementioned states [of health, disease, and in-between] point to one of three situations: a present condition, which according to Galen benefits only the patient as to what they have to do; a past condition, which Galen saw as benefiting only the physician, as it is indicative of the physician's progress in his profession and thus enhances the trust in his judgment; or a future condition, which he said benefits all since the physician realizes from it his progress in knowledge and the patient understands how to manage the illness.

Signs of Health

Some signs indicate an equitable temperament that we address under this topic. Some indicate structural soundness. Some signs are essential to be healthy, such as proper form, position, quantity, and number [of parts and organs], and these topics are defined [for definition of these terms, refer to the 3rd Section, 1st Lesson of the 2nd Art]. Some of the signs are nonessential, such as attractiveness and beauty; others are functional and insure the full and complete correct functioning of every organ; and every organ that completes its action is healthy. The functions are indicative of the health of major organs: for the brain by the quality of the voluntary actions, sensory functions, and instinctual actions (أفعال وهميه); for the heart by the pulse and breathing; and for the liver by the stool and urine since its weakness produces stool and urine that are similar to water or soft meat.

Symptoms Indicating Diseases

Some symptoms point directly to the disease, such as the variability of the pulse speed during fever, which indicates fever itself. Others point to location, like a sawlike pulse (نبض منشاري) when pain is in the chest; it indicates that the swelling is in the pleura and the diaphragm. Likewise, a wavy pulse (نبض موجي) indicates swelling in the lung itself. Other symptoms point out the cause of the disease, such as fullness in all of its forms; each form is indicative of its type.

Signs

Some are temporary, appearing and disappearing with the disease, such as acute fever (hyperpyrexia, حمى حاده), stabbing pain, dyspnea (shortness of breath, ضيق النفس), cough, and sawlike pulse (نبض منشاري) with pleurisy. Some do not follow, like headache with fever. Others appear at the end, like symptoms of a healing crisis (بحران), symptoms of [disease] maturity, or symptoms of permanent dysfunction (عطب); these appear mostly in acute diseases.

Symptoms

Some of these appear on the outside of organs, and these are observable measures [by the perceptive faculty] of colors and textures (solid, soft, hot, cold, etc.), and there are common, observable measures of an organ's structure, position, movement, and rest that may point to internal conditions (like trembling of lips [إختلاج الشفه] signifies vomiting), their amount (increase or decrease), and number. These may indicate the conditions of internal organs; for example, short fingers signify a small liver. The color of the stool is a visual indicator, whether it is black, white, or yellow. The sound of growling is an auditory indicator of bloating and indigestion. Similarly, using the smell and mouth odor and such. Hectic fever is visual and among the common observables.

External observations may point out an internal issue, such as redness of the cheek indicates pneumonia and convex nails, tuberculosis. We will simplify the indicators of movement and stillness as much as possible. Stillness symptoms may point out to sudden death (سكته), epilepsy, unconsciousness, and palsy. Those of the movement type are

goose skin, shivering, hiccups, sneezing, yawning, stretching, coughing, trembling, and spasm (as first symptom). Some of these are normal
actions, like hiccups; others are abnormal, like spasm and shivering;
a few are purely voluntary due to worry and insomnia, and some are
compound, normal involuntary and voluntary, like coughing and urination. Of these the involuntary precedes as in coughing; in others, the
involuntary follows if the voluntary action is not carried out, such as in
urination, defecation, and whatever is abnormal without the voluntary
movement. Sensory perceptions may feel some movements, such as shivering, but not others because they cannot be sensed, such as trembling.

Movements differ from each other in a few aspects. In strength,
coughing by itself is stronger than trembling, or by the number of
body parts involved, sneezing has more muscles involved than coughing because coughing is carried out by the parts of the chest while
sneezing is done by the combined movement of the chest and head
parts. Movements differ in their danger; the movement of dry hiccup is greater in danger than coughing even if the cough is stronger.
Differences in the supportive parts complement the movement by an
originating body part, like the use of abdominal muscles when defecat-
ing, or outside instrument, like air in coughing. There are differences in
the initial bodily parts of the movement, such as in coughing and nausea. They differ in the faculty deriving the movement; whereas trembling is derived by the involuntary physical faculty, coughing is derived
by the nervous faculty. Differences in the humor are involved, as when
coughing signifies the presence of sputum [phlegm humor] and trembling signifies the presence of gas. These above symptoms are evident in
organs and mostly indicate obvious conditions; they may indicate internal problems, like the aforementioned redness of the cheeks pointing to
pneumonia.

Some of the symptoms are indicative of internal diseases; however,
the examiner should have a good knowledge of anatomy to figure out
the nature of every organ: (1) whether it is fleshy or nonfleshy, (2) its
form to distinguish tumors and/or swellings if present, or (3) whether
it has the normal shape. Also, to know what an organ may or not retain
or discharge as a substance, like the jejunum. Also, to know its location

and judge whether the pain is in it or away from it; to know its closest organs and figure out if the pain originates from it or is shared by the other organs, and whether the substance is emanating from it or arrives from others, and whether what separates from it comes from its essence or if the organ is acting as a conduit for others. And to know the contents of the organ, thus to know if excreted matter belongs to it and know its function and trace its disease to the dysfunction. All of this is known through anatomy. The physician must manage the internal diseases from the anatomical point of view.

A physician who has knowledge of anatomy must rely on six laws to diagnose internal disease:

> First, dysfunctions; you have learned the types of functions, their quantity, and their primary effects.
> Second, the type of released substance, which is a consistent sign but not primary; it is consistent because its effect is seen and believed, and not primary because it signifies immaturity.
> The third is pain.
> The fourth is swelling.
> The fifth is position.
> The sixth is the suitable and obvious symptoms that are neither primary nor constant.

Let us detail each one of these.

Inferring from the functions. *When the organ function becomes abnormal then there is a problem with its energy and/or power* (قوة), *and a problem with an organ's energy causes a disease in the organ.* The harmful effects of the functions can be of three aspects:

- They diminish, like the eyesight becomes weaker and sees an object less defined and requires closer distance, or the stomach's digestion becomes difficult, slower, and lessened.
- The eyesight changes to seeing things that are not there or in different form than what is real, or the stomach corrupts food and misdigests it.

- Something stops completely, like the eyesight is extinguished, or the stomach ceases digesting.

Discharge and retention as indicators of disease. These have several possible aspects:

- They are an indicator of abnormal congestion of a substance that should be released, such as urine and feces.
- Discharge is an abnormal method of release; the released substance could be of the same nature of the organ or not. If it is from the same nature of the organ, then it signifies three things: the same nature indicates the disintegration of the tissue, like in the case of an expectorant throat; the quantity indicates the condition, as when the thick, dry tissue peels passing in the feces indicate the ulceration of the large intestine, and when they are thin they indicate the ulceration of the small intestine; color is an indicator, for example, red, flaky sediment signifying that the origin is from a fleshy organ like the kidney and white sediment signifying origin from nervous organs such as the bladder.
- Secretion that is not from the same nature of the organs signifies that it is abnormal secretion, for example, the secretion of normal humors and blood.
- The secretion is abnormal in quality, such as the putrid blood of normal or abnormal discharge, or of absolute abnormal nature, like a stone.
- The secretion is of abnormal quantity (above or below normal), even if it is normal in the method of discharge, such as reduction or excess of feces and urine.
- The secretion is of abnormal quality, even if the discharge is normal, such as black feces and urine.
- Abnormality in direction of discharge, as in an obstruction of the ileus, where the feces pass out of the mouth.

Pain as an indicator. It is of two types: the pain location indicates the affected organ, such as if it is on the right side then it is the liver and on the left side it is the spleen, or indicates the cause, as we have detailed in the lesson on causes; for example, if it is a heavy pain it indicates a swelling in an insensitive organ or loss of feeling, extended indicates excessive humor, and biting signifies sharp humor.

Swelling has three possible indicators. The nature of the swelling, such as yellow bile in the case of erysipelas and black bile in hard swelling. The location; right-sided swelling signifies closeness to the liver and left-sided to the spleen. The shape of the swelling also tells of its location; a crescent-shaped swelling on the right side signifies that it is in the liver, and if it is elongated then it is in the muscle above the liver (diaphragm).

Location indicators are either by primary localization itself or by colocation. The location by itself is obvious; however, in a colocation, sharing a pain in the finger indicates a previous injury to the sixth cervical pair of nerves of the neck.

SECOND SECTION

Difference between Single and Shared Diseases

Initially, diseases start in an organ or may be shared between or among more than one organ, as when the head and stomach share diseases. Therefore, we need to determine the difference between the two by clear signs. We say that we have to figure out which appeared first as the original and the other as the shared and which of the two will remain after the disappearance of the other, and thus, is the original disease, and by subtraction, the last disease to appear, or to recover simultaneously with the other, is the shared. This may cause confusion when the original disease is silent and painless at the beginning but becomes obvious only after the shared disease appears; then the two diseases are confused as being one, or only the latter is recognized and the original remains hidden. To avoid such a mistake, the physician should be knowledgeable about colocation, or sharing organs, through knowledge of anatomy and the diseases of every organ (palpable or silent) and does not judge a disease as original unless and until examining all the symptoms as belonging to it. Furthermore, the physician should ask the patient about the symptoms that may belong to the sharing organ of the sick organ or unfelt and painless symptoms that are not nearby but may show signs that are far from the organ. The patient perceives that the distant symptoms are not belonging to the diseased organ; it is the physician's knowledge that corrects this. The physician is mostly guided by the finding of harmful functions, and when these are found, the physician judges the disease as shared.

Organs vary in the appearance of their diseases; for example, the head may share its diseases with the stomach, but the opposite is unlikely.

We will put between your hands the general symptoms of the original and diseased temperaments, and those of each organ will be described in its own topic. As for the symptoms of the structural diseases, the obvious ones are perceptible, and some are internal. Symptoms other than fullness, obstruction, swellings, and discontinuity are difficult to include within the general description; therefore, we will be detailing them later.

THIRD SECTION

About the Signs of Temperaments

The types of indicators that define temperaments are ten.

The first is touch. The way to figure it out is by finding whether it is similar to the right touch of the equitable countries and weather; if it is identical then it is equitable. However, if a person with equitable temperament checking the temperament of a patient reacts by gaining or losing heat, or feels the patient was softer or harder than normal, or rougher than normal, and there is no other reason such as air or bathing to change the texture, then the patient has inequitable temperament. It is possible to know from the softness, roughness, or dryness of fingers' nails the state of the body temperament if they are not affected by another factor. Judging softness from hardness depends on the correct indicators of equitability in heat and cold, because heat softens the touch of the hard and rough and the equitable (by decomposition), thus they appear softer and wetter, while cold hardens the soft and the equitable by congealing and condensing, making them appear dry like ice and fat; ice congeals hard and fat thickens. Most of the people with cold temperament have soft bodies even if they are slim because they have excessive immature humors.

Second, good indicators of flesh and fat. Excess of red flesh [muscle] signifies moisture and heat, as well as compactness. If there is less flesh without excessive fat, then it indicates dryness and heat. Fats (soft and solid) point to coldness and there will be flabbiness; however, if this is accompanied with narrowness of vessels and reduced blood (circulation) as well as weakening by hunger due to weak circulation that supplies organs with nutrients, it points to a normal mountainous temperament, but in the absence of these other signs it indicates an acquired temperament.

Scarcity of fat indicates heat. Fats provide the fatty content of the blood, and its accumulation is caused by cold; therefore, it is less in the liver and more on the intestines, and it is more on the heart than in the liver because of its quantity, and not the temperament, the shape of the heart, or the nature of the fat. Accumulation of fats in the body increases and decreases according to the available heat.

The fleshy body without excess of fat is hot and moist; if it has a great deal of red flesh with little fat it indicates excess of moisture, and more overload of both indicates exceeding coldness and moisture, and the body is cold and wet.

Third, indicators of hair. It is considered from the following aspects: speed of growth or slowness, density, thickness, straightness or curliness, and color. Slow-growing hair or absence of its growth point out a very wet temperament if there is no evidence of anemia. If it is fast growing then it is not that wet but leaning to dryness, and its hotness or coldness can be determined by other means, as we have stated. Combined heat and dryness accelerate hair growth, density, and thickness. Density signifies heat, and density signifies smokiness [see our interpretation of smoke as ammonia] in youth and not children since the children have vapor and smoke, and the opposites produce opposites [coldness and wetness slow down hair growth, etc.].

As for appearance, curliness indicates heat and dryness and may also indicate the twisting of skin pores [and hair follicles], which does not change by a change in temperament because the first two [heat and dryness] change, and straight hair indicates the opposite.

As for hair color, black indicates heat, reddish-brown indicates coldness, blond and red indicate equitability, and grey indicates wetness and coldness, as in old age, or with excessive dryness, like a dry plant when its blackens, or when the green turns into white. This appears in humans after drying diseases. The cause of grayness, according to Aristotle, is the change in color to that of phlegm, and according to Galen, it is the excessive wetness [mustiness] of the food that goes to the hair when it is cold and moves slowly into the skin pores. If you examine both statements you find them to be very close, since the problem in grayness is the phlegm and the problem in the grayness of humidity is the same, the natural.

Furthermore, it should be noted that countries and climates have their effects on hair. It should not be expected that for the Negro [black African] to have blond hair in order to have an equitable temperament, or a Slav to have black hair to infer the hotness of their temperament. Age has an effect on hair; hair of the youth is like those in the southern countries, children like northern countries, and middle aged like middle regions. Hair abundance in a child signifies that their temperament will be melancholic in maturity and signifies a melancholic temperament for an elder.

Fourth, types of indicators taken from body color [complexion]. Whiteness of the skin is an indicator of blood scarcity with coldness. If it were with heat and yellow humor it would become yellow. Red skin is indicative of blood abundance and heat. Yellow and blond colors signify abundance of heat, however, yellow is more indicative of yellow bile, and blond color for blood or with choleric blood. Yellowness indicates scarcity of blood, even in the absence of yellow bile, as in the bodies of convalescents. Cloudiness is a sign of severe coldness that reduces the blood by congealing and turning it into black color. Change in skin and complexion color is a sign of heat. Purple color is a sign of coldness and dryness because it is a color that belongs to black bile. Chalky color is a sign of coldness and phlegm. Lead color is a sign of coldness and wetness with some black bile because it is white with little green, thus the white indicates phlegm or wet temperament and the green indicates congealed blood with blackness that is mixed with phlegm and gives it the green coloration. Ivory color is a sign of phlegmatic cold and little yellow bile. Most of the time, the color changes, because of the liver, to yellow and white; because of the spleen, to yellow and black, and because of the hemorrhoids, to yellow and green, but this is not fixed and varies.

Tongue color is an excellent indicator of the temperament of silent and pulsating vessels. The color of eyes is also a good indicator of the brain's temperament. It may be in one disease that the colors of two organs change, such as the tongue becomes white and the face darkens in jaundice, which has strong burning yellow bile.

Fifth, indicators of the shapes of organs. Hot temperaments produce broad chest and enlarged extremities, fullness without tightness, shortness, widening of vessels, and appearance of great strong pulse, as well as enlargement of muscles and their closeness to joints; all of this takes place because their proportional functions and compound structures are driven by heat. Cold does the opposite because of the insufficiency of these functions to complete the actions of building and synthesizing. Dry temperament produces dry and rough skin, pronounced joints, and pronounced cartilage in the trachea and nose; the nose is also straight.

Sixth, indicators of the speed of reactivity of organs. If the organ warms up fast without any difficulty then it has a hot temperament because it is easier to change to a suitable condition than to the opposite one, and if it cools down faster then it is exactly the opposite. Someone may say that it should be the opposite because we know that an object reacts to its opposite and not to its similar, but that is a discussion that I had presented and stated that the priority reaction should be from the similar. The answer to this is that for an object not to react to its similar, the similar has to be of the same quality in type and nature. A warmer object is not similar to a colder one, but rather two warm objects, one warmer than the other, differ in that the latter is colder than the first;

thus the first reacts to the colder second because it is not as warm, and also it will react to the ones that are less and less warm; however, one improves its quality and supports its strongest parts, and the other loses from its quality and thus changes to what increases its quality and is easier to support its strongest elements. However, there is an additional factor that is specific to the object sharing a quality but missing from the other; for example, the one that has a hot temperament in nature is accepted more easily because it has the warmth that opposes the cold, which lowers the heat of a hot temperament; therefore, when the two meet and neutralize the cold, they strengthen both of their qualities. If an external hot substance tries to annul the equitability, then the innate heat is the most resistant, and even the hot poisons are resisted, pushed out, and their nature corrupted by the innate heat. The innate heat is nature's mechanism that fends off the harm of an incoming hot substance by mobilizing the spirit [the modern respiratory apparatus and the vesication by the mitochondria] to expel it, remove its vapor, decompose it, and burn its substance, and resists the damage from the incoming cold by opposing it. This natural mechanism does not act on the cold; it resists and delays the incoming hot substance and does not resist the incoming cold substance.

Innate heat also protects the innate moistures from abnormal heat [discussed also in our introduction to the 2nd Lesson]; if the innate heat is strong it will enable nature to mediate its action on moistures by maturation, digestion, and preservation of health; therefore, the moistures act in the proper functions and do not follow the influence of abnormal heat, thus producing no putrefaction. However, if the innate heat is weak, nature cannot act on moistures due to the weakness of the instrument between it and the moistures, thus the moistures are taken over by abnormal activity that produces putrefaction.

Innate heat is an instrument for all faculties, whereas coldness is its antithesis, which is only indirectly beneficial. This is the reason it is called innate heat while there is no innate cold, and nothing is attributed to coldness like the body smokiness attributed to heat.

Seventh, state of sleep and wakefulness. Moderation in sleep and wakefulness indicates an equitable temperament, particularly in the brain. Longer periods of sleep denote moisture and coldness, and longer wakefulness indicates dryness and heat, especially in the brain.

Eighth, type of indicators taken from functions. If the functions run continuously in a normal manner until completion, then they indicate equitable temperament; however, if changed to excessive activity this indicates a hot temperament; also their acceleration denotes heat such as fast growth of hair and tooth. Dull, weak, inactive, and sluggish functions indicate cold temperament; however, this could also be the result of a hot temperament that also includes deviation from normal and weakness. Additionally, some of the normal functions may cease or decrease by heat, including normal functions such as sleep. For this reason, some normal effects of cold such as sleeping may increase, however, it is conditional, or by causes, and not from the absolute general normal functions since sleep is not needed for being alive, but health is an absolute necessity, and sleep is needed because the spirit cannot continue to function because of fatigue or the need to digest food and cannot do the two at the same time. Therefore, the need for sleep is due to insufficiency, and it is a deviation from the normal functions. This deviation is normal due to its necessity, and what is necessary is termed normal. The correct indication of this part's equitable temperament is moderate and complete function. However, sleep indications of hot, cold, dryness, and wetness are speculative.

Among the strong functions that are indicative of heat are voice strength and loudness, rapid and continuous speech, anger, fast movements, and fast blinking, even if these take place without any general cause but rather due to specific causes in the organ functions.

Ninth, the type of the body expulsion of waste and quality of discharge. Continuous expulsion of feces, urine, sweat, and others with warmth, strong odor, and characteristics that are similar to the originally ingested food indicates hot temperament, and the opposite denotes cold.

Tenth, indicators of psychological functions. These are taken from the psychological functions and reactions that, for example, include strong anger, anxiety, cleverness, understanding, courage, rudeness, open-mindedness, optimism, toughness, vigor, manly manners, lack of laziness, and lack of overreaction; they are indicative of heat and their opposites denote cold. The lingering of anger and satisfaction, imagined and memorized, indicates dryness, while the fast vanishing of reactions denotes wetness. Dreams fall within this category; a person with hot temperament dreams of the sun's heat, while a person with cold temperament dreams of coldness of ice or of being submerged in cold water. A person dreams of what is compatible with their temperament. All that, or most of it, we mentioned as characteristics of the original innate temperaments.

Hot accidental abnormal temperaments give the followings signs: harmful warmth of the body; harmful when in fever; loss of energy in movement because of increased heat and excessive thirst; inflammation of stomach mouth; bitterness in mouth; weak, very fast, and frequent pulse; distress from hot food; comfort by cold food; and adverse health condition in the summer.

Signs of abnormal cold temperament are lack of digestion, scarcity of thirst, laxity of joints, frequent phlegmatic fevers, adversity from catarrhs and ingestion of cold food, improvement with hot food, and adverse condition in the winter.

Signs of abnormal wet temperament are similar to those of cold temperament in addition to flabbiness, runny saliva and mucus, diarrhea, indigestion, adversity from moist food, excessive sleep, and puffiness of eyelids.

Signs of abnormal dry temperament are dry skin, insomnia, abnormal weight loss, adversity from dry food, adversity in winter, improvement from moist food, and quick and strong absorption of hot water and light oil.

FOURTH SECTION

Summary of Signs of Equitable Temperament

The signs of equitable temperament according to what we have mentioned are:

- Balanced texture in heat, cold, dryness, wetness, softness, and stiffness.
- Balanced color between whiteness and redness.
- Moderate shape between fullness and leanness with inclination to bulkiness.
- Veins are between sunken and superficially visible sitting on the flesh.
- Balanced hair in density and scantiness as well as curliness and straightness.
- Hair color tilting to blondness in youth and to black afterward.
- Balance between sleep and wakefulness.
- Organs carry their functions.
- Easiness and strong imagination, thinking, and remembering.
- Moderation of manners between conservative and excessive. (I mean a median between courage and cowardliness, anger and irresponsiveness, gentleness and harshness, irresponsibility and accountability.)
- Healthy and quality fast growth.
- Standing tall.
- Delicious, entertaining dreams that include pleasant odors, luscious voices, and enjoyable company.
- Lovable, with charming, smiley face.
- Balanced appetite.
- Good digestion in stomach, liver, and vessels.
- All of the body proportional.
- Balanced excretion through the normal exits.

FIFTH SECTION

Signs of Poor Constitution

This is a person with organs of incompatible temperaments, and the main organs may be antagonistic in their deviation from equitability so that one organ goes to a temperament and the other goes to the opposite. Therefore, if the person's constitution is disproportionate then their understanding and thinking is low like one with a huge belly, short fingers, round face and head, large head, or small head with fleshy forehead, face, neck, and legs with a semicircular face; however, if the jaws are large then he is very different. Additionally, if the person has a round head and forehead, excessively elongated face, very thick neck, and dull eyes and movement, then they are far from being good.

SIXTH SECTION

Signs Indicating Fullness (Repletion)

There are two types of fullness: fullness of vessels and fullness in relation to strength. Fullness of vessels occurs when the humors and "spirits," although good in quality, are excessive in quantity and fill the vessels and stretch them. A person with such a condition is in danger when moving because the vessels may rupture due to their fullness and their contents flow to congested areas, causing diphtheria, epilepsy, and apoplexy (sudden death). Fullness in relation to strength occurs when the harm is not only from the quantity of the humors but also from their bad quality since they weaken the strength by their quality and are not easy to digest or mature and the person becomes susceptible to diseases of putrefaction.

General signs of fullness: Heaviness of organs, lazy movement (sluggishness), redness of the body, puffiness of veins, skin distention, pulse fullness, coloration and thickness of urine, weak appetite, weakness of eyesight, and dreams that indicate heaviness, such as stillness, inability to stand, carrying a heavy load, or inability to speak. On the other hand, dreams of flying and fast movement indicate light humors in moderate quantity.

Signs of fullness in relation to strength: They share with the first type heaviness, laziness, and low appetite; however, if it is a simple fullness affecting strength then the vessels are not very engorged, the skin is not very extended, the pulse is not very full and large, urine is not very thick, and skin color is not very red; the person is weak and tired and appears as such after movement and activity, and their dreams include itching, stinging, burning, and malodors. There are also signs for the dominant humor that we will mention. *In most cases fullness in relation to strength causes the disease before the appearance of its symptoms.*

Signs Indicating Dominance of a Humor over a Humor

Signs of blood humor dominance are similar to those of the fullness of vessels; therefore, they may induce heaviness in the body, especially in the base of the eyes, head, and temples, accompanied with stretching, yawning, drowsiness, persistent sleepiness, fogginess of senses, slowness of thinking, fatigue without carrying out action, unusual sweetness in the mouth, tongue redness, pustules that may appear in the body, mouth sores, and bleeding in the soft areas, like nostrils, anus, and gums. Domination of blood humor is indicated by temperament, previous treatment, country, age, family, time since venesection, signs in dreams, like red objects, excessive bleeding, blood thickness, and the like.

Signs of phlegm dominance are increased whiteness in color, flabbiness, soft and cold skin, excessive sticky saliva, reduced thirst unless phlegm is salty, especially in old age, weak digestion, sour belching, whiteness of urine, excessive sleep, laziness, laxity of nerves, dullness, and slow irregular soft pulse, in addition to age, habits, previous treatment, occupation, country, and dreams that feature water, rivers, snow, rain, and thundering hailstorms.

Signs of yellow bile dominance are yellowness of skin and eye color, bitter mouth, rough dry tongue, dry nostrils, enjoyment of cool breezes, excessive thirst, rapid breathing, weak appetite, nausea, yellow and green bilious vomiting, burning (irritating) diarrhea, horripilation* like needle pricks, in addition to previous treatment, age, temperament, habits, country, time [of the year], occupation, as well as dreams

---

*The reflex of producing goose bumps is known as piloerection or the pilomotor reflex.

featuring fires, yellow flags and seeing objects that are not yellow with a yellow tint, inflammations, hot baths, sun, and the like.

Signs of black bile dominance are dryness and murkiness of color, blackness and thickness of blood, suspicious thoughts and thinking, burning in the cardiac orifice, false appetite, turbid thick urine of black and red color, skin black and hairy (rarely black bile accumulates in white short bodies), and frequent occurrence of vitiligo nigra, terrible sores, and spleen problems. Other signs include age, temperament, habits, country, occupation, time [of the year], previous treatment, and dreams featuring darkness, deep pits, black objects, and fears.

EIGHTH SECTION

Signs Indicating Obstruction (Blockage)

If the signs indicate congestion by substances and there is a feeling of distention without any sign of fullness, then there is an obstruction without doubt. Obstruction induces a feeling of heaviness when it is in ducts that carry large amounts through them; for example, congestion in the liver from food results in a large accumulation and a heaviness that is more heavy than a swelling and is distinguished from swelling by its heaviness and absence of fever. However, if the obstruction is not in such large ducts, there will not be a feeling of heaviness but the feeling of blood obstruction and distention. A person with obstruction of vessels will have yellow color because the blood is not going through to the surface of the skin.

NINTH SECTION

Signs Indicating Gases

Gases are felt by the pains they cause in the sensitive organs because of discontinuity they create. They are felt by the movement of organs, sounds, or touch. Extending pains indicate gases, especially if they are with lightness and moving pain; this is produced by discontinuity between sensitive organs [parts of the body]. However, in tissues like bone and glandular tissues, gases are not indicated by pain; there may be gases in the bones that break the bones or bruise them, but the pain is caused by their effects of breakage and not by the gases themselves.

However, investigating the gases from organ movement is like following trembles that indicate gases that are formed and move to disperse or decompose. Sounds that indicate gases are either like rumbling and alike, such as pain felt in the spleen from a stabbing gas, or detected by percussion, as is done to distinguish between ascites and tympanites. Using touch to investigate gases distinguishes between flatulence and tumor because the former has swelling that yields to pressure without trembling, runny liquid, or viscous humor. The difference between flatulence and gas is not in their natures but in their movement, stillness, and discomfort.

TENTH SECTION

Signs Indicating Swellings

Apparent swellings are observed by touch and vision, and internal hot ones by their associated fever and heaviness if the organ with the swelling has lost its sensation, or heaviness with stabbing pain if the swelled organ has sensation. Also, it helps to determine the problem with the organ or confirm the indicators of having a swelling in the area of the organ, as if the feeling of swelling leads to it. Cold swellings, without a doubt, are not associated with pain. It is difficult to point out all of their signs, and to make it easy will necessitate boring description; therefore, it is better to defer it to the particular description of each organ. Here it is said that the feeling of painless heaviness with phlegmatic humor signifies phlegmatic swelling. If the swelling has indicators of black bile humor then it is atrabilious, especially if it is solid to the touch; hardness is the best indicator. If the hot swellings are in the nerves they cause severe pain and strong fevers and lead to distention and mental confusion and disturb the movement of contraction and relaxation.

All swellings of the viscera cause thinning and weakness in the abdominal membrane. If the visceral swellings mature together and abscess they will cause severe pain, fever, severe roughness of the tongue, stronger insomnia, intense symptoms, greater heaviness, maybe a feeling of hardness and density, maybe the sudden appearance of weight loss, and sudden sinking of the eyes. However, once the swellings form pus, the fever foments, pain and throbbing decrease, and itching replaces pain; any existing redness is reduced and the exiting hardness becomes soft, all pain symptoms end, and heaviness reaches its fullness. If the abscess bursts it releases acrid pus that causes shivering, then fever, due to a burning of the pus; the pulse depletes and changes to weaker, smaller, slower, and irregular; there is also a loss of appetite and warming of extremities.

Pus moves according to its destination, either through expectoration, urine, or feces. The good signs after the release of pus are the complete cessation of fever, easiness of breathing, regaining of energy, and speed of pus excretion. The substance of internal swellings may move from one organ to another; the movement may be good or bad. The good movement involves transfer from a superior organ to an inferior organ, such as the movement of substance from brain swellings to behind the ears or from swellings of the liver to the groin; and the bad movement is the transfer to a superior organ from a lesser organ or to an organ that has less tolerance to the substance, for example, the transfer from the pleurae to the heart or lungs.

Movement of internal swellings and the transfers of their pus upward and downward have signs. Their movement to the epigastrium (شراسيف) causes distention and heaviness, and their movement to higher areas produces low-quality, constricted, and difficult breathing, tightness of chest, inflammation that starts from below and moves up, heaviness at the clavicle region, and headache that will affect the clavicle and arm. The upward movement is bad and dangerous if it reaches the brain, but it is better and will have a good prognosis if it goes to the soft tissue behind the ears. Nosebleed is a good sign in this situation and in all of visceral swellings. The details are provided after the discussion of swelling when we describe the swelling of each internal organ one by one.

ELEVENTH SECTION

Signs of Discontinuity

Discontinuity in apparent organs is identified by the senses, and if it takes place in the internal organs it will be felt by piercing, stabbing, and corroding pains, especially if associated with fever. Frequently, it is followed by leakage of humor, such as in hemoptysis into the thoracic cavity and discharge of pus after the maturation of the signs of swelling. One that takes place after the bursting of swelling could be after maturation or not; the one after maturation eliminates fever, discharges pus, and quiets and reduces heaviness, while the one without maturation intensifies and increases pain.

Discontinuity can be observed from the dislocation of the organ or its shift from its original location, as in hernia. Discontinuity is indicated from the congestion of excretions outside ducts in areas created by discontinuity, with separation from the normal tract, as in the case of fecal retention when the intestine is pierced.

Discontinuity may be hidden and cannot be diagnosed by the aforementioned general signs, and the specific signs of the organs are required. This situation occurs when the organ is insensitive, does not contain moisture to leak out, does not have the room for dislocation, or is not dependant on another organ such that its dislocation affects it.

Know that the most difficult swellings and discontinuities are those that take place within the sensitive nervous parts since they can be fatal and they are always followed by fainting and convulsions. Fainting is caused by severe pain, and convulsions by nervous effect within the organ. Affected joints are slow to accept treatment due to their excessive movement and the space around the joint that accepts flowing of matter into it. Because the pulse and urine are among the general signs of body conditions, we will talk about them next.

Pulse

(19 Sections)

FIRST SECTION

General Statement on the Pulse

We say that the pulse is a movement within the vessels of the "spirit" that consists of relaxation and contraction to cool down the "spirit" with air [look up the authors' commentary on aeration at the beginning of the 2nd Lesson]. Examination of the pulse is either general or specific according to each disease. Here we will discuss the general rules and postpone the specific to the discussion of particular diseases. A pulse is composed of two movements [systole] and two rests [diastole]. A beat comprises relaxation and contraction, then two rests between these two differing movements because it is impossible to immediately carry out a second movement after the ending of the first in distance and action, and this is illustrated by natural science. It is definite that each successive beat has four parts, "two movements and two rests," in this sequence: relaxation, rest, contraction, and rest.

Contraction movement according to many physicians is actually undetectable, and some others can detect it in a strong pulse due to its force, in a great pulse due to its height, in a hard pulse due to its resistance, and in the abdomen due to the long period of movement. Galen said, "For a while I was not detecting contraction but I continued looking for it until I detected some of it, then after a while I caught it and later I realized the many aspects of the pulse; those who follow my steps will reach what I did." Contractions most of the time are undetectable.

The reasons for examining the pulse in the left forearm are three: easy to access, very little difficulty in detecting it, and straightforward position near the heart. Examining the pulse should be done with the arm at the side since a resting arm increases the width and height of the pulse and decreases its length in thin individuals; a prostrated arm increases the height and length and decreases the width. At the time of pulse examination, the individual should be free of anger, joy, exertion, and other reactions; should not have overeaten or be hungry; and should have not quit long-term habits or acquired new ones. The exam should compare the pulse to that of a person of good equitable temperament.

Then we say that the types by which the physicians figure out the state of the pulse are ten, although they should have made them nine only. These are:

1. Amount of expansion
2. Strength as a force felt against the finger
3. Speed
4. Compressibility and/or elasticity
5. Turgor (volume): tension of the fullness
6. Temperature of the pulse
7. Duration of diastole
8. Constancy
9. Regularity and irregularity
10. Rhythm of the pulse (الوزن)

As for the amount of expansion, it is measured in three diameters: length, width, and depth. Therefore, the conditions of the pulse are nine simple and various compound varieties. The simple nine are long, short, and equitable; wide, narrow, and equitable; as well as low, high, and equitable. A long pulse is the one that is felt in its length as being longer than an absolute natural pulse, which is the true equitable temperament, or longer than the normal of that individual, which is the equitable that belongs to that person before, and you know the difference between them. The short is opposite, and the equitable is between them. By analogy you can figure out the other six. However, some of the compound varieties that are made of the simples have names and others do not. For example, the one that has excess of length, width, and depth is termed the great, and the one that is reduced in the three is termed the small, and between them is the equitable. The one with increases in width and height is termed the thick, the one reduced in both is the thin, with the equitable between the two.

The type based on the strength of the pulse against the fingers is of three subtypes. The strong is the one that resists the fingers during relaxation, the weak is the opposite, and the equitable is between them. The pulse type that is based on the speed of every movement is of three varieties: the fast is the one that completes the movement in a short time, the slow is the opposite, and the equitable is between them.

The compressibility (elasticity) of the vessel is of three subtypes: the soft can be easily pushed to the inside, the hard is the opposite, and then the equitable. As to the fullness of the vessels there are three subtypes: the full is the one with liquid that can be felt without pure space, the empty is the opposite, and the equitable is between. The one based on touch is of three subtypes: hot, cold, and equitable. As for the time of rest (diastole), there are three types: the first is the frequent, with short rests between the two successive beats (قرعتين), and it is also called the consecutive (المتدارك) or the condensed (المتكاثف); the second is the distant (متفاوت) or the long, and it is also called the relaxed (المتراخي) or the wobbly (المتخلخل); and the third is the equitable. The time of rest is determined by the contraction [between two systoles]; therefore, if the contraction is not felt then time is determined between two rests [diastoles], and if contraction is felt it is time between the two contractions.

The type taken from constancy (إستواء) may be also variable (إختلاف), as regularly variable (مختلف مستوي) or irregularly variable (مختلف غير مستوي) over several pulses, parts of a pulse, or one part of a pulse. The differences can be in five aspects: large or small, strong or week, fast or slow, frequent or distant, and hard or soft. One beat may have two fast rests due to high temperature or be weak due to general weakness. To simplify the discussion you can apply the same differences that are applied to constancy and variability to the other types. However, great consideration is given to constancy. The absolute constant pulse is the one constant in all of these features, but if constant only in one then you describe it as constant in strength or constant in speed. Similarly, the variable is variable in all or in one particular aspect.

The type taken from **order and disorder in irregularity** is of two subtypes: regularly irregular and sporadically irregular. The regularly irregular has a periodic schedule in two varieties: the first, it is absolutely regular and repeats only one irregular feature, and the second, it is periodically regular in two opposing features that work as a single cycle of complex irregularity. The sporadically irregular is the opposite. However, if you examine it you will find out that the latter is a subtype of the ninth type that falls under the variable subtype of the eighth type.

It should be known that the pulse has an existing musical nature. As music writing is carried out by writing notes with a ratio between them in pitch, weight, and rhythm of regularly recurring motion, so is the pulse. Music's time ratio in tempo (speed)* and frequency is the rhythm, and its ratio in strength, weakness, and amount is created; the rhythm and pitch could be synchronized or not, the asynchrony may be regular or irregular. Similarly, the ratios of the pulse are in strength and weakness, and the amount may be in synchrony or not, and this is outside of the regular type.

According to Galen the ratio of measured rhythm should be following one of these musical ratios [intervals]†: the total to the fifth base is a triple, one and a half times the fifth base, one-half of the total, one-half of the fifth base, as well as one-third and one-fourth of the fourth base; after that it is undetectable. I find it difficult to figure out these ratios by touch, and it is easier if one gets used to rhythm and its ratios by practice. Furthermore, one who is able to know music and compare the sound with its note can understand the pulse ratios by feeling the pulse.

I say that placing the subtypes of the regular and irregular type as one of the ten types, although beneficial, is not a correct classification because they go under the irregular as if they are in one of its subtypes.

The type taken from **rhythm** measures the ratios of the four times between the two movements and two rests. If touch fails to measure

---

*Tempo is measured in beats, and every heartbeat is in a group of four (two contractions and two rests).

†In music theory, an interval is a combination of two notes or the ratio between their frequencies.

all of the four, then one can measure the ratios of the rests' times to that between two rests or total time of movement to the time of rest. Those that bring under this topic measuring the time of movement to another time of movement or time of rest to time of rest are mixing two topics; however, it is permissible but not good. Rhythm is the one encompassing the musical ratios. We say the pulse is either having a good rhythm or an abnormal rhythm [dysrhythmia]. Abnormal rhythm has three subtypes: overrhythmic [pararhythmic], transcending the rhythm of an age group to the following age group, such as a child having the pulse of a young man; variable rhythm [heterorhythmic], such as a boy having the pulse of an old man; and out of rhythm [arrhythmic], which does not resemble the pulse of any of the age groups. A large departure of the pulse from rhythm indicates major changes in the body.

SECOND SECTION

Special Description of Constant and Variable Pulse

It is said that variable pulse is either variable in many beats or in one beat. The latter is either variable in many parts (i.e., the different locations of the fingers) or in one location of a finger. The pulse with continuous gradual variation (المختلف الجاري في الاستواء) is a subtype of the variable in many beats; it starts with one beat and changes to a stronger or weaker and continues like that to its minimum or maximum, vanishes, and starts again. Sometimes it completes its course, does not, or surpasses it. Other times, it pauses in the middle or skips the pause in the middle.

Intermittent pulse (ذوالفتره) is a variable subtype that has an unpredictable pause [see the eighth and ninth types on page 206] when a movement is expected. If more beats occur where a rest is expected then it is called a supernumerary pulse (الواقع في الوسط).

Variation of many parts within one single pulse may be in the location or movement of the parts. Variation in location pertains to a variable ratio of the artery according to directions, and since directions are six, then variations are six. Variation in movement means fast or slow, advanced or delayed (one part moves prematurely or late), strong or weak, and large or small. These variations may run in a constant order or variable order by an increase or decrease in two, three, or four parts (i.e., fingers' locations). Then you need to combine these variations and come up with conclusions.

Variation in one location may be of three varieties: intermittent [anacrotic] (منقطع), recurrent (عائد), and continuous (المتصل). The intermittent pulse is disconnected for one real period with both disconnected ends possibly differing in speed and similarity. The recurrent pulse is a large beat that becomes small and returns back gradually to its original. Under this variety is the coupled pulse (المتداخل), where a beat appears as if it is two beats due to differences or as two beats combined into one, according to those who opine on that. In the continuous, the change takes place gradually and is undetectable in its increase or decrease or when it changes to normal. This variation continues in such manner and may be very variable in some of its continuous parts, and less in others.

THIRD SECTION

Types of Special Compound Pulse

1. **Gazelle** (غزالي): It varies in one part. If it is slow, it becomes discontinued, then rapid.
2. **Wavy** (موجي): It is variable in regard to vessels, their width, thinness, height, and breadth. It also varies in being immature or late in starting the beat, with some softness. It is not that small and has some breadth. It feels like straight waves following each other with variation in their height, bottom, and speed.
3. **Wormy** (cordlike, twisting, دودي): It is like the wavy except it is smaller and of high frequency that erroneously implies speed, but it is not fast.
4. **Antlike** (نملي): It is much smaller with higher frequency

than the wormy, and they both differ in their height as well as advancement or delay, which are felt by touch and are the only distinguishing features between the two, but not the breadth.

5. **Sawlike** (serrated, منشاري): It is fast, frequent, solid, and varies in its large breadth as well as hardness and softness.

6. **Mouse-tail** (decurtate [shortened, curtailed], ذنب الفار): It gradually varies in its parts by decrease to increase and from increase to decrease. It could be in many beats, just one beat, or one to many parts of a beat. Its particular variation concerns its height, and may also be in speed and strength.

7. **Needlelike** (spindly, مسلي): It starts small but increases in size until it reaches it fullness, then decreases until it reaches its initial size; it is like two mouse tails fused at their bases.

8. **Double-beat** (dicrotic, ذو القرعتين): Physicians differ in defining this type of pulse; some make into one beat that varies in advancement and delay, others say that it is two successive beats. In general, the time between them is short to allow for a contraction and rest, and not all that feels like two beats is actually two; otherwise the returning intermittent pulse from its rest would have been considered two pulses. It should be considered two pulses only if starts, relaxes, and then gives a deep contraction followed by a relaxation.

9 and 10. **Intermittent** and **supernumerary** pulses have been described above. The difference between supernumerary and gazelle is that the latter has an extra stroke before the end of the first, while in the other the second beat appears in the resting time and after the passing of the first beat.

11, 12, and 13. **Spasmodic** (المتشنج), **trembling** (المرتعش), and **twisting** (المتلوي): The twisting behaves as if it is a thread that is twisting and wrapping with coils. These three varieties differ from each other in advancement and delay, position, and breadth.

14. **Cordlike** (متوتر) is a subtype of the twisting that resembles the trembling; however, the relaxation in the cordlike is more hidden, also its departure from consistency in height. Additionally,

the expansion in the cordlike is obvious and could be tilting to only one side. The cordlike is prevalent in dry diseases.

There is an endless and nameless list of compound pulses.

FOURTH SECTION

The Normal Types of the Pulse

The normal state of every one of these mentioned types of pulse that are irregular by an increase or decrease has an equitable state except the strong one since its normal is with an increase. When one of these types increases in strength and becomes strong (large), it is still considered normal in strength. However, the normal of other types that cannot tolerate an increase or decrease is the consistent, regular, and rhythmic.

FIFTH SECTION

Causes of the Mentioned Pulse Types

Causes of pulse: there are general, necessary, intrinsic causes that are responsible for the health of the pulse; these are called the retentive causes (أسباب ماسكه). There are causes that are not part of the pulse health; these are either the essential causes, whose alteration changes the pulse, or unessential alternative causes.

There are three retentive causes:

- First, the vital and/or animalistic faculty that creates the pulse in the heart, and you have known it under the animalist faculties.
- Second, the instrument of the pulse, pulsing crest, and you have known it when we mentioned the organs.
- Third, the need for cooling, which demands a certain amount of cooling that gets adjusted according to amount of charring, lack of it, and its equitability. These retentive causes get altered according to their association with essential or absolute altering causes.

SIXTH SECTION

Indicators of Retentive Causes

If the instrument [artery or arteries] is agreeable with its softness, its faculty is strong, and there is a great need for cooling, the pulse would be large. **The need for cooling is the instigator of the three.*** If the faculty is weak it will be followed by a weak pulse without a doubt. If the instrument is hard, even with a need for cooling, the pulse would be smaller. Hardening [of the artery] also diminishes the pulse; however, reduction that is caused by hardening is separate from that caused by the weakness because [the artery] is hard and not weak and it is not substantially short and low, as is the case due to weakness. Also, reduced need [for cooling] produces smallness, but there will not be weakness. Among these three, weakness is the producer of smallness. Slight hardening with strength is stronger than diminished need with strength. This is because strength without demand does not reduce much of the equitable since there is nothing that prevents the artery from expanding; it does not increase it much beyond what the equitable state needs.

If the need is great and the faculty is strong, but the instrument is hard and resists the large pulse [resists expansion], then the pulse compensates by becoming faster in order to offset that which is lost from the reduction of the pulse size. However, if the faculty is weak, then pulse enlargement and increase of speed will not take place; instead it becomes more frequent to compensate by the higher frequency for the large speedy pulse, thus the higher frequency replaces one to two sufficiently large pulses. This may resemble the case of one who wants to carry a heavy load; if they can carry it all at once they will do so, otherwise they will divide it into two halves or into several pieces and carry whatever they can slowly or quickly. They will not rest between loads even if they are slow; however, if they are very weak, they will rest, go back to move the loads with difficulty, and come back slowly.

When the faculty is strong and the instrument is pliable but the need is much stronger than the equitable, then the faculty provides

---

*The "need" can be interpreted as the demand for oxygen and transport of carbon dioxide to the lungs and out of the body.

speed in addition to a large pulse, and if the need is great then it causes higher frequency in addition to largeness and speed.

Length of the pulse is increased if enlargement and height are prevented by hardening and by thickness of flesh and skin that limit the pulse's height.

Breadth of the pulse is increased by slimness. The emptiness of the vessels increases breadth since the upper layer of the blood moves lower and pushes the vessels sideways. Also, the excessive softness increases breadth. Higher frequency is caused by weakness or frequent need for heat. Irregularity is caused by a strong need that has reached its maximum, severe cold that locked the need, or a cause that diminished the faculty and brought death closer. Weakness of the pulse is caused by worrying, insomnia, vomiting, excessive leanness, abnormal humor, excessive exercise, movement of humors into sensitive organs near the heart, and all decomposing things.

Causes of pulse [arterial] hardness are the dryness of the vessel body, its excessive extension, or freezing from severe cold. Carpenters' arteries may harden because of extreme labor and the distension of the organs in the direction of force. Softness of pulse is caused by the natural moisturizers, such as food, and moisturizing by disease, such as edema and sleeping sickness (ليثيارغوس), but neither by normal nor pathological causes, such as bathing.

Causes of pulse irregularity with the steadiness of strength are heavy substance from food or humor and struggle of the faculty with a disease when the faculty is weak. Other causes of irregularity include fullness of vessel, and this can be eliminated by venesection; low blood viscosity suffocates the moving "spirit" in the arteries, especially when this accumulation takes place near the heart; its occurrence in a short period is attributed to fullness of stomach and mouth and preoccupation of thinking. If the stomach contains abnormal humor, it will persevere the blood, causing the irregularity, and may lead to tachycardia.

The cause of the **serrated pulse** is the varying qualities of the materials infiltrating the vessel in putrefaction, maturity, and rawness; variability of the vessel in hardness and softness; and swelling or inflammation of nervous tissues.

The cause of **double-beat (dicrotic) pulse** is the extreme strength of the faculty, the need, and hardness of the instrument [vessels], thus it does not expand at once to accommodate the strength. It is similar to trying to cut something by one hit, and then when it does not work follow it with another. This pulse occurs in response to a sudden need.

The cause of **mouse-tail pulse** is the weakness of the faculty, thus the exhaustion leads to gradual rest, then from rest to exhaustion. The one with a fixed state is the best indicator of the weakness of the faculty. Mouse-tail and similar pulses indicate that there is still some strength and that the weakness has not reached its maximum. The worse of it is the **vanishing tail** and the **recurrent tail**. The reason for the same rest is the exhaustion and rest or a sudden disturbance that requires the immediate resources of the body. The cause of **spasmodic pulse** is abnormal movements in the faculty and defects in the structure of the instrument. The **trembling** is produced by a hard instrument and great need; otherwise, it should not occur.

The cause of the **wavy pulse** is mostly a weak faculty that cannot expand the arteries; however, softness of the instrument can be another reason, even if the faculty is not very weak, because the soft and moist instrument resists shaking and moving in its free part, unlike the dry and hard. Dryness prepares for shaking and vibration. The distant end of a dry hard object moves when its proximal end moves, however, no part of a soft moist object moves due to the movement of another part because of its quick acceptance of separation, bending, and alteration of shape.

The cause of **wormlike** and **antlike pulses** is extreme weakness until they gather slowness, higher frequency, and irregularity in the parts of the pulse because the faculty cannot expand the instrument at once but rather little by little.

The cause of **abnormal rhythm** when there is a deficiency in the time of rest is the increase of demand. On the other hand, if the increase is at the time of movement, then it is due to an increase in weakness or decrease in need. The case where there is a decrease in the time of movement due to fast expansion is different. The causes of full, empty, warm, hot, high, and low pulses are clear.

SEVENTH SECTION

Pulse of Males, Females, and Ages

Because of their strong vigor, higher need, higher strength, and need met with a large pulse, the male pulse is mostly slower and less frequent than that of females. Every pulse with constant strength and frequency will speed up without a doubt because the speed comes before frequency. Therefore, although men's pulse is slower, it has higher frequency.

Children's pulse is softer, weaker, and more frequent because their heat is strong but their faculty is not that strong since they have not completed their growth. Their pulse in comparison with the size of their bodies is large because their instrument is soft and their need is intense. Their faculty compared with their body size is not weak because their bodies are small in size but their pulse in comparison with that of complete growth is not large, but it is faster and more frequent due to need. Smoky vapor [carbon dioxide] accumulates in children for their excessive digestion and its abundance; therefore, they have high demand to get it out and aerate their innate heat.

Adults' pulse is large without an increase in speed (to the contrary, it is much less) or frequency, leaning toward irregularity. Those in early adulthood have a larger pulse, and those in the middle of their youth have a stronger pulse. We have explained earlier that heat in children and youth is very similar; therefore, their needs are also alike. However, the youth has excess of strength that reaches with a large pulse what substitutes for the lack of speed and frequency. The most important factor in making the pulse large is the strength of the faculty, whereas the need invites, and the instrument assists.

Pulse of the elderly is weaker and slower due to weakness and reduced need; therefore, it is very irregular. The pulse of advanced-aged elderly is small, irregular, slow, and may be soft due to abnormal moistures and not the normal innate ones.

EIGHTH SECTION

Pulse of Temperaments

Hot temperament has stronger need; therefore, if the instrument cooperates, the pulse would be large, and if one of them lags behind then look it up from the early description. If the heat is normal and not due to dystemperament, then the temperament would be strong and healthy and the faculty very strong. Do not think that an increase in the innate heat, no matter how high it reaches, necessitates a substantial reduction in the faculty; it puts strength in the essence of the "spirit" and nobility in the mind. The increase of the heat of dystemperament decreases the strength of the faculty.

In **cold temperament** the pulse tends to decrease in several aspects, such as smallness, in particular, slowness, and irregularity. If the instrument is soft, its width increases, it slows down, and it becomes irregular. A hard instrument does the opposite. Weakness is caused by cold; cold dystemperament is worse than hot dystemperament because the hot is more agreeable with the faculty.

Wet temperament induces the wavy and wide pulses, and **dry temperament** induces narrowness and hardness. If the faculty is strong and the need is great then they induce the double-beat, spasmodic, or trembling pulses. Then it is up to you to combine using the basics.

It may occur that a person's two sides have two different temperaments so that one side is cold and the other is hot, thus his pulse differs on each side where the differences are dictated by the heat and cold. The hot side will have the pulse of a hot temperament, and the cold side will have the pulse of a cold temperament. From this, one learns that pulse in its relaxation and contraction is not like the tide (ebb and flow) from the heart, but is like the relaxation and contraction of the arterial body itself.

NINTH SECTION

Seasonal Pulse

The pulse in the spring is equitable in everything, with an increase in the faculty. In the summer, the pulse is usually fast, frequent due to need, and small and weak due to the weakness of the faculty by the dispersal of the "spirit" by the excessive external heat. In the winter, the pulse is strongly irregular, slower, and weaker, although it is small because of the weakness of the faculty. In some bodies, heat gathers internally and strengthens the faculty; this usually happens when the hot temperament is dominant and resistant to cold, and thus the body does not react to it and cold does not go deeper. Autumn's pulse is irregular and tends to be weak. Its irregularity and weakness are due to the fluctuation of temperament between hot and cold. Temperamental fluctuations at any time are worse than the similar but constant, even if they are abnormal. And, also because autumn is a time that is antagonistic to the nature of life, where heat weakens and dryness increases. The pulse in the periods between the seasons follows the season that dominates it.

TENTH SECTION

On the Pulse of Countries

Some countries are temperate and springy, others are hot and summery, cold and wintery, or dry and autumnal. Therefore, the pulse of these countries follows that of the seasons.

ELEVENTH SECTION

Effect of Ingested Material on the Pulse

The ingested alters the pulse by its quality and quantity. By its quality, it may warm or cool, thus changing the pulse. As for quantity, a moderate amount transforms an equitable pulse to larger, more frequent, and warmer, and this effect lasts for a while. A large amount of food induces irregularity without order due to its exhaustion of the faculty strength; every type of heaviness induces irregularity. Archigenes* claimed that in this situation the speed is stronger than the frequency, and the effect continues as long as the cause is there. If the amount of food was less, then the irregularity of the pulse has an order; and if the food amount is even lesser, the pulse would be less in size and speed, and the effect does not last because the substance is small and is digested quickly. When the faculty collapses and weakens from excess or scarcity, the pulse becomes similar in smallness and low in frequency. However, when the faculty strengthens digestion and conversion, the pulse returns to its equitable state.

Alcohol has its specificity. Drinking a large amount of alcohol induces irregularity of the pulse, but its effect is less than that of food when comparing the same amount of both. This is because of its loose nature, gentle effect, and lightness. If alcohol is taken cold, its effect is that of a cold liquid, which reduces the size of the pulse, increases its frequency, and slows it down quickly due to its fast penetration [absorption] when it warms up in the body and the end of its effect as a cold liquid. If the alcohol is absorbed warm into the body, it is not distant from the innate faculty and it is broken down quickly. However, if alcohol is absorbed cold into the body, it is more harmful than any other cold drink because while cold drinks have to warm up before they are absorbed, alcohol is absorbed while it is still cold. When it disperses before it has warmed up to the body's temperature it causes severe harm, especially in the susceptible bodies, and this harm is not similar to its harmful effect if it is absorbed warm because it does not get warmed when it meets the body and the faculty has to be engaged to distribute it, break it down, and get rid of its waste. Cold alcohol weakens the faculty before it can work on distributing it or breaking it down. These are the effects of alcohol as to its quantity as well as its being hot or cold; however, as to its tonic effect, there are other rules because it is

---

*Archigenes ('Αρχιγένης) was an eminent Greek physician who practiced in Rome (48 CE–117 CE). He was born in Apamea (Arabic آفاميا) Syria and wrote several works, of which some portions are preserved.

strengthening to healthy people and revitalizing of strength by increasing the speed of the essence of "spirit."

Cooling and heating produced by alcohol, although harmful to most bodies, may be suitable or not depending on the temperament. Cold strengthens those with hot dystemperament, as Galen mentioned that pomegranate juice is a tonic for those with permanent hot dystemperament and honey water strengthens those with permanent cold dystemperament. Thus, drinking hot or cold drinks may strengthen one group and weaken another. However, our discussion here is about the strength that alcohol gives to the "spirit" because it is always a tonic; it is the properties of alcohol that may support the strength of the body or weaken it and accordingly affect the pulse. If it strengthens, the pulse will become stronger, and if it warms up then it increases the need, and reduces it if it cools. In most cases it increases the need (to increase the speed).

As for the water, it strengthens by assisting in food absorption, and it acts similarly to alcohol, and because it cools rather than warms, it does not reach the effect of alcohol in increasing the need.

TWELFTH SECTION

The Effects of Sleep and Wakefulness on the Pulse

Attributes of the pulse during sleep differ according to the phase of sleep and the state of digestion. The pulse in the early phase of sleep is small and weak due to reduction and inward movement of the innate heat, and not the expansion and outward movement, because it is focused on digesting food and maturing wastes, thus it is limited in its action. The pulse in this case is slow and less frequent because even if heat increases due to its internal concentration, it does not reach the same level as it does during wakefulness.

Movement strongly increases the innate heat and may tip it toward dystemperament. Moderate confluence and concentration are less conducive to increasing the innate heat and heat in general than sleeplessness (قلـة). You can tell from the fact that the breathing of a tired person and their sleeplessness is much more than that of the breathing and sleeplessness of a person with confined heat due to a cause that is similar to sleep. An example of this is the submergence in moderately cold water of an awake person, wherein their heat becomes confined inward and strong; but their breath will not reach the same amount as attained from fatigue and exercise, which in their effect are close to submergence. If you think about it, you will realize that there is not anything that induces heat like movement.

Wakefulness does not induce heat through body movement since cessation of movement does not stop heat production; however, it does that by the movement of "spirit" toward the body surface and its continuous connection to its place of generation. When food is assimilated during sleep, it strengthens the faculty because the blood that was used to transfer the food goes back to the exterior and to its original location; therefore, the pulse becomes large because the temperament becomes warmer by the food and the instrument becomes softer from the passing nutrients; however, the pulse speed and frequency do not increase since there is no increase in the need and the large pulse by itself is sufficient.

With prolonged sleep, the pulse becomes weak due to [inward] confinement of innate heat and the occupation of the faculty with waste products that will be eliminated by various ways (among these are exercise and other imperceptible methods) during wakefulness. Sleeping on an empty stomach without any food for digestion tends to cool the temperament and maintains a small, slow, and less frequent pulse that will continue to decrease in all three.

Wakefulness has a set of different rules. When waking up naturally, the pulse tends to become gradually large and fast and then returns to its normal state. However, one who is awakened suddenly may suffer a weakening of the pulse due to the absence of the faculty in the face of the sudden event; then a large, fast, frequent, and irregular trembling pulse kicks in, and since this is almost a compulsory movement it increases the heat. Also, because the faculty moves suddenly, with different movements, to deal with the event, it causes the pulse to tremble, but it does not stay like that for a long time, and it quickly becomes equitable since the cause, although it is strong, is not fixed, and its effect does not last.

Rules of the Pulse in Exercise

At the beginning of exercise, and as long as it is moderate, the pulse becomes large and strong due to the increase and strengthening of the innate heat; it also becomes fast and very frequent due to the excessive need that is generated by movement. If the exercise is continued and prolonged, intensive, or even shortened after that, it cancels the faculty's effect; thus the pulse becomes weak due to dissipation of innate heat. However, it can become fast and frequent for two reasons: first, excessive need, and second, weakness of the faculty to induce a large pulse. The speed continues to decline and the frequency increases at the same amount of the faculty's decline; then at the end if the exercise continues and induces fatigue, the pulse becomes antlike due to weakness and intense frequency, and with extreme exercise that brings a person close to death, it causes what all breakdowns do, namely, a wormlike pulse tending to be irregular and slow with weakness and small size.

Rules of the Bathers' Pulse

Bathing may be done with hot or cold water. The hot water bath initially increases the faculty strength and the need; therefore, its excessive decomposing effect weakens the pulse. Galen said, "The pulse is then small and slow." We say the weakness and smallness of the pulse are inevitable, but if the hot water produces temporary warmness in the body it will soon become dominated by its cooling nature, which may stay on for a while. Therefore, if the effect of the temporary quality dominates the pulse it becomes fast and frequent, and if its true natural effect dominates it becomes slow and irregular. If the temporary heating becomes excessive, it increases the decomposition of the faculty to an almost unconsciousness level, and the pulse becomes slow and irregular as well.

Bathing in cold water weakens the pulse and induces irregularity and slowness. If the coldness does not sink deep but instead gathers the heat, it increases the faculty and thus the pulse becomes large and decreases in speed and frequency. In bathhouses, astringent water increases the hardness of the pulse and decreases it size; warming water increases the pulse speed but decreases the faculty according to that we mentioned above.

FIFTEENTH SECTION

Specific Pulse of Women: Pulse of Pregnant Women

The need increases in pregnant women due to sharing by the fetus of the inhaled air, thus it is as if the woman is breathing in for two needs and two beings. The faculty strength, without a doubt, does not increase, or it may decrease slightly according to the fatigue of the pregnancy. Therefore, moderate faculty and intense need dominate and produce a large, fast, and frequent pulse.

SIXTEENTH SECTION

Pulse of Pains

Pain affects the pulse because of its intensity, for being in a main organ, or when it lasts for a long time. Initially, pain excites the faculty and instigates it to resist and defend, and ignites the heat; therefore, the pulse is large, fast, and very irregular because the need requires largeness and speed. When the pain overwhelms the faculty because of the factors that we mentioned, the pulse starts to turn around and weakens until it loses its largeness and speed; this is followed by high frequency first, then smallness and wormlike and antlike pulses. If the pain becomes worse, it increases irregularity and leads to death after that.

SEVENTEENTH SECTION

Pulse of Swellings

Some swellings cause fevers, and because of their size or location within a vital organ their fever changes the pulse in the whole body; we will explain it in its place. Other swellings do not induce fever, thus they change the pulse of the organ where the swelling is located; they may change it in the whole body indirectly, not as swelling, but as a pain. Pulse-changing swelling causes changes according to its type, phase, size, location within an organ, or by the effects it causes.

Change is according to the type of the swelling, such as when hot swelling causes a **sawlike pulse** that is trembling, fast, and frequent, and if it is not opposed by a moisturizing factor, the sawlike turns into a **wavy pulse.** Trembling, speed, and frequency are always associated with swelling, and there are causes that prevent a sawlike pulse or that promote it and make it appear.

Soft swelling makes the pulse wavy, and if the swelling is very cold it makes the pulse slow and irregular. Hard swellings increase a sawlike pulse. Pustules that accumulate pus turn a sawlike pulse into a wavy pulse due to the moisturizing and softening that follows; pustules also increase variability because of their heaviness. The speed and frequency of the pulse decrease with the subsiding of temporary heat due to the maturation of the abscess.

The pulse changes according to the phase of swelling. A hot swelling in its initial phase and increasing will have a sawlike pulse with its associated signs all on the increase, as we have mentioned; it also increases in hardness due to the increase of extension and is jerky due to pain. When the swelling reaches its end [full maturity], all signs increase except those of the faculty, which weakens the pulse and thus increases its frequency and speed. However, if the swelling persists, the pulse ceases to be fast and turns into antlike. When a swelling declines, disintegrates, or ruptures, the pulse becomes stronger due to the unloading of the faculty, and its trembling effect is reduced because of the decline of the extending pain.

As for the size of the swelling, a large swelling makes these conditions greater, and a small swelling makes them small and less.

As for the affected organ, a swelling in the nervous organs increases the hardness and sawlikeness of the pulse; a vascular swelling makes the pulse larger and unequal, especially if the arteries are dominant, as in the spleen and lung. This large pulse is maintained as long as the faculty is strong, and the soft moist organs make the pulse wavy, as in the brain and lung.

There are examples of the effects on the pulse by the changes in a swelling, such as inflammation of the lung [pneumonia] induces a pulse of suffocation; hepatitis gives a wilted pulse, inflammation of the kidney gives a confined pulse; and inflammation of very sensitive organs like the stomach, mouth, and diaphragm gives a spasmodic-to-fainting pulse.

EIGHTEENTH SECTION

Pulse Rules of Psychological Conditions

Anger stimulates the faculty strength and expands the "spirit" instantaneously, thus causing the pulse to be very large, fast, and frequent. The pulse should remain uniform because the reaction is consistent, except when it is mixed with fear, then the two states may alternate in dominance. Similarly, if anger is associated with shyness, mental anguish, or a restraint from showing anger to another person, then the pulse would be unequal.

Pleasure's outwardly gentle stimulation does not reach that of anger in causing a fast and frequent pulse since a large one may be sufficient, and also it is slow and irregular. Similarly, joy gives mostly a large soft pulse that is slow and irregular.

In sadness, heat is congested and sinks in, and the faculty strength becomes weak, therefore, the pulse becomes small, weak, irregular, and slow. Sudden fear makes the pulse fast, trembling, unequal, and irregular. A prolonged and gradual state of fear affects the pulse the same way as sadness.

NINETEENTH SECTION

Changes Produced by Issues
Contrary to the Nature of the Pulse

These causes change the pulse by producing a dystemperament (the pulse of each temperament is known) by compressing the strength of the faculty, thus changing the pulse, and if the pressure is severe then the pulse becomes disorderly or arrhythmic, and the presser is usually an excess of substance that may be a swelling or not; or by disintegrating the faculty, thus weakening the pulse, and like severe pain and psychological pains, all three are associated with strong dispersion.

Urine and Feces

(13 Sections)

*Acidic urine is produced by cold temperament that is
affected by abnormal metabolism, but extreme acidity is a
sign of death due to diminished innate heat.*

FIRST SECTION

General Statement about Urine Indicators

There should not be a trust in urine examination unless certain conditions are followed:

- It must be the first collection in the morning.
- It has not been left out for a long time.
- It is over-the-night urine.
- No food or drink was consumed.
- The patient has not taken any coloring in food or drink, such as saffron, pomegranate, purging cassia (golden shower tree, *Cassia fistula*), since this will color the urine to yellow and red, and legumes color it red and blue, *al-muri** colors it black, and alcoholic drinks color it to their color; skin colorings like henna may color the urine.
- The patient has not taken something that will push out a humor through urine, such as yellow or phlegm humors.
- The patient has not carried out movements and works.

---

*Al-muri (also *murri*) is an old Arabic drink made from honey, bread, flour, anise seeds, fennel seeds, nigella seeds, celery seed, carob, quince, saffron, and lemon juice. This mixture is fermented and then diluted to make a drink.

Some of the out-of-the-ordinary external states change the urine color, such as fasting, lack of sleep, fatigue, hunger, and anger, which all change the color to yellow or red. Intercourse markedly increases the oiliness of the urine. Also, vomiting and evacuation change the original color and texture of urine.

Urine should be examined fresh; this is why it is said not after six hours because its indicators become weak, its color changes, and its density dissolves, changes, or becomes thicker. However, I say not to look at it after one hour.

The complete volume of urine should be taken in a large bottle without decanting any of it. The examination of urine should not start immediately but after it has settled in the bottle without exposure to the sun, wind that stirs it, or cold that freezes it, until settling has been recognized and examination carried out. Not all urine precipitates or is completely very mature. The bottle should not be used again until it is washed well.

Children's urine has fewer indicators, especially that of infants, because it is affected by the milk and the persistence of coloring material within it due to their weakness and prolonged sleeping; therefore, it lacks indicators of maturity.

The container for examining the urine should be of a transparent and pure material such as clear glass or crystal. Be aware that the closer you look at the urine, the more thick it appears to you and the more distant, the clearer it becomes; this is a distinguishing property for adulterated specimens that physicians examine. Once the urine is taken in a bottle it should be protected from cold temperature, the sun, and wind, and looked at without direct exposure to sunlight.

Let it be known that the initial indicators of urine are the states of liver and urinary tracts, as well as the conditions of the vessels, and when these are in moderate condition urine could indicate other diseases. The most accurate indicators of the urine are these of the health of the liver, especially its functions. Indicators of the urine are derived from seven types: color, texture, clarity, sedimentation, quantity, odor, and foam. Others include touch and taste, but we have dropped them due to their repulsiveness.

We mean by the color that which the eye distinguishes of colors; I mean the black and white and that in-between them. The texture means the density and lightness. Clarity and turbidity mean the easiness or difficulty to see through the urine. The difference between the latter and texture is that a thick urine may be clear like egg yolk, fish glue, or oil, and it may be thin textured but turbid like murky water, which is much thinner than egg yolk, and the cause of turbidity is the admixture with parts of strange colors or colors that are difficult to detect with transparency; therefore, it cannot be detected alone. Sedimentation differs in that it may be distinguished by the senses, but color permeates throughout the nature of moisture and is very much mixed with it.

SECOND SECTION

Indicators of Urine Color

Of urine colors are the various **shades of yellow** in the following order: straw-yellow, citron-yellow, blond, flame-yellow, fiery-yellow (similar to saffron, which is saturated yellow), saffron-yellow (similar to blond, also called bright red). All after the citron-yellow indicate heat, differ according to their degree, and may result from hard movement [exercise], pain, hunger, and thirst.

Yellow shades are followed by the **shades of red** such as reddish-brown, rosy, dark red, and blackish-red, and they all indicate the dominance of blood; however, a tilt toward saffron indicates yellow bile. A tendency toward darkness points out blood dominance. The fiery-yellow is a better indicator of heat than the red or black-red as the yellow bile itself is warmer than blood.

Urine color in acute burning diseases [i.e., excessively hot fevers] tends to be saffronlike and fiery, therefore, if the texture is light it indicates maturity that has started and is not fully obvious in the texture; if the yellowness becomes intense toward fieriness, or its end, then the heat has increased; on the other hand, a bright-blond indicates clarity and decrease of heat.

In acute hemorrhagic diseases, the urine may be as red as blood without the rupture of a vessel, which is rather indicative of extreme fullness of blood. If the urine comes out little by little and is associated with a foul odor it is a dangerous sign of possible blood accumulation in the cavities. The worst of this urine is the thinnest in color, condition, and texture. A large quantity of urination has a good prognosis in acute and mixed fevers because it is indicative of a healing crisis and recovery, except if the urine becomes thinner before a healing crisis; then it is indicative of a relapse, and also if it gradually thins after a healing crisis.

In jaundice, it is better when the urine is dark red to almost black, permanently stains the clothes, and is more in quantity. Thus, if the urine of jaundice is white or slightly reddish and the disease remains the same, it is feared that edema may develop. Starvation colors urine and substantially increases the intensity of the color.

Shades of green include, in this order, pistachio-green, verdigris, sky-green, emerald-green, and leek-green. Pistachio-green is indicative of cold, and so are those that have green, except the verdigris and leek-green because they indicate a severe charring. However, the leek-green is safer than verdigris, and the latter after fatigue indicates convulsion.

Among children, the green urine denotes convulsion. Their sky-green urine is an indicator of severe cold, and most of the time is preceded by green urine. It has been said that it is also signifying poisoning, and if the urine has sediment then the prognosis is good, otherwise death is a possibility. The verdigris urine is very good indicator of damage.

Shades of black include a black color that comes from saffron-colored urine, such as in jaundice, and it indicates the condensation of yellow bile and its charring, or the black bile develops from yellow bile, indicating jaundice. Dark black or reddish-black denotes sanguineous black bile. Black with a hint of green or emerald-green denotes pure black bile. Black urine in general signifies either severe charring, severe cold, the extinguishing of innate heat and decline, or a healing crisis and the expulsion of black bile waste. Black urine signifies severe charring if the preceding urine is yellow and red with slow sedimentation of immature and limited residues, and it is not very black but leaning to saffron, yellow, or reddish; if it is yellowish then it indicates jaundice. Cold is exposed when the early urine is greenish and cloudy and the residue is little and condensed with a dry appearance, and the blackness of this urine is pure. It may help distinguish between two temperaments. When the black urine has an odor it is indicative of heat, while an odorless or weakly odorous urine indicates cold since the steep decline of nature is odorless. Black urine signifies the decline of innate strength when it is followed by a drop in and disintegration of strength. Black urine may signify cleansing and a healing crisis when it takes place at the end of spring, and the resolution of spleen illness, backaches, uterine issues, fevers of black bile (daily and nightly), and temporary illness such as amenorrhea and constipation, especially if nature or medicine assisted in excretion.

Black urine occurs in women with amenorrhea where the nature of the body expels the blood waste, which is preceded by immature watery urine; the body after that feels light since the urine is plentiful and comes out in a large quantity. Other than that, black urine is a bad sign, especially in acute diseases and in particular when its amount is small. Its small amount indicates that moisture has been dissipated by charring. Thick black urine is worse, and the thinner it is the better. Sometimes black or dark red urine is from a drink that has the same color, which the natural processes did not affect; if it comes out with the same color, there is no harm in this. Black urine can be a good indication of a healing crisis in acute diseases as well, such as when the patient urinates thin urine with sediment in all of its parts it indicates headache, insomnia, deafness, and mental confusion. This is especially true if urination is in small amounts over a long period of time and has an acute odor. If these signs are present in fevers then they strongly signify headache and mental confusion, and if there is insomnia, deafness, mental confusion, and headache it indicates nosebleed. Black urine possibly signifies a kidney stone.

According to Rufus,* black urine is preferred in disease of the

---

*Rufus of Ephesus (ca. late first century CE) was a Greek physician who wrote treatises on dietetics, pathology, anatomy, and patient care. He was particularly influential in the Middle East, and some of his works survived only in Arabic. His teachings emphasized the importance of anatomy and sought pragmatic approaches to diagnosis and treatment.

kidney and the hyperactive diseases of thick humors, and it is a sign of mortality in acute diseases. We say that black urine is also bad in kidney and bladder diseases if there is severe charring; therefore, always examine all the symptoms. Black urine in the elderly is a sign of great corruption, and there is not any fix as far as is known, and similarly in women. Black urine after fatigue indicates spasms. Generally, black urine at the beginning of a fever is a sign of death (blackwater fever), and also the one at the end of a fever if it is not accompanied by relief or healing crisis.

The term *white urine* may have two meanings: one is light and transparent, and people may call it the *white transparent,* as they call white the clear glass and crystal. The second is the *true white,* with a color that scatters the light, such as yogurt and paper; this type is not transparent, and the vision cannot penetrate it because transparency in fact is the absence of all color. Transparent white urine is indicative of cold in general and lack of maturation, and when associated with thickness signifies phlegm. True white urine is always with thickness. Mucus-white denotes an excess of phlegm and lack of maturation, fatty-white signifies digestion of fat, and greasy-white (اهلي) indicates phlegm and diarrhea (present or to take place); bubbly-white that is thin and accompanied with pus signifies open pustules in the urinary tract, however, if it is devoid of pus then it indicates the dominance of excessive raw humor. The latter may be associated with a stone in the bladder.

White urine may resemble semen and could be the result of a healing crisis from phlegmatic swellings or flabbiness in the viscera and illnesses caused by glassy phlegm. When semen-white is not due to a healing crisis of phlegmatic swellings and happens at the beginning then it indicates apoplexy or paralysis. If the urine is white throughout a fever, it is on the verge of becoming a quartan fever. Lead-white urine without sediment is very bad. Milky-white urine in acute disease has a fatal prognosis. Whiteness of urine during acute fevers, after the disappearance of color, indicates that the yellow bile has gone into an organ that is undergoing swelling or diarrhea (gone toward the bowels), and most of the time means that it has gone toward the head. Furthermore, if the urine is light during fevers then turns suddenly white it indicates

a mental disturbance. Persistent white urine during a healthy state signifies a lack of maturation. Greasy-white urine that is oily in fevers is a
sign of close death or hectic fever.

Be aware that there could be white urine with hot bilious temperament and red urine with cold phlegmatic temperament. When yellow
bile moves away from the urinary tract and does not mix with urine,
the urine stays white; therefore, the white urine should be examined to
see if its color is bright, its density is high, and its texture is thick, then
this whiteness is produced by cold phlegm. On the other hand, if the
color is not that bright, the sediment is meager and not separating, and
the white is not cloudy, then know that it is due to the concealment
of yellow bile. However, if urine is white in an acute disease and there
are indicators of safety that lethargia (cerebral disturbance) is unlikely,
then the acute substance has turned toward the intestine and may cause
abrasion.

The cause of red urine in cold disease is one of the following reasons: severe pain that disintegrates yellow bile, such as that in cold colic;
a problem that takes place in the duct between the gallbladder and the
intestine so that the bile does not go into the intestine as usual, and thus
goes out with the urine, as it happens in a cold colic; or weakness of the
liver that makes it unable to distinguish between watery and bloody
substances, as it happens in cold edema and mostly in diseases of liver
weakness that give a urine that looks like the wash of a soft flesh. The
decongestion caused by obstruction changes the color of the phlegm in
vessels due to its putrefaction. Its symptoms are that the water fraction
of urine and density are as mentioned, the color weak and not bright
(bilious urine is usually bright), and in most of the cases the urine starts
as white and turns into black with offensive smell, as in jaundice.

Urine after a meal is white and remains so until the food is digested
and its color taken in; this is also the reason for the whiteness of insomniacs' urine, in addition to the wasting of their innate heat; it is also not
bright and turbid due to lack of maturation.

Red coloration in acute diseases is better than watery, and the
white's texture is better than the watery. Sanguineous red urine is much
safer than bilious red, and the latter is not that scary if the yellow bile is

calm, but it is frightening if it is on the move. Dark red urine in kidney diseases is bad because in most cases it is indicative of hot swelling, and in headaches it is a warning sign of mixing.

In acute diseases, if the urine starts red and remains as such without sediment it is a sign of impending death and indicates a kidney swelling. However, if it is turbid with red and remains as such, it indicates a swelling in the kidney and weakness of innate heat.

Some of the **urine colors are compound**. One of these colors is the color similar to the wash of soft flesh and resembles blood diluted in water, which may indicate a weakness of the liver or excess of blood. However, in most cases, it results from the weakness of the liver due to a dominant dystemperament; this is indicated by weakness of digestion and other faculties. Therefore, if the faculty is strong, then it is due to excess of blood and overabundance above the needed amount to be distinguished as such. Among the compound colors of urine is the oily, which is bilious mixed with scalded humor and resembles the blood color in its viscosity; it has transparency with fatty reflection, its texture varies from the transparent to the thick. In most cases it has a bad prognosis, and in rare cases it indicates the evacuation of fatty substances in the course of a healing crisis if followed by an odor. The one that is a sign of death is the one with malodorous fat with little-by-little urination. If this urine is mixed with something resembling the water of soft flesh then the situation is worse. This takes place mostly in edema, tuberculosis, and bad colic.

Sometimes oily urine is followed by mature black urine, and this is a good sign. In many cases of acute diseases, an oily urine on the fourth day means that the patient will die around the seventh day. In general, the oily urine is of three types: it is fatty throughout, fatty in its bottom, or fatty on the top. It may also be oily in its color only, as in tuberculosis, and particularly in its beginning. It may be oily in its texture or in both color and texture, as in the kidney diseases and the peak and decline of tuberculosis.

Among the compound urines is the purple urine. This is a fatal sign because it indicates the charring of the yellow and black biles. Also, it may be a red color mixed with some black, which indicates compound fevers and fevers arising from thick humors. If the urine is clearer with blackness at the top, it indicates pleurisy.

THIRD SECTION

Urine Texture: Its Characteristics and Turbidity

Urine texture is light, thick, or medium. The very light indicates lack of maturation in all the situations; obstruction of vessels; weakness of the kidney and urinary tract, thus attracting the light or only expelling the thin that is easily pushed; excessive drinking of water; or very cold temperament with dryness. In acute diseases, it indicates weakness of the digestive faculty, lack of maturation, and maybe weakness of all other faculties; thus nothing is expelled out with water, but rather it goes out as it comes in. This type of light urine is considered to be worse in children more than in youth since the normal urine of children is thicker than that of youth and because their bodies are more moist and more attractant to moist substances, as well as their production of waste material from growing. If their urine becomes very thin in acute fevers, then they have become very far from their normal state. Continuity of such a state is indicative of damage and a sign of death unless accompanied by good signs and persistence of strength; in this situation, an abscess forms, especially under the liver. If this type of urine persists in healthy individuals then it indicates a swelling in the location of the pain. In most cases, they feel the pain in the loins and kidney, which shows susceptibility to forming a swelling; if this pain is not localized but generalized all over the body, then it indicates pustules, smallpox, and swellings all over the body. Thinning of urine during a healing crisis indicates a relapse.

Very thick urine is indicative of lack of maturation in most of the cases, and in a minority of cases it points out the maturation of thick humors during the decline of humoral fevers or the rupture of swellings. Thick urine in acute diseases is a bad sign; however, thin urine is still worse. Thick urine shows that there is some digestion that appears in the urine texture; thus, it is a sign that digestion and the faculty are contributing to evacuation. It may also be a sign of corruption and excess of matter, and therefore, its lack of specific sedimentary maturation is a bad sign. Distinguishing between these two situations follows whether a comfort develops or an increase of weakness. The passing of large quantities of thick urine in fevers is a good sign, while the passing of small quantities is a sign of excessive humors or weakness of the faculty. The beneficial thick urine is the one followed by comfort. If the thin urine becomes thick without comfort in acute diseases it is an indication of wasting away. In a healthy person, when the thick urine persists and is accompanied with pain in the head area and weakness, then it is an early sign of fever. This can be due to evacuation, rupture, or sores in the urinary tracts. Both the thin and thick urines are indicative of low maturation because maturation of thick urine turns it into moderate texture. The thick is digested into thinness, and the thin matures by digestion into warm urine. Thick urine may be clear and transparent, as we mentioned earlier, and may be turbid, and the difference between the thick transparent urine and the thin urine is that when the first is stirred in a wavy motion, its waves do not diminish in size but rather form bigger waves that move slowly, and if it is foamy, its foam contains many bubbles that burst slowly; this type is formed from a well-digested phlegm or yolky-yellow bile when yellowish in color; however, without color it indicates the disintegration of glassy phlegm, which is usually found in epileptic patients.

Thin urine with lots of color is not due to maturation because maturation would improve its texture first, but rather due to the admixing with yellow bile. The first action of maturation is improvement of texture, then coloring of urine, therefore, maturation of texture [normal texture] is healthier than [normal] coloring. For this reason, the persistence of thin yellow urine during an acute disease has a bad prognosis and indicates weakness of the digestive faculty. If you see thin urine with different parts of red and yellow you may guess a fiery fatigue, and thin urine without illness-containing particles like wheat bran denotes the charring of phlegm. Thick urine in acute diseases is generally indicative of excessive humors, and it may indicate wasting of the body if it solidifies and turns very thick upon standing for an hour.

In general, urine's earthy **turbidity** is caused by the admixing of air and water, and by their separation from each other the clarity is restored. It must be looked at as three states. First, the thickening of thin urine indicates a struggling nature in trying to mature the matter but is unsuccessful in doing so completely, and this indicates a wasting of organs. Second, the urine comes out thick, then clears up by the precipitation of the thick part; this indicates that the nature has managed to overcome the matter and matured it. The faster and plentiful the sedimentation, it is a better evidence of maturation. Third, if an intermediate state between the two is persistent and accompanied by strong nature and faculty, then the complete maturation will take place. However, if the faculty is not stable then it is of concern that deterioration will take place before maturation happens; the prolonging of such a condition (without any scary sign) forewarns of headache because it is indicative of overactivation and vapors.

A urine that converts the thinness into turbidity and remains as such is better than one that remains turbid most of the time. Often, the urine becomes thick and turbid due to weakness rather than the elimination of waste.

Urine that comes out watery and remains watery indicates a total lack of maturation. The best type of thick urine is the one that is easy to pass out and has lots of sediment; this type has a good prognosis for palsy and alike. The gradual thinning of thick urines accompanied by large quantity is a good sign. Similarly, the scarcely turbid and thick urine that becomes suddenly profuse is a good sign; this causes the dissolution of the illness, especially in acute fevers and other diseases of fullness that have not yet shown any symptoms, and this is a rare type of urine. When the normal urine becomes excessively thick it indicates an extreme shortage of material and maturity by its ease of passage; sometimes it indicates damage due to the presence of excessive humors, weakness, difficulty in urinating, and scantiness of quantity. Good thick urine is a sign of healing in diseases of the spleen and mixed fevers where maturation is not expected and nature works on pushing out. In general, frothy urine indicates excessive humors that engage nature in maturing them. Thick urine with oily sediment indicates the presence of a stone.

Thick urine that indicates the rupture of swellings is known from its content or its earlier characteristics. It may contain pus that is malodorous with flakes of white, red, or straw color or other material that indicates the condition. Earlier signs are those that point out swelling or sores in the bladder, kidney, liver, or areas of the chest by the rupture of the swelling. If earlier signs include urine that resembles the wash of soft flesh, then the pus is from the convex part of the liver; however, if the urine resembles feces, then it is from the concave side of the liver. If this urine is preceded by chest tightness, dry cough, and stabbing pain in the chest parts, then it is pleurisy's empyema* that ruptured and moved toward the aorta. If the pus is mature, then it is a good sign. If the urine is thick to black and accompanied by pain on the left, then it is the spleen; if it is above the naval and the upper parts of the abdomen then it is the stomach; and most of the cases are in the liver and urinary tracts.

When a healthy, unexercising person passes urine that looks like pus or ichor, it cleanses the body and removes its flabbiness. Even if it exists in the liver and causes obstruction, the thick urine indicates the dissolution of an obstruction and its discharge; urine thickness in this case is not due to pus, however, the type coming out of a rupture contains pus.

Turbid urine mostly indicates the loss of strength, which leads to the dominance of cold, like an outside coldness. Turbid urine with a color resembling bad-quality wine or chickpea water is seen in pregnant women and individuals with chronic hot swellings of the viscera.

Urine resembling the **urine of donkeys and cattle** that looks wobbly due the busting of its bubbles is a sign of corruption of bodily humors. This urine is mostly generated due to heat acting on raw materials and producing a thick gas. It is also a sign of an existing headache or impending one. Its persistence is a sign of tremor.

---

*An empyema (a Greek word) is a collection of pus within a naturally existing anatomical cavity, such as the lung pleura, which is different from an abscess, which is a collection of pus in a newly formed cavity that does not represent a normal anatomical space or potential space.

The persistence of urine with a color resembling the color of an organ indicates the presence of a problem in that organ. Some have said that if the bottom of the urine resembles cloud or smokiness, then it is a sign of a prolonged illness, and if it is throughout an illness then it is a fatal sign. Rawness differs from pus in that the latter is malodorous. Urine of various-sized particles usually indicates a more active and strong nature, with open pores when its large particles are dominant. Urine with entangled threads indicates a recent sexual intercourse; you may figure that by experiment.

FOURTH SECTION

Indications of Urine Odor

It has been said that the urine of a patient never has the same odor as that of healthy individuals, and we say if the urine has no odor at all it indicates a cold temperament and excessive rawness [i.e., lack of maturation], and in acute diseases signifies the death of the innate nature. Urine with foul odor with signs of maturation is an indication of scabs and sores in the urinary tracts, and can be inferred by their signs. However, in the absence of maturation, the malodor may be the result of scabes and sores; it may also be due to putrefaction. In acute fevers, when the malodorous urine is not due to problems with the urinary tract, it is a bad sign. The acidity of the urine is a sign that the putrefaction is in cold humors that are dominated by abnormal heat; if the disease is acute, it is a sign of death because it indicates the extinction of innate heat, the dominance of coldness with abnormal heat.* Urine of sweet odor indicates the predominance of blood humor, very rotten

---

*Avicenna infers here that acidity of the urine is a sign of death because the innate heat that is necessary for the function of cells, organs, and the body is diminishing. In modern biology, we may say that the acidity occurs because of the accumulation of lactic acid and the malfunction of the mitochondria, where the acids of the Krebs cycle (a.k.a. tricarboxylic acid cycle) are accumulating in the tissue and blood and are being excreted out in the urine rather than completing their cycle to produce energy (in the form of ATP and heat), carbon dioxide, and water. So, the energy necessary for normal cellular functions and differentiation is not sufficient for the cells to carry out their specialized functions.

odor for the yellow bile, and acidic rotten odor for black bile. Persistent malodorous urine in healthy individuals indicates fevers caused by putrefaction or the expulsion of putrescent matter that should give a feeling of improvement after its release. In acute diseases, when malodorous urine becomes suddenly odorless without any accompanying sign of improvement, then it indicates the loss of faculties.

FIFTH SECTION

Indications of Urine Foam

Foam is caused by the air mixed in the water; the froth is formed during the passing of urine due to the separation of air from the urine, especially if the air is mixed with the water, as in individuals with many gaseous distensions. The foam may indicate by its color, such as pointing out by its blackness and blondness to jaundice; by its bubble size, as their largeness indicates high viscosity; by its amount, where its abundance denotes high viscosity and excess of air; and by the speed of which its bubbles burst, where a slow burst indicates viscosity and persisting water from kidney disease, and it is a sign of a prolonged illness due to the existence of air and viscosity. In general, the viscous humor in kidney diseases is a bad sign that indicates bad humors and cold.

SIXTH SECTION

Indications of Urine Sediments

We say first that physicians' usage of *sediment* and *residue* has departed from the commonly known; this is because they use these terms not only for materials that do precipitate but also for those that are denser than the water and differ from it, even if they are suspended or floating. The sediment can give indication by its nature, quantity, quality, shape, place, time [of appearance], and the nature of its affinity.

The nature of sediment as to whether it is normal indicates healthy digestion and maturation; this is usually white, cohesive, homogeneous, and flat sediment, and it must be round shaped, smooth, consistent, and similar to the precipitation of rose water. The white sediment indicates the ratio of maturation in the whole body, just as the white smooth pus indicates the maturation of a swelling; however, the pus is thick, while the white sediment is light. Sedimentation is a good sign even without a color. According to ancient physicians, the consistency of the sediment is a better indicator of maturity; hence, a smooth, consistent, and red sediment is better than the white rough one. Most of the sediments have the same color as the urine, and the best other than the white is the red, followed by yellow and arsenic [bluish-gray]. Colors indicating abnormality begin with lentil color [usually green]. Do not pay attention to others' opinion, since white color may not indicate maturation and consistency is always due to maturation; some white may be produced by excessive mixing with air.

Abnormal sediment is better dispersed than uniform, and it is easy to identify from a close distance. The good normal sediment that we mentioned above resembles the pus and raw material in its lightness; however, pus has an added malodor, and raw material aggregates particles, and the normal sediment differs from both by its gentleness and lightness. This type of a sediment [i.e., the abnormal sediment] is found in sickness and not in healthy conditions because the patients have dregs in their veins and their lack of maturation points to the corruption, while the healthy individuals do not have in their veins bad humor but rather undigested food that will show up in the urine as mature or immature.

Lean healthy individuals have less sediment, especially those who exercise and work in physically demanding professions. Sediment occurs mostly in the urine of obese sedentary individuals. Also, it should not be expected in the urine of sick thin individuals; the sediment that occurs in the urine of sick obese individuals is not the same as in sick lean individuals, who may recover before showing any sediment in their urine. Additionally, the sediment in their urine is so very little that it rarely precipitates, and some of it may be floating or suspended. It is incorrect that all urine has a sediment except the very mature; this should be given time to [produce] sediment. In most of the time, the color of the precipitation is the same as the urine, and best other than white is the red, then the yellow.

Abnormal sediment may be flaky (husky, red *kersannah* [Arabic],* porridge [like red arsenic], or saturated yellow), fleshy, fatty, purulent (pus-like), mucoid (slimy), yeasty (resembles soaked yeast), bloody leechy (like a leech), hairy (filamentous), sandy gravely, and ashy. The flaky (like peel) sediment with large flakes that are white and red indicates that they separated from the urinary organs. White sediment denotes sores, scabs, or erosion in the bladder. The red fleshy is from the kidney. Dark cloudy flakes like fish scales are the worse type of sediment among the ones mentioned above and indicate the peeling of the lining of the original organs. Most of the time, the first two types (flaky and fleshy) are not harmful at all, and they may cleanse the bladder. It was told that a man was given "Spanish fly" (cantharides) and his urine had white flakes like that of the outer white membrane of an egg; these flakes were the type that dissolved in water and gave red color, which was a good sign, and the man recovered and lived.

Among the flaky type is one whose flakes are thinner and denser than the others; when it is red it is called red kersannah (bitter vetch), or husky when it has other colors. The red kersannah one may indicate charred parts of the liver or charred blood in it; also it may have originated from the kidney; however, this one is more cohesive and fleshy, while the other is not fleshy and dividable. When the color is deep yellow, it is without any doubt from the kidney since that emanating from the liver is dark and sometimes is also shared by material from the kidney.

Husky [or scaly] sediment may be due to scabs from the bladder or wasting of organs. If there is itching within the base of the penis, malodorous urine, pus preceding urine, and urine maturation that is indicative of sound upper vessels, then the bladder is the source of the sediment; however, it is due to humoral liquefaction if it is associated with fever, weakness, sound urinary organs, and dark color.

Floury and porridge sediment is mostly due to blood charring if its color is reddish and could be attributed to organ wasting and shedding if the sediment color is white or from the bladder's scabs. You can tell the difference from what you have learned.

---

*Red kersannah (*Vicia ervillia*) is also called bitter vetch; its grain resembles red lentils when split.

Sediment that is blackish denotes blood charring in the spleen. All flaky sediment that is not from bladder, kidney, and urinary tract is a sign of a bad prognosis and death in acute diseases.

You have known from this section the condition of **fleshy sediment** and that most of it is from the kidney, and when it is not from the kidney then it is from healthy flesh without any decomposition in the body. Mature urine [i.e., urine signifying complete digestion] indicates healthy arteries since kidney problems do not prevent urine maturation because the process takes place before it gets to the kidneys.

Fatty sediment indicates decomposition of soft and hard fat as well as flesh. In an extreme case it resembles gold water. Its indicators are the quantity and whether it is mixing or not. Its excess and purity indicates an origin from kidney fat, and its scantiness and excessive integration indicates a further-up source. If you see in the urine a white piece like a pomegranate seed then it is from the kidney fat.

Puslike sediment indicates a ruptured sore in the urinary organs, especially if there is benevolent sediment. **Mucoid sediment** indicates the presence of raw thick humor, either in the body as a whole, from the urinary organs, or from the recovery of varicose vein and joint pain, which produces lightness of symptoms [recovery] afterward. Its ameliorating effect may indicate that it is benevolent sediment; however, in diseases one should not be fooled by the benevolent sediment if the time and evidence of maturation are absent. It may also indicate very cold temperament in the kidney. The difference between the puslike and raw [mucoid] sediments is that the first is malodorous, indicating a swelling, easy to aggregate and disperse its parts, mixes with water, and some of it separates, while the raw is turbid and thick, and difficult to aggregate and disperse. Urine with lots of mucus and at the end of gout and joint pain is a good sign.

Hairy sediment results from the action of heat on prolonged gripping moisture. It may be white or red. Its thickening takes place in the kidney. It has been said that it could reach several hand spans in length. **Yeasty sediment** resembling soaked yeast indicates weakness of the stomach and intestine and indigestion in both. Its cause could be eating yogurt and cheese. **Sandy sediment** indicates a stone that has either formed, is still forming, or is dissolving. **Red sediment** means that it has a kidney origin, while the nonred points to the bladder. **Gray sediment** mostly indicates phlegm or pus that changes color and fragments after a while. It may also be due to a passing charring.

Leechy sediment that is very mixed indicates weakness of the liver, or in organs below it [after the material has passed the liver], and indicates cuts in the urinary tract and discontinuity within the urinary organs. If the sediment is distinct then it points to the bladder and penis. We will discuss this with the partial diseases in the section on urinating blood [hematuria]. If the urine contains something similar to a red leech and the patient has spleen illness, then it indicates the disintegration of the spleen. Also note that in bladder illness there is not much blood that comes out because its vessels are deeply embedded, slightly tight, and a few in numbers.

Indicators of the quantity of sediment are taken from its excess or scantiness; they point out the magnitude of the cause. As for the sediment particle sizes, they were discussed under the flaky sediment.

Indicators of the quality are taken from the sediment's color, odor, composition, location, speed of sedimentation, and mixing. Black-colored sediment is bad in the types that we mentioned, and the safest of all is where the sediment is black but the water is not. Red indicates the presence of blood and dyspepsia. Yellow indicates severe heat and serious illness. Some of the white are safe, as we have said, and some are bad, like the mucoid, pus, and foamy, which is antagonistic to maturation. The green is a step toward the black. As to its odor, it is as stated above. The sediment **composition** is in the texture and dispersal; smoothness and constancy of the benign sediment are good, and are bad in the malevolent one. Dispersal denotes gas and weakness of digestion. As for **location,** a floating sediment is called cloudy, one hanging in the middle is suspended, which is more mature than the first, and the better of them is the one with its load pointing downward. The one settled at the bottom has better maturation in the benign sediment, while in the malevolent one is lighter, like the black, which is better, especially in severe fevers and when the humor is phlegmatic or melancholic. The cloudy is better than the precipitant because it indicates amelioration, unless the cause of floating is excessive gas; if it is not then the floater of the cloudy type is better than the suspended, and the worse is the precipitant. The cause of floating is elevated heat and gas.

Distinct sediment floats in the thick urine, especially if it is light, and settles at the bottom if it is heavy. If the suspended and floating appear early in the sickness and persist, it is a sign that recovery will occur when the abscess is excreted. However, skinny people recover from sickness with benign floating or suspended residue sedimentation, as we mentioned before. Fatty floating or suspended that resembles a cobweb or accumulation of protein is a bad sign. Most of the time, the appearance of a floating bad residue is dreaded, however, it is a sign of early maturation. If it turns into good quality, gets suspended, and then settles, it is a good sign. However, if it is followed by malevolent sediments then early fear is justified.

Fast-settling sediment after urination is a sign of good maturation. However, slow settling or unsettling is a sign of lack of maturation according to its amount. As for mixing, we have mentioned that in hematuria and fat in the urine, and you know all of it.

SEVENTH SECTION

Indications of Urine Quantity

Low quantity of urine signifies the weakness of faculties. Less urine than the intake of liquids indicates excessive decomposition, diarrhea, or propensity for edema. Large quantity of urine signifies disintegration, evacuation of humors of disintegration, and the state of the faculty from the difference between the two.

Heavy discharge of urine with a color signifying problems is better. Intermittent urine discharge is a bad indicator, such as the black and the thick. Urine discharge of varying quantities (a lot, scant, and retained) indicates an exhausted faculty, which is a bad sign.

If heavy urine discharge in acute disease does not produce relief, then it is a sign of hectic fever or a spasm produced by inflammation, and so is sweating. Urine passing drop by drop without flow in acute diseases is sign of a brain disease that affects the nerve and muscle. If the fever is not raging and there are other signs of recovery, then it is forewarning of nosebleed, otherwise, it indicates mental confusion and corruption of thinking.

When the urine of a healthy individual becomes persistently scant and thin, with a feeling of heaviness and pain in the loins, it indicates a solid swelling and/or tumor in the kidney region. If the urine flow is heavy in colic, it may forecast a special release if it is white and easily discharged.

EIGHTH SECTION

Good, Mature Healthy Urine

It is of moderate texture, gentle in color, leaning toward citron color, and with healthy sediment that is white, light, smooth, consistent, and round shaped. Its odor is moderate, neither stinky nor odorless. If this type of urine appears suddenly in a case of acute diseases, it is a sign of recovery in the following day, and you know that.

NINTH SECTION

Urine of Age Groups

Infants' urine tends to be milky and white due to their food source and their wet temperament. Children's urine is thicker and denser than that of youths, with more froth; we have mentioned that before. Youths' urine is fiery-yellow and moderate in texture. Urine of middle-aged individuals is whitish and thin, and could be thick due to excreted waste. Urine of the elderly is very thin and white, and may rarely become thick, as mentioned. When their urine is very thick it is because of the presence of [kidney] stones.

TENTH SECTION

Urine of Women and Men

Women's urine is thicker, much whiter, and less thin than men's urine due to their excessive waste, weak digestion, the wideness of their excretory ducts, and the uterine waste that comes out with urine. Notice that when you shake men's urine it becomes turbid and its turbidity moves upward, while women's urine does not become turbid when shaken due its well-mixed constituents; most of the time it has round foam at the top, and it may become only slightly turbid.

Men's urine after intercourse will contain intertwined filaments. Urine of pregnant women is clear with cloudiness at the top; its color could have the color of chickpea water [light brown] or trotters' water [boiled feet of cattle], which is yellow with a tint of blue and has a cloud at the top that is always seen as fluffed cotton, is frequently like granules, and goes up and down. Very pronounced bluishness appears in the beginning of pregnancy, and redness signifies the end of it, especially if it becomes cloudy by moving. The urine of a puerpera is mostly black, as if it has ink or soot.

ELEVENTH SECTION

Urine of Animals for Examination and Showing Its Difference from Human Urine

The physician may benefit from the examination of animals' urines when experimenting; however, it is difficult to get it right. It has been said that the urine of the camel in a glass container looks like melted ghee [clarified butter], with turbidity and thickness. Urine of livestock resembles that of camels, but it is clearer and seems that its upper half is clear and the lower half is turbid. Sheep's urine is white with yellowness and close to that of people but without texture; its residue is like fat or the residue of fat. The better quality the feed, the clearer it is. Urine of deer resembles that of sheep and people but does not have texture or residue and is clearer than sheep's urine.

TWELFTH SECTION

Fluids That Resemble Urine and the Distinction between Them and Urine

Note that waters of oxymel, honey, fig, and saffron seem clearer the closer to the eye you hold them, but it is the opposite with urine. Honey water has yellow foam. Fig water residue settles on the side of the container and not in the middle, without order or movement. This amount on the states of urine is sufficient, and there are more details in the other specific books.

THIRTEENTH SECTION

Indicators of Stool

The **quantity** of the stool when compared with the amount of ingested food may be less, more, or equal. It is known that its increase in quantity is due to the excess of many humors, its reduction due to decline in humors or their retention in the cecum and the colon or the fascia, and that is the beginning of colic, which indicates weakness of the faculty.

Its **texture** has some indicators. A moist stool indicates obstruction, indigestion, or weakness of the mesentric vessels and their inability to absorb moisture from the food. It may also be due to catarrh from the head or due to the ingestion of something that moisturizes the stool. Viscosity associated with moist stool indicates the wasting of organs; this is usually coupled with stinky odor. It may also be a sign of excessive bad viscous humors when it is not associated with malodorous humor or the ingestion of a large quantity of viscous food coupled with strong hot temperament that disabled digestion. Foamy stool indicates excessive heat or admixing with a lot of gas. Dry stool indicates fatigue and decomposition or excessive urination, fiery heat, dry food, and extended retention in the intestine (will be described under its own topic). If the hard dry admixes with moisture, it indicates that its hardness is due to a prolonged retention in moistures that prevented its release and the absence of a bitter biting substance to push it out. In the absence of extended retention and signs of moisture in the intestine, the cause is the flow of burning pus waste from the liver into its succeeding organs, where the pus's action started before mixing.

The **color of the stool** has its indicators. Its natural color is fiery light; its increase of intensity indicates excess of bile [from the gallbladder], and its reduction indicates rawness and lack of maturation. If the stool color is white it may be due to an obstruction in the bile duct, which indicates jaundice, and when associated with pus and pus odor it signifies the rupture of an abscess. Very often, the stool of a resting healthy individual who has given up sports may contain pus; in this case it is a cleansing and healthy evacuation that eliminates the flabbiness that has developed by quitting sports, as we have said in the urine.

Note that the excess fieriness of the stool is frequently an indication of maturation at the decline of the disease, and very often signifies a bad condition.

Black stool has the same indicators as the black urine. It indicates strong charring, the maturation of melancholic disease, the ingestion of a colorant, or the drinking of an inducer of black bile evacuation. The first indicator is the worst. The color of the one produced by black bile is not sufficient as an indicator; however, it can be confirmed by its acidity, acridity, and the frothing upon its contact with earth. It is bad as a stool or vomit, and it has a distinctive sparkle. Generally, the excretion of black bile humor is mostly fatal (i.e., a sign of impending death). *Black chyme is frequently excreted; however, the excretion of the original black bile is an indicator of excessive charring and the disappearance of moisture.* **Green stool,** as well as the darker one, signifies the diminishing of innate heat.

Compression and distension of the stool are also indicators. Stools that are expanded like cow dung are a sign of gas. The stool's **turnaround time** is also an indicator. Stool that exits fast or prematurely is a bad sign that indicates excess of bile and weakness of retention. Slow-exiting stools are indicative of weak digestion, coldness of intestines, and excessive moisture. **Sound** denotes puffing gas. Stools of unpleasant and mixed colors are bad, and we will mention them in detailed books [Books 3–5].

The best of stools is cohesive, homogeneous, well hydrated, dense like honey, exits with ease without burning, yellowish in color, slightly odorous, and without pressure, bubbling gas, rumbling, or froth. It has the proper turnaround time with a quantity comparable to that of the ingested food. Note that not all stool consistencies are good, as well as smoothness; they may be produced by excessive digestion and maturation of all parts; however, they may be due to charring and disintegration, and both are bad signs.

Note that stool of moderate texture that leans toward softness is benevolent if it is not associated with rumbling and without sporadic excretion, bit by bit. Its excretion should not be due to its association with pus that prevents it from aggregating. Attention should be directed to signs that appear in vessels and other parts. However, this talk is more suitable in the detailed discussions you will find on stool and urine, as well as others; therefore, understand what we have illustrated thus far.

◆

HEALTH, DISEASE, AND THE NECESSITY OF DEATH

Introduction and 5 Lessons

There are two faculties that the physician treats: one of them is natural, which is the nutritive faculty that replaces whatever decomposes in the body, and it has earthy and watery nature; the other is animalistic (vital), which is the pulsating faculty that replenishes the "spirit" [oxygen and energy], and it's airy and fiery in nature.

AVICENNA

At the beginning of the 1st Art, Avicenna divides medicine into three parts; the first two are the theory and practical knowledge, and the third is the practice. He considers the first two Arts of the 1st Book as the theoretical part of medicine and the rest of the *Canon* as the practical knowledge. The latter consists of knowledge of health preservation and health restoration (or treatment). Avicenna starts the 3rd Art by explaining, in Unani terminology, the formation of the zygote from the male and female gametes, then he lists the challenges that face the new life-form, namely, the loss of moisture as well as putrefaction and its resulting abnormal moisture. He further explains the interplay between moisture and innate heat. Moisture supports innate heat because it supplies the innate heat with the necessary ingredients (i.e., nutrients and oxygen) to maintain it. Abnormal moisture is the antithesis to innate heat because it sequesters nutrients and produces toxic intermediates. Avicenna returns here to moisture production by innate heat, a point that was explained earlier in the authors' comments on the "Hydration in Relation to Health and Aging" section at the beginning of the 2nd Lesson of the 2nd Art.

According to Avicenna, longevity is predetermined by the primordial temperament if it is properly managed; therefore, health management should aim to prevent putrefaction and protect moisture, thus preserving strength. The foremost consideration should be on managing seven factors:

- Maintaining the temperament near equitability
- Eating healthful food

- Cleansing from waste
- Maintaining physical fitness
- Breathing clean fresh air
- Maintaining a healthy environment
- Improving the physical and psychological practices, including sleeping and wakefulness

After covering zygote formation and issues related to its survival in the introduction of the 3rd Art, Avicenna moves to the next topic in the 1st Lesson on raising children and managing their health. He covers the regimens for a baby from birth until standing up, and for nursing and weaning, as well as diseases that afflict infants and their treatments, and then the regimen for childhood. Avicenna follows with a lesson on the common regimen of adults.

He starts with exercise as the prime necessity for maintaining a healthy body. He goes on to explain this necessity as the best measure to prevent the accumulation of fullness, when properly practiced, and to renew the innate heat and instill lightness in the body. Additionally, Avicenna details the process he calls waste accumulation in the body; he attributes this to the residual amount that is left over in the body from every digestion and the body systems' insufficiency to get rid of it by natural evacuation. Waste buildup in the body causes diseases of putrefaction, swellings, gases, and dystemperament and therefore has to be eliminated. For this purpose exercise is preferred over using drugs. Drugs can flush out some of the good humors and innate moisture and affect respiration, while exercise does not. Exercise induces a gentle heat that decomposes the daily accumulation of waste. Thus, exercise increases the innate heat, strengthens the body, removes stiffness, reduces moisture, opens skin pores, and makes the organs ready to accept food by the loss of waste.

Avicenna explains the benefits and potential harms of massage, the different types of massage, preparing for the massage, and its proper times. He states that the purpose of massage is to solidify loose bodies and firm up soft bodies, to loosen the dense, and to soften the hard.

Avicenna proclaims that healthy people who are free of metabolic waste, thus having an equitable temperament, are not in need of bathing. It is beneficial for others, who will benefit from gentle warmth and moderate moisturizing. There are rules to follow in the bathhouse, such as moving gradually to rooms of higher temperatures, leaving the hot room at the early signs of discomfort, bathing only after complete digestion, avoiding entering the bath on an empty stomach first thing in the morning, and avoiding cold and hot drinks while in the bath. Additionally, he lists the benefits and harms of the bath. He follows the topic on bathing with a section on washing with cold water, its rules and benefits, and uses after exercise.

Avicenna provides some guidelines on the best type of food that can be eaten. He strongly favors the meat of young goat, beef, and lamb; wheat; drinks of aromatic herbs; and rich fruits, such as figs and dates. He is not in favor of green, leafy vegetables and calls them medicinal food. (They are currently given as the preferred diet for cancer patients for their low sugar content, and they also contain many phytochemicals strongly associated with a reduced risk for cancer.) He advises to eat only when feeling hungry and not to prolong hunger, and to select the food that is appropriate for the season. He lists the harmful consequences of indigestion of hot and cold foods and ways to treat them, the suitable foods for the temperaments, the order of consumption for food types, the approach to eating full meals, the treatment of corrupted appetite, the proper time for drinking after eating, the treatment of indigestion, and the harmful effects of hot and cold foods. Furthermore, Avicenna writes about moist fruits and bitter green, leafy vegetables, as well as acidic, bitter, dry, fatty, pungent, and sweet foods. He also lists a number of rules for the mixing of foods and drinking water and wines. Among the benefits of wine, Avicenna mentions its facilitation of food penetration to all parts of the body, stopping and breaking down phlegm, excreting yellow bile, antagonizing black bile and bringing it out, and loosening condensed humors. He also outlines the rules for drinking wine and the treatment for overdrinking and drunkenness.

Avicenna discusses normal and abnormal sleep and their opposites, wakefulness and insomnia, the ways to induce or diminish each of them, as well as the indications of each, and benefits of sleeping, sleeping after eating, sleeping on an empty or full stomach, and sleeping positions. In a brief section, he describes the strengthening of weak organs, as well as fattening them and increasing their size.

In an extensive treatise on fatigue that follows exercise, Avicenna details the three main types of fatigue that follow exercise—soreness, expandedness, and swelling—and adds a fourth possible one: dryness. He describes the causes, symptoms, and treatments of each type. He follows with a section on stretching and yawning and their probable causes. He also explains the causes of looseness and over-hydration and their treatments.

The elderly face two major health issues that should be attended, according to Avicenna; these are dehydration and coldness. These are managed with the combined application of moisturizing and warming foods, drinks, and baths; extended sleep; constant induction of urine; evacuation of phlegm from the stomach; gentle massage with oil rubs; and walking or riding. Additionally, Avicenna has sections on wine drinking for the elderly and preventing and removing obstructions in various organs, as well as massaging and exercising the elderly.

In the 4th Lesson, Avicenna tells us that the two goals for managing individuals with hot temperament are to bring them back to balance and to preserve their health. As for cold dystemperament, there are three types: balanced in wetness, wet, and dry. The lesson also includes discussions on the treatment of susceptible bodies, fattening of the skinny, and thinning of the obese.

On the management of seasonal changes, Avicenna tells us in the 5th Lesson that in the early spring one should abandon warming and moisturizing meats and drinks, simplify the diet, exercise less rigorously, eat less in quantity and frequency, and imbibe cooling drinks that are not bitter, acrid, or salty. The same trend should continue in the summer. However, one should reverse this trend in the fall and winter.

On management of early symptoms of illness, Avicenna

lists a good number of symptoms and their foretelling of disease. He also has a comprehensive set of instructions and precautions on the management of travel, diet regimen, drinking and thirst management, and preparations before departure, as well as resting and exercising. In his section on the precautions for hot weather, especially for travel, he advises to protect the head and the skin from the sun's heat, not to start the travel on an empty stomach to avoid becoming weak, and to take oils of rose and violet to sprinkle them each hour on the head. He also gives advice on traveling in hot sand storms, the *samoum,* and the treatment of heat stroke. Avicenna follows with a section on the precautions for travelers in cold weather and frost, a section on protecting the extremities from the harmful effects of cold, a section on protecting skin color during travel, a section on protecting the traveler from the harmful effects of various waters, and ends the Lesson with a section on precautions for the maritime traveler.

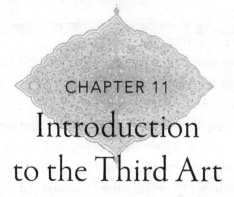

CHAPTER 11

Introduction
to the Third Art

Introduction to the Third Art

• Avicenna's Introduction

Note that medicine has two parts: theory and practice, and both are knowledge and theory. However, what is meant by theory is that it contains opinion without the benefit of practical knowledge at all, such as the parts that teach about the temperament, humors, faculties, types of disease, symptoms, and causes. What is meant by practical knowledge is practice and management, such as the part that teaches you how to preserve the health of a body that is in a certain condition or how to treat a body with a certain disease. Do not think that this practical knowledge is itself the practice and work; it is the part that delves deeply into practice and work. We have explained this before [in the 1st art], and we are done with the 1st Art of the general theoretical part of medicine. We will focus in the remaining parts on the practical part in a general approach.

The practical part divides into two: knowledge of managing healthy bodies (i.e., how to preserve them), called the knowledge of health preservation. The second part is the knowledge of managing the sick body (i.e., how to restore it to a healthy state), called treatment.

We start by writing in this Art a summary on health preservation, and we say the initial formation of our bodies encompasses two things: one is the semen from the man, which is properly in the *active* role, and the second is the woman's gamete, and the blood [that comes out] of menstruation, which is properly in the *substance* role. These two substances are similar in that they both are moist liquids, even if they differ later. In the woman's gamete and blood, watery and earthy temperaments are dominant, while the airy and fiery temperaments are dominant in man's semen. The first fusion of these two is a moist fusion, which is the result of the earthy and fiery temperaments if they exist. The firmness of the earthy temperament and the maturation effect of the fiery temperament interact to harden the fusion and make it the best hardening and fusion (its hardening does not reach that of solid objects like stone or glass), so that nothing is lost from them, or only a negligible amount, and they will be safe from being exposed to a total destructive cause or over a very long period.

Our bodies are exposed to two types of problems, and each of them has an internal cause and an external cause. One is the gradual disappearance of our primordial moisture—dispersion. The second is putrefaction of the moisture and its corruption and its inability to sustain life; this is different than the first, although it is as harmful as desiccation, by first corrupting moisture and by destroying its beneficial nature to our bodies. Furthermore, the disintegration of putrefaction, which initially benefits moisture, produces gray, dry material. These two problems are different from other causes like freezing cold, poisons, fatal discontinuity, and all diseases, and they produce thickness.

We need to consider these two problems in health preservation. Each of them occurs due to external and internal causes. External causes include air that produces dehydration and putrefaction. Internal causes are such as our internal innate heat that disperses our moisture and the abnormal heat that is produced from putrefied food and other sources.

All these causes together act to dehydrate us as we begin to complete our growth and become mature. This dehydration enables us to carry out our functions. Dehydration continues until the end of life. However, this dehydration to which we get exposed is important because we are initially [at the formation of the zygote] very wet, and, without a doubt, our heat is fully in control of this wetness, otherwise it would cause congestion, and thus heat always is acting on it and drying it. The first sign of dehydration is equitability, then when our bodies reach the equitable level of dehydration and heat, the dehydration increases, more than at first because the matter is lessened and more accepting of heat; thus causing the dehydration to go beyond the equitable, and it will keep increasing until all moisture vanishes. Hence, the innate heat becomes the accidental cause for extinguishing itself by evaporating its moisture like the lantern (oil lamp) that goes out when its supply declines; the less it lights up, the more its heat decreases, thus causing a continuous decline to accelerate. Additionally, there is a failure to replace the lost moisture.

Therefore, there are two ways to the increased dehydration; one is the decline in supply, and the other is due to the evaporation by the heat, which weakens the innate heat by the increase of dryness in the organs. The decrease of innate moisture is like matter and like the oil to the lantern because the lantern has two moistures: water and oil; one lights it up, and the other extinguishes it. The same with innate heat; it is supported by moisture and suffocates with the abnormal. The increase in the abnormal moisture that is generated by weak digestion resembles the moisture in the lantern. If dehydration is complete, the innate heat gets extinguished, and natural death takes place. However, the body stays alive for its period not because the natural, initial moisture resists the desiccation by the outside heat, the internal innate heat, and the body's movements to resist desiccation; rather it is due to substituting whatever is lost of moisture from the breakdown of food [this point has been explained earlier in the authors' comments section "Hydration in Relation to Health and Aging," at the beginning of the 2nd Lesson of the 2nd Art]. We have illustrated that food is used by the "power" [metabolic health] up to a point.

The profession of health preservation does not include protection from death and the saving of the body from external problems. It does not also bring to the body the absolute longevity that humans seek. It includes two issues: preventing putrefaction and protecting moisture from loss by evaporation thus preserving the strength to the period that is dictated by the primordial temperament. This is done by the proper management of replenishing whatever has been lost.

Management prevents the dominance of the causes that accelerate dehydration without affecting the proper natural causes of dehydration. Precautious management for putrefaction protects the body from the takeover of abnormal heat, whether it is internal or external. Bodies are unequal in the strength of their primordial moisture and heat; they are different in these, and every body has its limitation in resisting normal desiccation so that it does not exceed and is dictated by its temperament, innate heat, and the amount of innate moisture. However, this natural resistance to dehydration can be overcome by causes that accelerate dehydration or are fatal in other ways. Many say that natural deaths are these [i.e., dying from natural causes] and that the accidental ones are the others [i.e., dying from unnatural causes], as if the profession of health preservation brings the human to such an end that is called normal death by preserving the suitable conditions. There are two faculties that the physician treats: one of them is natural, which is the nutritive faculty that replaces whatever decomposes in the body, and it has earthy and watery natures; the other is animalistic (vital), which is the pulsating faculty that replenishes the "spirit" [oxygen and energy] and is airy and fiery in nature. Since food is not exactly like the person eating it, the assimilative faculty changes the ingested food to a real food. For this purpose there are instruments and channels that attract, push, retain, and digest. Therefore, we say that the prime issue in the profession of preserving health is the modification of the mentioned general causes. Prime attention should be on modifying seven issues:

- Bringing the temperament to equitability
- Ingesting good food
- Purifying from waste
- Preserving structure
- Breathing good air
- Improving the environment

- Improving the physical and psychological practices, including sleeping and wakefulness

You know from the previously discussed topics that there is not one set limit for equitability and health, and not every temperament is healthy and equitable at the same time, but between the two.

Let us start with the regimen for a baby with an absolute equitable temperament.

CHAPTER 12

Raising Children

First Lesson of the Third Art: Raising Children

FIRST LESSON OF THE THIRD ART

Raising Children
(4 Sections)

FIRST SECTION

Regimen for a Baby from Birth to Standing Up*

When the baby of equitable temperament is born, it has been said by a group of respectable physicians that the first thing to do is to cut the

---

*The regimen for pregnant women and those close to delivery will be addressed in the specific discussions.

umbilical cord at a measure of four fingers above, tied with a wool thread that has been gently woven so that it will not cause pain and covered with an oil-soaked cloth. It is also strongly encouraged to dust the naval with a mixture containing equal parts of greater celandine (*Chelidonium majus,* عروق صفر), *Dracaena cinnabari* (دم الأخوين), *Astragalus sarcocolla* (الانزروت, العنزروت), *Cuminum cyminum* (الكمون), *Muscus arboreus* (اشنه), and myrrh (from *Commiphora myrrha* or related species, المر).

Very early after birth, the skin of the baby should be washed with lightly salted water to firm up the skin and strengthen it. The most suitable salts are the ones mixed with bloodstone* (شادنج), *Costus speciosus* (قسط), sumac (*Rhus coriaria,* سماق), fenugreek (*Trigonella foenum gracum,* حلبه), and thyme (*Origanum* sp., زعتر). The nose and the mouth should not be washed with salty water. The reason for our preference to firm his body is that the baby is harmed from the touching of hard and cold objects because of the sensitivity of the skin and its warmth, which feels everything as colder and harder. If needed, the washing with salty water may be repeated, especially when the baby has an excess of dirt and humidity, followed by a rinse with lukewarm water. The nose openings should be cleaned with nail-trimmed fingers. Place a few drops of oil in the eyes. The anus should be cleaned with the little finger (the fifth) to keep it open. Care should be taken to prevent the baby from getting chills. If the terminus of the umbilical cord falls off after three to four days, then the most proper action to take is to sprinkle the ash of sea shells, ash of calf heel's tendon, or the powder of lead oxide dissolved in alcohol.

To begin the swaddling (تقميط) of the baby, the midwife should gently touch the baby's parts by gently pressuring them in the proper direction and shape of the part by widening the ones that should be wide and narrowing the ones that should be narrow, all of this by gentle pressuring with the tips of the fingers (غمز), and this should be repeated. The eyes should repeatedly be wiped with a soft clothlike silk. A gentle pressure by the tip of the finger should be applied on top of the

---

*"Bloodstone" is made of hematite, which is the mineral form of iron oxide (Fe_2O_3), one of several iron oxides.

bladder to encourage the exit of urine. The hands should be spread, the arms placed next to the knees, the head covered with a hat or wrapped, and the baby placed to sleep. The sleeping room should have moderate temperature, neither hot nor cold, and slightly dark without direct sunlight entering it. The head of the baby should be higher than the rest of the body while sleeping, with care taken that none of the body parts get twisted, such as the neck, arms, and the trunk.

Washing the baby should be done with moderately warm water in the summer and hot, but not burning, in the winter. The best time for washing is after the baby's longest sleep. Washing can take place two or three times a day, and gradually move to lukewarm water as the summer approaches. During winter, the water should be moderately hot at all times, and the bathed baby reaching warmth, and care taken to prevent the water from going into the ears. The following steps should be followed for handling the baby: catch the baby with the right hand and rest the baby's chest (not the belly) on the left arm, with the baby's hands to the back and the legs and the head hanging gently. Dry the baby gently with a soft cloth and place it face down first, then on the back, continuing wiping, massaging, and shaping the body parts. Wrap tightly with a cloth and place a few drops of virgin [olive] oil in the nose since it washes the eyes and their lids.

SECOND SECTION

Regimen for Nursing and Weaning

As to breast-feeding and feeding, the baby should be breast-fed the mother's milk as soon as possible since it is very similar to the feeding in the womb. It had the same nutrients that become milk. The baby is more accepting of the mother's milk, and it also feels familiar to the baby. *Experience has shown that sucking on the mother's nipple is very beneficial in pushing away harmful diseases.* The baby should be breast-fed two to three times a day. Initially, the amount of breast-feeding should not be excessive. It is desired that a woman other than his mother initially breast-feed the baby until the mother's temperament becomes balanced. The best is to let the baby suck on some honey before nursing. Before the first breast-feeding of the day, two to three squeezes of the milk should be pushed out before giving the baby the nipple to suck; this should be applied if the milk has a problem. If the milk of a breast-feeding woman is of low quality or sour, then she should eat something first in the morning before nursing the baby.

There are two beneficial things for the baby to strengthen the temperament: gentle movement as well as music and singing that are used to put babies to sleep. The degree of the baby's acceptance to these two practices shows the body's physical and mental development.

If some reason prevents the mother from breast-feeding the baby, such as her weakness, corruption of her milk, and/or its thinness, then a wet nurse should be selected according to the conditions that we describe. These conditions include her age, physique, manners, breast shape, quality of her milk, the time since she delivered her baby, and the gender of her baby. If she fits the conditions, her meals should include wheat, Roman barley (*Triticum romanum, Triticum spelta,* خـنـدروس), meat of sheep and lamb, and fresh fish. Also considered good food are lettuce, almond, and hazelnut. Arugula (جـرجـيـر), mustard (خـردل), and basil ([Persian] بـادروج) are considered bad because they spoil the milk, and mint has the potential to do that as well.

We will mention the characteristics of a good wet nurse. We start with her age. The best age is between twenty-five and thirty-five years of age since this is the age of youth, health, and complete growth. As to her physique and structure, she should have a good skin color, strong neck, wide shoulders, solid muscular development, moderate weight, and fleshy not fatty. She should have good manners and good temper without excessive reactions of anger, depression, and cowardliness, and other such reactions since all of this could spoil the baby's temperament and get transferred to the baby. For this reason, it is prohibited to use a mentally ill woman as a wet nurse since her erratic behavior may prevent her good treatment of the baby. The shape of her breasts should be large and full, not hanging or excessively large, and should be moderate in firmness and softness.

Her milk should be of moderate texture, moderate amount, and white in color without darkness or green, yellow, or red colors. The milk's odor should be pleasant without sourness or putrefaction. The milk's taste should be sweet without bitterness, saltiness, or acidity. The milk should be homogeneous and not thin or thick like cheese, without too much froth. It can be tested by placing a drop of it on top of a fingernail; if it runs then it is thin, and if it stays then it is thick. It can also be tested in a glass by adding to it a little of myrrh and stirring by fingers, and from its coagulation one can know its amount of cheese and water. The recommended milk is the one with balanced cheese to water.

When the milk of a wet nurse lacks the proper characteristics it has to be managed, either by modifying the feed or by treating the wet nurse. The thick and stinky milk should be squeezed out and left to air for a while before feeding it to the baby. If the milk is very hot then it should not be given to the baby the first thing in the morning. As for treating the wet nurse, when her milk is thick she should drink the seeded oxymel that has been ameliorated by cooking it with pennyroyal (*Mentha pulegium,* فودنـج), hyssop (*Hyssopus officinalis,* زوفـا), and Persian thyme (*Thymus capitatus,* حـاشـا); and she should eat mountain thyme (*Origanum,* صـعـتـر جبـلي) and sweet lemon (*Citrus medica,* طـرنـج). Also, she should add to her meal some radish, induce vomiting by drinking hot oxymel, do light exercise, and eat food that produces thick blood. She may also drink a sweet drink such as grape syrup if there is not any contraindication. She should prolong her sleep. If her milk is scant, it is hoped that it is due to hot dystemperament in all of her body or only her breasts. This may be figured out from the symptoms mentioned in the previous chapters. If touching her breast indicates heat, she should be fed barley milk (كشـك الشـعـيـر), spinach (إسـفـانـاخ), and the like.

When signs indicate cold temperament, obstruction, or weakness of attractive faculty, then increase her gentle warming food and gently perform cupping under the breasts; carrot seeds and carrots are beneficial in this condition. When the cause is her lack of appetite, she should be fed soups of barley, bran, and other grains. Her soups and food should include the root and seeds of fennel (*Foeniculum vulgare,*

[Persian] رازیانج), dill (*Anethum graveolens,* شبت،شبث), and nigella (*Nigella sativa,* شونیز). It has been said that eating the breast of sheep and goat, including their milk, is very beneficial in this regard due to their homology [in location] or a specific property [of function]. It has been proven to be effective to take one dram* of termites (أرضه) or dried earthworms (خراطین) in barley water for several days, and the boiling of salty fish heads in dill water. Also effective in inducing more milk is to take one *oka*† of cow's ghee and mix it with a pure beverage, to be drunk by the wet nurse, or take tahini (sesame seed paste), mix it with a beverage, filter, and drink. Spread an oil mix of spikenard (also known as *jatamansi, nardin,* or *nard; Nardostachys jatamansi,* ناردین) and milk of female donkey (she-ass). Take one oka of boiled eggplant pulp, mash, and mix with water, and drink. Boil bran and radish in water and drink. Take three okas of dill seeds, one oka of blue fenugreek seeds (*Trigonella caerulea,* حندقوقی), one oka of leek (*Allium porrum,* کراث), two okas of alfalfa (*Medicago sativa,* رطبه) and fenugreek, mix with the juice of fennel, honey, and ghee, and take as a drink.

If the milk is in excess and harmful due to its congestion and condensation, then reducing it should be done by reducing the food intake and food of low nutritious value, as well as tying to the breasts and the body cumin and vinegar, or pure mud and vinegar, or lentil cooked in vinegar, followed by drinking salty water. Also, the use of a lot of mint induces milk. Stinky milk can be treated by consuming basil drink and food of pleasant odor.

As to the time since the wet nurse has delivered her baby, it must be very close to that time, only a month and a half to two months. She should have delivered naturally a boy and never had a miscarriage. The wet nurse should exercise, eat food that has good chyme, and not have intercourse since it corrupts the odor of the milk and reduces its amount and may get her pregnant, which has deleterious effects on the baby by losing gentle milk that will go to the fetus and on the

---

*A dram is an ancient unit of weight that varied over centuries from three to four grams.
†An oka equals forty drams, or dirham (plural darahem), which is approximately 123.5 to 128 grams.

fetus by having insufficient food, which is shared with the baby as a milk.

Before every breast-feeding, some of the milk should be squeezed out and the breast poked to assist the baby in sucking without hurting the throat or esophagus. Giving the baby a spoon of honey before breast-feeding is beneficial, and it is all right to mix it with some drink. The baby should not breast-feed a lot of milk at once, but rather little by little since a large amount of milk at once may produce distention and gas, as well as white urine. If these occur, then the baby should be held from breast-feeding and allowed to undergo excessive hunger or allowed to sleep until full digestion takes place. The baby breast-feeds a lot in the first few days, about three times a day. It is better that the baby breast-feeds from a woman other than his mother on the first day, as we have mentioned. If the wet nurse gets a dystemperament, painful illness, lots of diarrhea, and harmful retention, then another wet nurse should breast-feed the baby until the first regains her health. The same should be done if it is necessary to give her a medication of dominant strength and temperament. If the baby sleeps after a breast-feeding, refrain from strongly rocking the crib so that the milk inside the baby's stomach does not get shaken; the crib should be rocked gently. A little bit of crying before breast-feeding is beneficial for the baby. The normal period of breast-feeding is two years. If the baby desires food other than milk, it should be given gradually without pushing. When the baby's incisors appear, the baby should be introduced gradually to harder food that is not difficult to masticate. The baby could start with bread soaked with water and honey, a drink, or milk, followed with a drink of water or sometimes mixed with a drink. The baby's stomach should not get full, and if that happens and the baby develops fullness, distention, and white urine, then feeding should be stopped [until the dissolution of fullness]. The best feeding time is after an oil rub and a bath. When the baby is weaned, the food should be soups and light meats. Weaning should be gradual and not all at once, and the baby distracted with balls [acorns in the original] of bread and sugar. If the baby misses and cries for the breast, then the breast should be coated with a paste made of one dram of myrrh and one dram of the seeds of purslane (*Portulaca oleracea,* بقله، فرفحين، فرفج). We say in general that the child's regimen is about moisturizing since it is compatible with his temperament and the need for it in food, growth, and excessive moderate movement. This is normal for them, as if nature shares with them, especially when they move from infancy into childhood.

When the infant starts to move and stand, they should not be allowed to do hard movements and should not be forced to walk or sit before they are ready, otherwise they may develop problems with their legs and back. When the baby starts to crawl on the floor, they should be placed on a leather carpet so that they are not hurt by the roughness of the floor. Objects of sharp edges like knives, wood, and the like that may poke or cut should be removed from around the baby. Also, the baby should be protected from falling from a high place.

When the canine teeth start to come out, all solid objects that cannot be chewed on should be removed from around the baby so that they do not damage their canines. At this time, the depth of the gum should be coated with rabbit brain and chicken fat because it eases their emergence. During the emergence of the teeth, the head and neck should be massaged with oil mixed with hot water, and drops of oil put in their ears. If the teeth emerge to the point where the baby starts to bite their fingers, then the baby should be given a piece of soft licorice root that has not yet dried or its extract. Licorice is beneficial for the sores and pains of the gum. Also, the gum should be rubbed with salt and honey to prevent gum pains. Once the teeth are fully emerged, the baby should be given licorice extract and a piece of licorice root that is not dry yet to hold in the mouth. It is also beneficial during the emergence of the incisors to massage the neck with virgin oil or virgin ghee; if the baby starts to talk, then they should extend this to the root of the tongue.

THIRD SECTION

Diseases That Afflict Infants and Their Treatments

The primary goal in treating infants is to treat the mother or the wet nurse by undergoing venesection or cupping if she has blood fullness or elimination if she has an abnormal humor. She should also be treated with the appropriate medications if needed to stop diarrhea or induce it, prevent a vapor from going to the head, heal respiratory organs, or change her dystemperament. If the mother develops a diarrhea or induces it, or vomits or induces it, then another woman should nurse the infant on that day.

Let us mention localized diseases that afflict the infants. Of these are the **swellings of the gum** during dentition and the **swellings at the tendons** near the jaws and their spasm. In the latter, the tendons should be gently massaged with fingers and rubbed with oils that were mentioned in the section on dentition. Some use a mouthwash of honey mixed with chamomile fat, or turpentine resin (*Pistacia terebinthus,* علك الانـبـاط، علك البطم); also, shower the head with a decoction of chamomile and dill.

Infants may develop **diarrhea** during dentition. Some claim it is because the infant is ingesting some of the salty pus from the gum with the milk; however, it may instead be due to the occupation of the system with creating an organ rather than digestion or to the presence of pain, which prevents digestion in weak bodies. A little diarrhea should not be of concern; however, if an escalation is feared, then a fomentation* of rose seeds, celery seeds, anise seeds, or cumin seeds should be applied, or wrap the infant's belly with cumin and rose soaked in vinegar or millet (*Panicum miliaceum,* جاورس، دخـن) cooked in a little vinegar. If these treatments are ineffective, take one-sixth dram of lamb's rennet† in cold water and give it to the infant; care should be exercised that the milk does not turn into cheese inside the stomach by feeding the infant a

---

*Fomentation is the application of warm, soft, medicinal substances to ease pain by relaxing the skin.

†Rennet is a natural complex of enzymes produced in any mammalian stomach to digest the mother's milk.

milk substitute such as the yolk of a half-boiled egg, cooked bread pulp, or the cereal of roasted wheat or barley flour in water.

Infants may develop **constipation**. This may be treated with mouse dung or by using suppositories of solid honey alone or mixed with penny-royal or orrisroot (*Iris florentina* or *I. germanica,* إيرسا، سوسن اسمانجوني), as is or roasted. Also, the infant may be fed a small amount of honey or turpentine resin in the amount of a chickpea. Furthermore, gentle rubbing of the infant's belly with oil or coating their naval with cow's bile and Persian cyclamen (*Cyclamen persicum,* بخور مريم) can be applied as treatments of constipation. Inflammation of the gums is treated by a fomentation with oil and wax and can benefit from salty, rotten meat.

Infants may develop **spasms** (convulsions) during dentition, mostly due to weak digestion and the weakness of nerves, especially those with a moist, bulky body. This can be treated with oils of orrisroot, henna, or wallflower (*Erysimum cheiri,* خيري). Trismus* may also afflict them. This can be treated with a tincture of squirting (exploding) cucumber (*Ecballium elaterium,* قثاء الحمار) or a mixture of the oils of orrisroot and squirting cucumber. If the spasm is associated with dryness due to its occurrence after a fever, severe diarrhea, or gradually taking place, the joints should be topically treated with fat of viola alone or mixed with clarified wax, and pour on their heads a lot of oil and fat of viola. Also, use the same treatment for a dry trismus.

When infants develop **cough and nasal congestion,** it has been ordered to pour a lot of hot water on their heads, place a lot of honey on the tongue, then pressure the tongue base with a finger to induce vomiting. The vomiting brings out a lot of phlegm, thus helps in the recovery. Or, make a mixture of gum arabic, extract of milk vetch (extracted from *Astragalus gummifera,* كثيراء تستخرج من القتاد), quince seeds, licorice extract, and sugar, mix with some milk, and give daily as a drink.

If the infant develops **difficulty in breathing (dyspnea)**, then the roots of the ears and the tongue root should be rubbed with oil, and induce vomiting. Squeezing the tongue with fingers is very beneficial.

---

*Trismus is the inability to normally open the mouth due to one of many causes.

Also, dropping hot water in the mouth and licking some flax seeds mixed with honey.

Stomatitis and aphthae* are frequent among infants because the linings of their mouth and stomach are very soft and sensitive to touch and are hurt by the passage of milk. The worst kind of aphthae is the charcoal black, which is fatal, and the safest are the white and red. Therefore, they should be treated with specific drugs for stomatitis as mentioned in the specific book [Books 3–5 of the *Canon*]. The viola alone may be sufficient to treat it, or mixed with roses, some saffron, or carob alone. Also, the juice of lettuce, European black nightshade (*Solanum nigrum,* عنب الثعلب), and milk vetch could be good enough. However, if it is stronger, then the ground licorice root. Gum ulcers and aphthae can be treated with myrrh, astringent [from oak tree], and the finely ground bark of frankincense mixed with honey. Also, the extract of sour mulberries or sour grapes may be sufficient by itself. Washing with honey water or a drink mixed with honey is beneficial and should be followed with a drying agent. If something stronger is needed, then take six drams of each of pomegranate peel, flower (جلنار), and leaf midrib, sumac, four drams of oak, and two drams of dill; grind all, sieve, and sprinkle.

The infant's ears may **discharge liquid;** this is due to their moist bodies, especially their very moist brains. For this, take a small piece of wool, shape it as a wick, and dip it in a mixture of honey and wine that has in it a small amount of alum, saffron, and natron, and place the wick in their ears. It may be sufficient to dip the wool wick in an astringent drink, or add some saffron to astringent drink and use it as a drip.

Frequent **earaches** may happen due to gas or moisture. This can be treated by boiling any of the following: boxthorn (*Lycium afrum,* عوسج، حضض), thyme, rock salt (الملح الطبرزد), lentils, myrrh, seeds of bitter gourd, and savin (*Juniperus sabina,* أبهل), and place a few drops in the ear.

Sometimes, infants develop hot swelling in the brain called **meningitis** (العظاس), with its pain frequently reaching to the eye

---

*An aphthae is a small ulcer occurring in groups in the mouth or on the tongue.

and throat and causing yellowness of the face. In such a case, the brain should be cooled down and moistened with the peels of pumpkin and cucumber, water of European black nightshade, specifically the juice of purslane, oil of rose with little of vinegar, and egg yolk with rose oil. This is done by replacing one with the other.

The brains of the infants may accumulate **"water on the brain"** [hydrocephalus]. We have mentioned its treatment in the diseases of the head. For their swelled eyes, spread on the exterior boxthorn mixed with milk, then wash the eye with a chamomile decoction and basil water. Excessive crying of infants may cause whiteness on the pupils or inflammation of the eyelid [blepharitis]; both conditions can be treated with European black nightshade. When fevers occur, the nursing mother should stop breast-feeding and be given, and the infant as well, pomegranate juice with oxymel and honey or cucumber juice with [a] little camphor and sugar. Then they should sweat by wetting their heads and legs with the juice of green reed, and then be wrapped [for warmth].

In the case of **colic,** the infant may twist from pain and cry. The belly should be fomented with hot water and lots of hot oil mixed with wax. Excessive **sneezing** indicates a swelling and/or inflammation near the brain; if so, it should be treated with cooling agents such as rubbing with cooling juices and oils. If the sneezing is not due to a swelling, then the powder of basil should be blown into the nostrils.

Boils may develop in the infants' bodies. The ones that are black are fatal, but the white and red are safer. Thrush could be fatal, especially if it gives boils [probably Avicenna meant systemic mycosis here]. The appearance of boils may have good benefits. The treatment of boils includes washing with astringents prepared by boiling roses, myrtle leaves, mastic tree leaves (*Pistacia lentiscus,* مصطكي), and tamarisk (*Tamarix gallica,* طرفاء). These may also be used as rubs [in oil]. Intact boils should be left until they ripen, then treated; if they open, use the ointment of white lead. Washing should be done with honey water containing some natron. In thrush, when the boils become dense, the wash should be done with borax water mixed with milk so that it can be tolerated; if their skin becomes spotty, they should be bathed with a decoction of myrtle, rose, lemongrass (*Cymbopogon schoenanthus,* إذخـر), and leaves of mastic. However, the most important thing is to fix the diet of the nursing woman.

Excessive crying in infants may cause umbilical **hernia** or other forms of hernia. In this case, it has been prescribed that the infant be given bishop's weed (*Carum copticum,* نـانـخـواه) as a drink or mixed with egg white and placed at the hernia with a piece of linen, or mix the ashes of bitter lupin with wine and apply and wrap to the herniated spot. Stronger than the last are the hot astringents, such as myrrh, bark and fruit of cypress (*Cupressus sempervirens,* سـرو), fruit juice of gum arabic (*Acacia arabica,* أقـاقـيا), and aloe, as well as others mentioned in the section on hernia.

Occasionally after the severing of the cord, a swelling and **inflammation of the naval** may develop. For this condition, alkanet (*Alkanna tinctoria,* شـنـكـال) and terebinth resin should be dissolved in sesame oil, drunk by the infant, and rubbed on the naval.

The infant may become **sleepless**, cry, and moan; this requires the use of the peel of the capsule of the opium poppy and its seeds, lettuce oil, and poppy oil, by placing them on the temples and top of the head. If stronger medication is needed, then follow this formula: take [equal parts] of hemp seeds, mangosteen (*Garcinia mangostana,* جوز كندم), yellow poppy, linseed, walnuts, milk vetch seeds, grand plantain seeds (*Plantago major,* لـسـان الـحـمـل), lettuce seeds, fennel seeds, anise seeds, and cumin seeds; boil on slow flame and then mash the mix; add one part of fried *Plantago stricta* seeds but not ground; mix with an equal amount of sugar; and give two drams of it to the infant to drink. This formula can be fortified by adding to it one-third of a part of opium.

Treat the infant's **hiccup** with coconut mixed with sugar. In case of **severe vomiting** treat with a half denim* of cloves, and it could be beneficial to wrap the belly with weak preventers of vomiting. **Stomach weakness** [indigestion] is treated by washing the belly with licorice water, rose water, or myrtle water, and by giving the infant quince water

---

*A denim is 0.525 gram (the weight of eight grains of barley).

with cloves and *sek** (سك) or one carat of sek with a little water.

Frightening dreams are mostly due to stomach fullness, which is the result of the infant's strong appetite. If food corruption is felt by the stomach, the felt harm is transferred from the sensing faculty to the imaginative faculty, which induces bad dreams. The infant should not be allowed to sleep with this fullness discomfort, but should be given a spoon of honey to help digest the food in the stomach and push it down.

Inflammation of the throat between the mouth and the esophagus could spread to the muscles and cervical vertebrae; therefore, the bowels should be softened with a suppository, then treated with the syrup of mulberry and the like.

Heavy **snoring** during sleep should be treated with a spoon of ground linseed mixed with honey or ground cumin seeds mixed with honey.

The treatment of infantile **convulsions** has been described in the section on the diseases of the head; however, we mention here a treatment that may work better. Take equal amounts of thyme, castoreum, and cumin, mash and mix with water, and give it as a drink made of three grains.

For treatment of **anal prolapse,** take one dram of the following: pomegranate peel, soft myrtle, acorn's soft peel, dry rose, burnt horn, alum, goat's hooves, pomegranate flowers, and French tamarisk; boil well to extract their astringent power; then sit the infant in the lukewarm water.

Infants may develop **enteritis** due to exposure to cold. To treat enteritis, take three drams of watercress seeds and cumin seeds, grind, sieve, and mix with aged cow ghee. Give with cold water.

Small harmful **threadworms or pinworms** (*Oxyuris vermicularis*) may infest the belly of the infant, mostly near the anus. Also, giant **roundworms** (*Ascaris lumbricoides*) may riddle them, but rarely **tapeworms** (*Taenia solium*). Roundworms are treated with wormwood (*Artemisia judaica,* بعثران) water mixed with milk in quantity, depending on the infant's tolerance, and they require that the belly be wrapped

---

*Sek is a powder made from the fruit of Indian gooseberry (*Phyllanthus emblica* [syn. *Emblica officinalis*], الأملج).

with absinthe, or wormwood (*Artemisia absinthium*), false black pepper (*Embelia ribes*), ox bile, and fat of bitter gourd. As for pinworms in the anus region, take one part of common inula (*Inula helenium*) and greater celandine, add sugar in equal part to both, and mix in water.

Abrasion of the thigh should be dusted with the powder of myrtle and root of white lily (*Lilium candidum*), or powder of roses, cypress, barley flour, or lentil flour.

FOURTH SECTION

Regimen of Childhood

In the phase of childhood, most of the care should be focused on adjusting manners. To protect the child from severe anger, grave fear, depression, or insomnia, attention should be paid to find out his likes and bring them closer and keep away things that the child dislikes. There are two benefits: (1) in themselves, so that they have good manners that are permanent, and (2) to their bodies, since bad manners are due to dystemperament, and a prolonged habit will generate its related dystemperament. For this reason, anger generates excessive heat, depression dehydrates, and mental dullness weakens the psychological faculty and tilts the temperament to phlegmatic. Therefore, improving manners preserves mental and physical health together. When the child wakes up, it is better to bathe and play for one hour, then give something light to eat, and allow them to resume play for a longer time. After play, the child should be bathed and fed. It is better not to let them drink water with food to prevent the absorption of incompletely digested food.

By the age of six years, children should be introduced to a teacher and gradually introduced to education, without forcing them to read for a long time. At this age, they should be bathed less, and their exercise lengthened before meals. They should avoid wine, especially for those with hot and moist temperament, because of the harm it inflicts to increase bile. This wine effect to induce the bile or moisten the joints is not needed in children because the increase in bile is diuretic and their joints do not need moistening. Cold, pure water increases appetite. This is the regimen to fourteen years of age, taking care to follow the specific individual requirement for every child, such as the decrease of moisture, dehydration, and hardening. Therefore, they should gradually decrease sports, especially violent ones, from childhood to youth, and stick to moderate exercise.

After this age, their regimen should be for growth and preservation of the body. We introduce our statement on the subjects that matter in the regimen of healthy adults, starting with exercise.

CHAPTER 13

Common Regimen
of Adults

Second Lesson of the Third Art:
Common Regimen of Adults

- Exercise (3 sections)
- Massage (1 section)
- Bathing (2 sections)
- Food Regimen (1 section)
- Regimen of Water and Wine (1 section)
- Sleep and Wakefulness (1 section)
- Topics That Are Mentioned Here but Should Be Delayed (1 section)
- The Strengthening of Weak Organs, Their Fattening, and Size Increase (1 section)
- Exercise and Fatigue (5 sections)
- Management of Bodies' Dystemperament (1 section)

Common Regimen of Adults

(17 Sections)

FIRST SECTION

General Statement on Exercise

Since most of health preservation is to exercise, then diet, and then sleep, therefore, we should start with exercise. We say that exercise is a voluntary movement that induces deep, frequent breathing. Its proper, moderate use prevents physical illnesses as well as diseases of dystemperament that follow and are produced by them, that is, if the exercise is managed properly.

This is explained as follows. We are required to eat, and the preservation of our health is by proper diet that is moderate in quantity and quality. *Not all the food potential is converted to actual use by the body, but rather, there is a residual amount from every digestion that is left over in the body, and the body systems try to get rid of it.* Natural evacuation is not by itself sufficient to complete the evacuation; therefore, there is waste that is left from every digestion. By repetition of this cycle, there is an accumulation of waste that is harmful to the body from several aspects. Its putrefaction causes the diseases of putrefaction; its accumulation in a body part induces swellings; its gases corrupt the temperament of the "spirit." These waste products have to be removed from the body, a process that is induced in most cases by poisonous drugs, which without a doubt exhausts the body systems, and even if not poisonous, they still affect the nature of the body. Hippocrates has said that the drug purges and deranges because it also flushes out some of the good humors, innate moisture, and the "spirit," which is the essence of life. This weakens the strength of the main organs and the supporting ones. Therefore, these are the harms of fullness if left untreated and if pushed out. Exercise is the best measure to prevent the accumulation of fullness if practiced properly to renew the innate heat and instill lightness in the body. This is because it induces a gentle heat that decomposes the accumulated waste every day. The movement should be precise in its direction to move the waste out, thus preventing accumulation of significant amounts of waste. As we have said, exercise amplifies the innate heat and strengthens the joints and tendons, thus it:

- Enables action and prevents reaction
- Makes the organs ready to accept food by the loss of waste
- Stimulates the attractive faculty
- Removes stiffness from body parts and softens them
- Reduces moisture
- Opens skin pores.

Frequently, a person who abandons exercise develops hectic fever because the organs' faculties weaken due to the reduction of the movement that brought them the "spirit" and its subsequent innate heat, which is the instrument of life of every organ.

SECOND SECTION

Types of Exercise

Some exercises are part of regular human activities, others are pure exercise done for one purpose, the sake of exercise, and one gets from them the benefits of exercise. The latter have several forms; they can be brief or lengthy, tough or relaxed, fast or slow, strenuous and fast or relaxed. There is always moderation between the extremes.

Among the types of exercise are wrestling, grappling, boxing, running, brisk walking, archery, dance, hanging by hands, hopping on one leg, sword fencing, javelin throw, horseback riding, and fast clapping front and back while standing on toes—a fast exercise. Gentle sports include swinging on a swing or cradle in standing, sitting, or lying positions, and sailing in small and large boats. Harder sports include riding horses, camels, howdahs, and carriages.

Among the strenuous exercises are field workouts, such as running fast in a field to a point in the field and running back, and each time reducing the distance until one ends up standing in the middle of the original distance; shadow chasing; clapping; jumping; throwing; playing with small and large balls; playing with the scepter; playing with racket or bat; wrestling; weight lifting; and running along horses and catching them.

There are a few grappling techniques, such as clinching and applying the bear hug, take down, collar tie, and joint lock. Fast exercises include the quick exchange of places between two individuals, jumping backward and forward with or without order, and sticking in the ground two long stakes on each side of the individual, then taking the one on the right out and planting it on the left side and the one on the left in the right side as fast as one can.

Strenuous and fast exercises are rotated with periods of rest and soft exercises. Different types of exercise should be practiced and do not fixate on one in particular. Every organ has its specific exercises. The exercises of arms and legs are obvious. The chest and respiratory organs are exercised by alternating between deep loud and sharp sounds or a mix of the two, thus they exercise the mouth, uvula, tongue, and eyes as well. These exercises improve the skin color and cleanse the chest. Taking a deep breath, holding it, and then exhaling exercises the whole body and enlarges its passages. Enlarging the voice for a very long time is dangerous, and prolonging it requires lots of inhaling and exhaling, and both are dangerous. It should be started with an easy reading, and then gradually raising the voice. When the voice is stressed, enlarged, and stretched, then this should be for a moderate time, which then benefits greatly; however, its prolonging is dangerous for equitable healthy people.

Every person should practice suitable exercises. Soft exercise such as swinging is suitable for a person who has been weakened by fevers and is incapacitated, is recovering from illness, or is weakened from drinking hellebores and alike, and in individuals with a disease in the diaphragm. Gentle swinging brings on sleeping, breaks down gases, improves the recovery of head diseases such as absentmindedness and forgetfulness, and improves appetite and desire. Swinging while lying down is more suitable for people who have semitertian fever, compound or phlegmatic fevers, and gout and kidney diseases, since this swinging encourages the harmful humors to move and leave. Soft is for soft, and hard is for the stronger. Riding a carriage may also have the same benefits, and it has stronger effect. The carriage may be ridden facing backward, which greatly benefits the weak and vanishing eyesight.

Sailing in small and large boats near the shore benefits people with leprosy, edema, and apoplexy, as well as with cold and distended stomach. An episode of vomiting followed by relief is good for the stomach. Riding the sea in high waves has a stronger effect on recovery from these diseases because it puts the individual in different moods of happiness and sadness.

The digestive organs are exercised when whole-body exercises are performed. Eyesight is exercised by looking at small objects and then gradually and gently looking at distant ones. Hearing is exercised by listening to faint sounds, and rarely by listening to loud sounds. The details are mentioned in the preservation of the health of each organ in the detailed volume on the topic [in a different source].

The exercising individual should take care that the exercise does not reach the weak organ except in a secondary way. For example, a person with varicose veins should not excessively move their legs, but reduce the legs' movement and exercise the upper body parts such as the head, neck, and torso so that the effect on the legs comes down from the upper body. The weak body needs soft exercise, and the strong body needs strong exercise. Note that every organ has its specific type of exercise, such as looking at tiny objects to exercise the eye, gradually raising the voice to exercise the throat, and there are exercises for the tongue and ear as described in their sections.

THIRD SECTION

Time of Starting and Stopping Exercise

To start the exercise, the body should be free of raw and bad chyme in the viscera and vessels because exercise will spread it throughout the body; the food of the previous evening should have been digested in the stomach, liver, and veins, and the time of another meal has arrived. The latter is evident by the maturation of urine in texture and color, which is the first phase of digestion. After some time, the digestion is complete, and the yellowness of urine becomes darker than normal due to an increase in its fieriness [no nutrients are available in the body]; exercising at this time is harmful because it drains the innate heat. For this reason, it has been said that if the exercise is necessary then it is better if some food is in the stomach and it is not totally empty. The food should be dense in the wintertime and light in the summertime. It is preferred to exercise with a full stomach rather than an empty one and while warm and moist rather than cold and dry; however, the best is moderate. Exercise may cause diseases to individuals of hot and dry temperament, and their cure will occur when they quit the exercise.

A person wanting to exercise should start by cleansing the intestine and the bladder and getting massaged in a manner that refreshes the metabolic vigor and widens the skin pores. Massaging should be done with a rough scrubber, followed by rubbing sweet oil and gradually and gently pressuring the organs, but not deeply. During the massage, lots of strokes should be applied with different directions to reach every part of the muscles. After the massage, the individual should be left to start the exercise.

The **best time to exercise** in the spring is the middle of the day in a house of moderate temperature, and in the summer it should be done earlier. However, during the winter, it should be done in the evening, removing any obstacles, such as warming up the house to become moderate in its temperature. As mentioned above, the exercise should be performed according to the suitable time of digestion and elimination.

There are three factors that should be followed when deciding on the **duration of exercise**. The first is color; as long as it is improving then the person can continue exercising. The second are the movements; as long as they are light then one can continue exercising. The third is the condition of the organs [body parts] and their swelling; as long as they are continuing to swell then one can continue exercising. However, if these conditions start to reverse and the sweating turns from vapor to liquid then one should stop exercising and rub diaphoretic oil (inducing perspiration) in a confined room. If the length of exercise and amount of food are determined for a person, then only the amount of food should be adjusted the next day and the length of exercise kept the same.

FOURTH SECTION

Massage

Hard massage firms up the body, and soft relaxes it. Excessive massage reduces weight, and moderate increases fertility. Combinations of these conditions produce nine variations of massage. Rough application of massage can be carried out by a rough piece of tissue; this brings the blood quickly to the surface. Smooth massaging is done with the palm of the hand or a smooth piece of tissue; this collects the blood in the body part and confines it there. *The purpose of massage is to solidify loose bodies and firm up soft bodies, loosen the dense and soften the hard.*

There is also **sports massage**, or prepping massage, which prepares the person for exercise; this starts soft and becomes hard to firm up the body before commencing the sport. After exercise, there is **restorative massage**, also called calming massage; its purpose is to break down and disperse waste that is trapped in the muscle that was not eliminated by the exercise and to refresh the tissue and prevent fatigue. This massage should be gentle and moderate; it's best when oil is applied and should not be finished with hard or rough rubbing to avoid hardening the organs. This type of massage should not be given to children because it hinders their growth; however, it's harm in adults is less.

It is better to err by giving a hard massage rather than erring by giving a soft one because the dispersing effect of hard massage is easier on the body than the soft massage that prepares the body to accept the waste. Excessive hard massage for children prevents their growth. You will find more explanation after the section on the time of massage and its conditions; however, we wanted here to state the fact that restorative massage is a kind of exercise.

Restorative massage should be started hard with oil, but should not be finished with the same strength of application. It is better to use more that one masseur at the same time. After the massage, the person should stretch out the massaged body parts to disperse the waste from them, and then follow that by wrapping them with bandages while stretched. The breath should be held as much as possible and the abdominal muscles relaxed while wrapping the body parts. Stretching should start with the thoracic muscles if possible and end with light stretching of the abdominal muscles in order to give the viscera some restoration. In between these activities, the person should walk, lie down, and entangle their legs with another person.

Individuals who excel in sports apply breath holding between their exercises. They may also use restorative massage in the middle of exercise (stop and resume) if they want to prolong the exercise. There is no need for excessive restorative massage, especially for those who have no complaints or problems and will not resume exercising. For fatigue, one should do a gentle rubbing of oil as we describe. When some body parts are hard, they should be massaged until they become moderate, between softness and hardness. Hard massage and pressure are beneficial for sleeping because they dry the body and prevent moisture from seeping into the joints; take a note of this.

FIFTH SECTION

Bathing and Bathhouses

The individuals whose regimen we are discussing here have no need for a dispersing bath because their bodies are free of metabolic waste. The bath is needed for people who will benefit from gentle warmth and moderate moisturizing. If they use the bathtub, they should only stay until their skin becomes red and puffy, and leave at the start of the dispersion of their bodily waste. The air around them should be humidified by the pouring of pure water, then they should rinse quickly and get out. An exercising person should not go into the bath until they have rested completely.

The conditions for bathhouses have been described earlier. What must be said here is that the bather should move gradually between the rooms of different temperatures. One should not stay in the hot room [sauna] beyond discomfort, thus benefiting from the dispersal of waste and preparing the body to accept nutrients, at the same time being careful against weakening the body and developing a cause for putrefactive fevers.

A person who desires to add weight should bathe after a meal, knowing that they will not develop indigestion and obstruction. However, as a prophylaxis against obstruction, a hot temperament individual should drink oxymel, and a cold temperament individual pennyroyal and pepper. A person desiring to lose weight should bathe while hungry and prolong their stay. A person desiring to preserve their health should bathe after a complete digestion of food in the stomach and in the liver, and to prevent the excitement of the gallbladder if bathing in the morning before breakfast, one should eat something light. The latter should be taken by a hot temperament person with gallbladder problems, and he should not go into the hot room of the bath. The best for such an individual is to eat bread soaked in fruit juice or rosewater.

After getting out of the bath or while in the bath, avoid drinking a cold drink since the pores are already open and the cold will rush into the main organs and weaken their faculties. Also, avoid all very hot things, especially water, because drinking will cause heat to accelerate into the main organs, thus causing tuberculosis and hectic fever. One should avoid leaving the bath suddenly, then uncovering the head and exposing the body to cold; rather, one should leave the bath during wintertime while bundled up. Individuals with fevers or with discontinuities should not enter the bath.

You have learned earlier that *the bath may be warming, cooling, moisturizing, dehydrating, beneficial, or harmful.* Its benefits include inducing sleep, opening of tissues and pores, dispersal and elimination, maturation, and attracting food to the outer tissues of the body. It also assists in decomposing the material that needs elimination and should naturally be eliminated, holding diarrhea, and eliminating fatigue. Its harmful effects include weakening of the heart if bathing excessively, inducing nausea and fainting, stirring stagnant materials, exposing them to putrefaction, and moving them into cavities and weak organs, thus causing swellings in the surface and inside of these organs.

SIXTH SECTION

Washing with Cold Water

This can be performed for the individual with proper regimen of all aspects and who has the proper age, strength, physique, and season. This person should also be free of indigestion, vomiting, diarrhea, insomnia, and catarrh and should not be a boy or an elderly person. Washing with cold water should be carried out when the body is active and movements are easy. Cold water may be followed with hot water to strengthen the skin and confine the innate heat; for this the cold water should not be very cold but rather moderate.

Cold-water washing may be done after exercise; however, the massage that precedes should be harder than usual. Oil rubbing should be as usual, and exercise after the massage with moderate rubbing is slightly faster than usual. Washing with cold water should start immediately after exercise, and the water should touch all the body parts at the same time up to the point of tolerance and before developing goosebumps. After the wash, the person should be massaged as we have mentioned and given an increased portion of their food and reduced portion of their drink, and the time to regain their normal skin color should be observed. If the normal color returns quickly, then the length of the cold-water wash is moderate, but if it takes longer, then the wash was longer than it should be. Therefore, the next day the cold wash should be adjusted. One can return to the cold wash a second time after the massage and will later regain color and warmth.

One who wants to do the cold wash should do it gradually by starting on the hottest day of the summer at noontime, and there should not be wind. Cold wash should not be done after sexual intercourse, eating (also not before the food has been fully digested), vomiting, evacuation, cholera, or insomnia; additionally, it should be avoided if one has general body weakness or stomach weakness or after exercise, except for those who are very strong, then it should be used according to the limit mentioned. The sudden use of cold washing as we outlined pushes the innate heat internally [i.e., it is greatly reduced at the surface], then strengthens it multiple times.

SEVENTH SECTION

Food Regimen

One who is seeking health preservation should endeavor not to have the essence of their food as medicinal foods such as green, leafy vegetables and fruits, and alike. The attenuant food chars blood [i.e., oxidizes], and heavy food causes phlegm and weightiness of the body. Food should be composed of meat, especially that of the young goat, young beef, and young lamb; wheat that has been cleaned and is free from contamination and from healthy fields that have not been affected by disease; sweets that are suitable to the temperament; and good drinks made of fragrant herbs. Other than that is used for treatment and preservation. Fruits that resemble food are figs; whole, mature, and very sweet grapes; and dates in the countries that usually grow them. If eating these [food types] produces superfluity, then evacuation should be carried out.

Eating should be done when one is hungry, and appetite should not be resisted unless it is a false appetite like that of drunk or dyspeptic people with indigestion. Prolonging hunger fills up the stomach with bad putrescent humors. Foods of hot effect should be eaten during winter, and the cold or slightly warm foods during the summer; the hot and the cold should not get to such a level that cannot be tolerated.

Note that there is nothing worse than fullness during the fertile, plentiful season followed by hunger in a drought, and *vice versa*. The opposite is worse, and we have seen people that went through a scarce season, and later, during a plentiful season, they filled up, became full, and died. Excessive fullness in all situations is fatal, whether it is by food or drink. There are men who filled up, suffocated, and died. If a mistake occurs and some of the medicinal food was eaten, then it should be managed through digestion and maturation, and precautions should be taken to deal with expected dystemperament by taking an antagonist afterward until it gets digested. For example, if it is within the cold food category, like Armenian cucumber, cucumber, and pumpkin, fix with an opposite, like garlic or leek; if it is within the hot food, fix with an opposite, like Armenian cucumber and purslane. Obstructive food should be treated with something that will open and evacuate; the individual should then fast and not eat until fully recovered, feeling a real appetite, and until the stomach and upper intestines have emptied, since the most harmful thing to the body is to pile new food onto old food that has not been digested and matured.

Indigestion from low-quality food is the worst. Indigestion caused by heavy food will give joint ache, kidney problems, asthma, shortness of breath, gout, induration (hardening) of the spleen and liver, and phlegmatic and melancholic diseases. However, if indigestion is due to light food it causes acute malicious fevers and bad acute swellings, and it may be necessary to feed with food or foodlike medication, as in the case of individuals who eat spicy, hot, and salty foods; in this case, if they follow a period of indigestion with simple moist food, it will fix the chyme of what they have eaten. For these individuals, this regimen should be sufficient and there is no need for exercise. For the opposite of this situation, one should follow the heavy food after a while with fast-digestible hot food. Light exercise should be equivalent to the amount of food in the stomach, especially for those who want to sleep. Excessive psychological excitement and physical moves prevent digestion.

Food with little nutritive value, like green, leafy vegetables, should not be eaten in the winter season, but rather rich, large grains. In the summer it is the opposite. The stomach should not be filled up so that there is no space for the food's waste; rather, one should stop eating while there is still some room left in the stomach. Any feeling of hunger after that will dissipate within an hour. This should be customary since the most harmful food is the one that is heavy on the stomach, and the most harmful drink is the one that exceeds moderation and floats in the stomach. When individuals overeat one day, they should fast the next day and prolong sleep in a moderate place without excessive hotness or coldness; sleep can be stimulated by a long, light stroll without stopping or resting with little drinking. Rufus said, "I am thankful for the walk, especially after lunch, because it prepares a good place for the dinner."

Sleeping should be first on the right side for a while, then left side, and then right side. Note that covering the body and raising the pillow assists digestion. In general, the body should be tilting downward and not upward.

The **amount of food** should be according to the regular habit and strength; its amount in healthy individuals should be equal to their strength so that it does not produce heaviness, distention of the abdomen, bloating, rumbling, floating, nausea, bulimia, collapse, dullness, and insomnia; its taste should not appear in belching after a while; and the longer its taste lasts, the worse it is.

A sign that the food is suitable is when it does not amplify the pulse while reducing the breath size. If this happens, it indicates that the stomach is pushing against the diaphragm, thus causing small frequent inhalations. Small inhalations do not meet the heart demand and lead to weakness. A person who becomes hot and feels warm after a meal should not eat their food quickly, but rather slowly, so that fullness does not give shivering that is followed by a strong fever when the food causes the warmth. A person who cannot fully digest the food should reduce its amount and eat several times.

The melancholic person needs moistening food that is slightly warming. The choleric needs moistening and cooling food. The sanguine needs cold, less-nutritious food. A phlegmatic person needs less-nutritious food that warms and ameliorates.

There is an order for the use of food that should be followed by the person desiring to preserve health. One should be cautious not to eat a light and easily digested food after a strong and harder one, since the second will get digested before the first while it is floating on top of the first without a way to exit the stomach, which leads to putrefaction and corruption with anything that mixes with it. There is an exception to this that we will mention. Also, food that slips easily through the digestive tract should not be followed by a strong and hard food because it may slip with the first into the intestine before it has been full digested, such as fish and the like, which should not be eaten after an exhausting exercise because it gets corrupted and corrupts the humors. Some individuals with a weak and relaxed stomach that allows food to go through quickly without proper digestion may take something that has astringent power and should always check the condition and temperament of their stomach. The stomach of individuals with fiery stomach corrupts light, gentle, easily digestible food but digests hard, strong food; there are people who have the opposite, and each should have their own regimen.

Countries have their own characteristic traditions and temperaments, and some depart from the rules, thus this should be noted and experience followed in this case, rather that the rules. Sometimes a popular but harmful dish is more suitable than a good but unpopular one [i.e., a popular dish in one area that is harmful in another is sometimes better than the known good dish from the latter].

For every body type and temperament there is an appropriate diet, thus changing it may produce harmful effects. Individuals who are harmed by good foods should keep them out, and those that like bad foods should not be indifferent because they will eventually accumulate bad humors that develop fatal diseases. Frequently, people with bad humors are allowed to expand their diet with good food, especially if they cannot tolerate diarrhea due to their weakness. Individuals who have a loose body with fast dispersion should feed on moist, easily digestible food, even though they can tolerate various thick foods and are far from being harmed by external causes.

When living affluently and eating lots of meat, one should resort to venesection (bloodletting, or bleeding). A tendency for cold temperament of the stomach should be opposed with *jawarish* and *attrefel* (*jawarish* and *attrefel* are two sets of compound medicinal preparations) and others that cleanse the stomach, intestines, and surrounding ducts. One of the most harmful is to accumulate several types of foods over a long, extended meal where successive foods follow food that has already been digested, resulting in a heterogeneously digested mass of food. Most agreeable is delicious food since the stomach and the retentive faculty work strongly together on food if it is of good nature and all major organs are sound and harmonious in their temperaments; however, it should be of significance if there are dystemperaments within the organs (for example, liver abnormally different from stomach). The drawback of delicious food is that one may overeat.

The best way to eat **full meals** is to eat only one a day and two the day after (morning and evening). This schedule should be strongly followed since a person who gets used to two meals will become weak and lose strength. A person with weak digestion should eat two meals and reduce the amount of food each time. Also, when getting used to one meal and then eating twice, it brings on weakness, sluggishness, and looseness. Holding back the food at night weakens, and a supper that has not been digested and assimilated will cause acidic burping, malicious breath, nausea, bitterness of the mouth, and soft bowels because the stomach is not used to having food at this time, causing the signs of indigestion. Additional signs include cowardice, fear, and pain; burning in the stomach and mouth; a feeling of suspension of the stomach and intestine due to emptiness of the stomach and its contraction; burning urination; and burned stool, and there may be coldness in the fingers and toes due to seeping of bile into the stomach (this is more frequent in choleric individuals and those with only choleric stomach) and insomnia and restlessness. Frequent accumulation of bile in the stomach requires the intake of several quick meals, and always long periods before bathing. Others should exercise, bathe, then eat, and not eat before bathing. Whoever feels hungry before exercise should eat bread alone in amounts that will be digested before starting the exercise. Exercises, before and after meals, should be gentle and soft.

The best treatment for a **corrupted appetite** that favors hot and despises the sweet and fat is to induce vomiting by the use of oxymel or radish after fish. Overweight individuals should not eat after getting out of the bath, but rather they should wait by taking a short nap; the best for them is one full meal a day. One should not sleep while there is floating food in the stomach. One should completely avoid strong movements after eating so that the food does not pass or slip into the intestines before digestion or its temperament become corrupted by the shaking, also one should not drink an excess of water that will create a barrier between the food and the stomach, thus extinguishing it [i.e., preventing digestion].

Drinking water should be postponed until the food moves down from the stomach, indicated by lightness of the upper belly. However, if thirsty, then sucking a little cold water should be fine; a little cold water satisfies better and flattens and contracts the stomach. In general, drinking water after, not during, the meal, in an amount that is good for digestion, is acceptable.

Sleeping thirsty is beneficial to individuals with coldness and wetness [i.e., phlegmatic] and harmful to those with warmth and biliary conditions, and the same is true for tolerating hunger. In fasting biliary individuals, the gallbladder will pour its bile into the stomach; therefore, if they do eat, the food will not get digested and will cause them the same symptoms of indigestion. The loss of appetite may happen; in this case, a light drink that counteracts it and softens the bowels should be taken, such as pear juice or little *manna* [exudate from *Atraphaxis cotoneaster*], so that if appetite returns, the person eats. Individuals with an excess of natural humidity in their bodies are prone to fast decomposition of their nutrients, and therefore cannot tolerate hunger as well as those with drier bodies, unless their organs are filled with moistures that differ from their natural one, and these moistures [nutrients] are good and the body is able to convert them to complete food by action.

Drinking water with food is very harmful because it is quickly digested and absorbed, thus it assists food absorption before it has been fully digested; this causes obstruction [deposition of large molecules into the arteries], putrefaction, and sometimes scabies. Sweets accelerate obstruction due their fast absorption before their digestion. Obstruction causes many diseases, such as edema and heaviness of air and water, especially during the summer, which corrupts food. In this case, take a glass of wine mixed with water or a decoction of agarwood (*Aquilaria agallocha*) and mastic resin.

Dense food in a hot, strong stomach will frequently cause gas to bloat the stomach and its neighboring areas and produce related illness. Eating light food on an empty stomach is safe, but following it directly with dense food upsets the stomach and causes indigestion and putrefaction; waiting awhile helps avoid this problem. The best practice here is to eat the dense food little by little, so that the light food gets digested first.

When a problem occurs due to overeating, excessive churning, or drinking, then immediate **emesis** is required. If emesis is delayed or is difficult to induce, then slowly sipping hot water will help in reducing fullness, and it will induce sleepiness, which one should follow. If this is not enough or is not attainable, then let nature takes its course by pushing it through; otherwise, give it some assistance by a gentle laxative. A person feeling hot should be treated with attrefel and laxative galangal mixed with some thyme jam. A person feeling cold should be treated with cumin, *shahrabzani* (dense preparation of dates, الشهربزاني), and dates—as mentioned in the pharmacopoeia. It is better to fill up with drink rather than with food. It is beneficial to take aloe (the amount of three chickpeas) after such food, or half a dram of turpentine resin and a minim* of borax (or the amount of two chickpeas of the light kind of borax), or mastic with one-third of borax. Also very favorable is taking some dodder (*Cuscuta epithymum*) with a drink. If it is ineffective, then take a long sleep and fast for one day. If relief of symptoms happens, then the person should bathe, bundle up, and eat light food. However, if, in spite of all this, fullness persists and heaviness and laziness settle in, then the vessels have gotten filled up with the by-products of the food, since an excessive amount of food, even when digested in the stomach, is rarely broken down further in the vessels. It stays raw, stretches, and may break the vessels, and causes laziness, stretching, and yawning; this should be treated with vessel laxative. However, if only weakness develops, then the

---

*A minim is one-sixth of a dram, equal to 0.521 gram.

individual should rest for a while and be treated for this type of weakness, as we will mention below.

The older the person gets, the less the body will accept what it was used to in youth; therefore, the food will produce more waste, and the person will eat less. A person who is used to dense food when switching to lighter food permits the air to go into the areas where the thick food used to be, which are occupied by the light food; then when switching back to dense food, it produces obstruction.

Harmful effects of **hot food** are treated with seedy oxymel (سكنجبين بزوري). The most beneficial oxymel is sugary, and if honey was added to it, then this simple formula should be sufficient. Harmful effects of **cold food** are treated with honey water and its mixed drinks as well as the cumin decoction. **Dense food** that is followed by a hot temperament is treated with seedy oxymel, heavy on the seeds; however, if followed by cold temperament then treatment should be with decoctions of pepper and pennyroyal.

Light food is better for preserving health but less supportive of "power" and the skin, and dense food has the opposite effect. Thus, a person who eats food with strong chyme to promote skin growth should not eat until becoming very hungry and then eat a digestible amount (i.e., not excessive). People who are in sports and manual labor are more tolerant to dense food. They are aided in their digestion by their deep sleep; however, because of their excessive sweating and decomposition, their livers have to deal with undigested food, which exposes them later, or early in life, to fatal diseases, especially when they stay up at night successively for periods of time and when combined with bathing.

Moist fruits are agreeable with nonexercising choleric people in the summer, and they should be eaten before meals. These are like apricots, mulberries, watermelons, peaches, and pears. It is preferred that they manage with alternative fruits because these make the blood watery. They ferment inside the body the same way the fruit juice ferments outside, and although they are initially beneficial, they will induce putrefaction. Similarly, they fill up the blood with raw humor, although this may be beneficial, like Armenian cucumber and cucumber. For this reason individuals who eat large amounts of these become susceptible to fevers, although they initially have a cooling effect. Also, note that the watery humor may turn into watery pus if it does not disintegrate and remains in the vessels. If these individuals have been exercising before the accumulation of watery humors and do so when they eat fruit, the watery humors break down and their harm lessens. Also learn that when the raw and watery humors are prevented from attaching to the body they will diminish, and a person who eats fruits should walk afterward, and then eat to push them out.

Foods that produce watery, thick, viscous, and bilious humors cause fevers because the watery humor putrefies blood, the viscous and thick blocks vessels and ducts, and the bilious warms up the body and produces sharp blood. **Bitter green, leafy vegetables** are beneficial in winter, and the tasteless are good in the summer. If one is eating low-quality food, they should reduce the number of times they eat it, make it less frequent, and use that which antagonizes it. For example, when **sweet food** harms a person, then they should have with it acidic substances like vinegar, pomegranate, oxymel of vinegar, quince, and alike, and induce emesis. If **acidic food** is harmful it should be followed with honey and aged wine before digestion and maturation of the food. Additionally, to avoid the harmful effect of **fatty foods** they should be eaten with **pungent foods** such as chestnut, true myrtle, carob, Christ's thorn jujube, and azarole; also with **bitter** foods such as bitter inula, salty foods, and pungent foods like pickles, garlic, and onion. The opposite is true as well.

An individual with bad humors and skinniness should eat plenty of good food; one with fast decomposition must feed on moist and easily digestible food. Galen said, "Moist food has no quality as if it is tasteless; it is neither sweet, sour, bitter, hot, astringent, nor salty."

A loose body is more tolerant to heavy food than is a dense body. An excess of **dry food** ruins the appetite, damages skin color, and dries the body. Fatty food causes sluggishness and diminishes appetite. Cold food induces sluggishness and coldness. Acidic food brings on senescence. Hot and salty food harms the stomach; salty harms the eye. Good fatty food gets ruined if followed by low-quality food. **Viscous food** is slow in moving down. Unpeeled cucumber goes down faster than peeled. Bread with bran goes down faster than the one without. If a fatigued person is gently well managed but later breaks a fast with dense food like rice with milk, it causes them irritation in the blood that requires venesection, even if they had done that a short time ago. The same applies to the angry person. Sweet food is quickly absorbed by the body before its maturation and digestion, therefore, it causes abrupt corruption of the blood.

There are **rules for the mixing of food**. Experienced Indians have said that milk should not be mixed with acidic food or fish because this causes diseases that include leprosy. They also said that about yogurt with radish and bird's meat; also rice mixed with milk should not be followed with flour-roasted wheat or barley. Fat or ghee stored in a copper container should not be used in food. Meat grilled on charcoal of the castor oil plant should not be eaten.

Mixed foods are harmful in two ways. First, their variation in digestion and the variation of the digested and undigested. Second, they may be consumed more than needed. Athletic people of old times got around this by eating only meat for lunch and only bread at dinner.

The best time for eating in the summer is the coolest. Trying to prevent hunger may fill up the stomach with bad pus [i.e., bad humor]. Digested kabob is considered the most nutritious of foods, and it is slow moving in the caecum. Soups are good food; when they are mixed with onion they expel the gas, and without it, gas accumulates. Some people think that following roasted [lamb] heads with grapes is good, but to the contrary, it is very bad. Similarly, wine should be followed with pomegranate seeds without their residue [the hard part of the seed].

Note that the **partridge** is dry and causes constipation, while **chicken** is moist and loosens the bowels. The best-roasted chicken is one that has been roasted inside of a young goat or a lamb and thus kept its moisture. Also note that the soup of a chick (young chicken) is an excellent corrector of humors, even more than that of chicken soup. However, the chicken soup is more nutritious. The cold young goat is tastier due to the immobility of its moisture. The hot lamb is tastier due to the melting away of its offensive odor. *Zeerbaj** cooked for

---

Zeerbaj is a meat stew cooked with cinnamon, chickpeas, salt, sesame oil, vinegar, sugar, ground almonds in rose water, dry coriander, pepper, mastic, and saffron.

individuals feeling warm should be without saffron, and for those feeling cold with saffron. Sweets that are made with sugar, like *falouthaj** (*falouzaj*, Turkish delight) are bad due to their obstructive and dehydrating effects. Also note that the harmful effect of undigested bread is immense, and that of undigested meat is less, thus you may use that for comparison.

EIGHTH SECTION

Regimen of Water and Wine

The best water for equitable temperaments is moderate in the severity of its coldness, or its cooling was accomplished by freezing from outward [by placing ice around it], especially if the freezing was not done well. Water from melted ice is harmful to nerves and breathing organs as well as most of the internal organs; it is only tolerated by those of extreme sanguine temperament, but even if it does not affect them immediately, it will over the longer term and in old age.

Experienced people have said that one should not combine the waters of well and river unless one of them is running. We have explained the methods for selecting water and the way to fix the low-quality sources, as well as its improvement by mixing it with vinegar.

Note that it is harmful to drink on an empty stomach first thing in the morning and after exercise and bathing due to false thirst during the night, as happens to the drunk individual; similarly, when the body is busy digesting harmful food. Excessive drinking is very harmful; instead one should be exposed to cold air or wash the mouth with cold water. If this does not help, then drinking should be done from a bottle with a narrow nozzle. However, a drunk may benefit from drinking a good amount of water and may even benefit by drinking early in the morning. If after exercise one feels the strong need to drink, then start by drinking a mixture with hot water. One afflicted with false thirst should know that sleeping and tolerating thirst will calm it because

---

*Falouthaj is a sweet made of sugar, starch, and water.

eventually the body will decompose the substance causing the thirst.

Drinking to quench the demand of thirst will diminish the digestive and maturation process, and later thirst will appear due to the formation of dehydrating humor. A person with false thirst should not sip the water but rather should suck it little by little. Drinking cold water is harmful, but when necessary it should be taken after a sufficient amount of food. Lukewarm water causes nausea, and warmer than that, if drunk in excess, weakens the stomach and sometimes washes the stomach and releases the bowels.

Gentle **white wine** is more agreeable with individuals feeling warm. It does not cause headache, and it may moisten, thus alleviating headaches caused by inflammation of the stomach. The one clarified with bagel (cake) and bread can be its alternative, especially if it is mixed two hours before drinking. **Thick sweet wine** is for individuals who want to gain weight and strength; however, one should be watchful for any obstruction. **Aged red wine** is suitable for an individual with phlegmatic temperament.

Drinking wine after every type of meal is bad, and we have given the reason. Drinking should begin after the food has been digested and moved into the intestine. Drinking wine on food of bad chyme, and after it has been digested, is bad because it allows the bad chyme to go through the body; similarly, drinking wine on fruits, especially watermelon. It is better to start with small glasses rather than large. However, drinking two to three glasses with food for those used to it is not harmful, and the same after venesection of the healthy. Wine is beneficial to those with yellow bile by stimulating the gallbladder and to those with excess moisture in their bodies by accelerating its maturation. The more aromatic the tastier and better the wine. *Wine is the best facilitator for food penetration to all parts of the body.* It stops the formation of phlegm and breaks it down, and gets yellow bile out in the urine. It slips out black bile easily and antagonizes its effect; it loosens every condensed material without excessive abnormal heating. We will describe its characteristics in the proper section.

A person with a strong mind does not get drunk easily, and their brain does not accept the ascending harmful fumes; only the suitable heat of the wine reaches their brain and clears their mind like no other substance. Individuals with the opposite characteristic [i.e., weak mind] will get the opposite effect. A person with tightness and weakness of the chest in the winter should not drink in excess. Those who would like to drink a lot should not fill up on food and should have something diuretic in their food. If fullness of food and drink takes place, then one should stop, start drinking honey water, vomit, wash their mouth with vinegar and honey, and their face with cold water. If the harmful effect of drinking appears as warmness of the body and liver fever, then they should eat sour unripe grapes and the like; it also gets reduced by pomegranate water and sour citron (*Citrus medica*). When the harmful effect is in the head, one should reduce drinking and drink wine that has been clarified and settled and eat quince with it. When the harm appears in the stomach as heat, one should eat the roasted seeds of ilex and suck on disks of camphor and other materials that have astringency and acidity. If the wine-induced harm is stomach coldness the person should eat galingale (*Cyperus longus*), clove, or citron peel.

Know that aged wine is like medicine and not a type of food. Fresh wine is harmful to the liver and causes its excitement and hyperactivity due to effects of distention and bowel movement. The best wine is moderate in age between old and fresh, clear white to red, moderate in odor, and moderate in taste between acidic and sweet.

The good drink, known as the washed (المـغـسـول), is made by taking three parts of the [grape] juice and one part of water, boiled, and reduced by one-third.

When wine causes biting [in the stomach] it should be followed with sucking on pomegranate, cold water, drinking of absinth the next day, bathing, and reduced intake of food. The mixed drink [with water] relaxes the stomach and moistens it. It causes drunkenness faster due to the fast penetration of its watery portion; however, it clears the skin and the mental faculty. A smart person avoids drinking wine first thing in the morning, or before the organs have absorbed moisture in individuals with moisture, or after excessive movement, since these are harmful to the brain and the nerve and may cause spasm, confusion, hot humors, or diseases of hot humors.

Repeated drunkenness is very bad; it causes dystemperament of the liver and the brain, nervous weakness and diseases, dropsy, and sudden death. Excessive drinking of alcohol causes abnormal yellow bile in some stomachs and acidic vinegar in others; both are very harmful. Some are with the opinion that drunkenness once or twice a month is beneficial for the psychological faculty, relieves by inducing urine and sweat, and decomposes waste, especially from the stomach.

Note that most of the harmful effect of drinking is in the brain, thus a person with brain weakness should not drink unless it is little and mixed [i.e., diluted with water]. The right thing to do for someone who has drunk excessively is to induce vomiting if it is easy; otherwise, have them drink a lot of water, alone or with honey, then bathe in a bathtub, spread oil on the skin, and put them to sleep. Youth drinking is like adding fire to fire in a weak stove. The elderly may drink up to their tolerance. Young adults should drink moderately. It is better for young adults to drink aged wine mixed with pomegranate juice or mixed with cold water to stave off harmful effects and avoid dystemperament. Cold countries are suitable for drinking while hot countries are not.

One who intends to drink a lot should not fill up on food and sweets, but rather should drink fatty soup, eat porridge of bread or pasta in fatty soup and fatty meat cut into small pieces (all in moderation), avoid fatigue, and snack on salty almonds and lentils, as well as pickled capers. Also, eating cabbage and drinking olive water and alike are beneficial and helpful to drinking, furthermore, all that absorb vapor, like the seeds of common cabbage (*nabati*), cumin, dry common rue, pennyroyal, black salt (*nafty*), bishop's weed, and the foods that are viscous and nutritious. These foods concentrate the [alcohol] vapors [in the stomach], like viscous sweet and fatty foods, and prevent drunkenness, even though they do not absorb a lot of alcohol due to their slow absorption.

A weak brain is the reason for fast drunkenness, or due to excess humors in it. It may also be due to the strength of the drink, scarcity of food, and mismanagement of related matters.

Drinks to slow down drunkenness: mix one part of white cabbage water, one part of acidic pomegranate juice, and half part vinegar, boil, and drink one oka before starting drinking alcohol. Also, make pills from salt, common rue, and black cumin; dry and take one pill after another. Also, take cabbage seeds, cumin, peeled bitter almonds, pennyroyal, absinth, black salt, bishop's weed, and dry common rue; for those who will not be adversely affected by this drink's heat, they should drink two drams in cold water first thing in the morning.

To sober a drunk, give them water and vinegar three times in row, or onion juice and sour milk, also, sniffing camphor and sandalwood or placing repercussive coolers, like rose oil mixed with red wine vinegar. The treatment of hangover is mentioned in the particulars.

To get drunk quickly without harm, soak in the drink lichens or agarwood. One who requires heavy drunkenness in order to undergo a painful treatment of an organ should add an equal part of darnel water to their alcoholic drink or take one and a half dram of the following: fumitory, opium, and henbane, as well as one carat of nutmeg, gooseberry, and pure agarwood. The mixture is added to the drink as needed. Alternatively, boil the mixture of black henbane and mandrake peels until it becomes red; mix with the drink.

NINTH SECTION

Sleep and Wakefulness

The discussion of normal and abnormal sleep and their opposites, wakefulness and insomnia, and the actions to bring them on or to push them off, as well as the indications of each one of them and other topics, have been mentioned previously and will be also mentioned in the particular medicine. What is said here is that moderate sleep is empowering to the faculties' functions, soothing to the psyche, and a lot of sleep gives relaxation and prevents the disintegration of "spirit"—any type of "spirit" [i.e., promotes respiration in all body parts]. Therefore, sleep helps digestion and recovers the body from weakness due to the abnormal breakdown from fatigue, sexual intercourse, anger, and the like.

Moderate sleep, when it meets moderate humors in quantity and quality, induces moistness and warmth; this is best for the elderly since it preserves moisture and brings it back. For this reason, Galen mentioned that he eats *boqaileh** of cooked lettuce; the lettuce to induce sleep and the warmth of the cooking to balance the coldness caused by the lettuce. Galen said, "I am keen on sleep now." He meant that he is now an old man who needs the moistening benefit of sleep. This is the best regimen for insomniacs, and it is best if preceded with a bath (after the completion of food digestion) and with excessive pouring of hot water on the head; it is the best enhancer. However, the regimen that is stronger than this will be mentioned in the treatments.

Healthy individuals should sleep moderately and not excessively and should not harm their brains and faculties by staying up for long periods. Sometimes an individual stays up to prevent loss of consciousness and the fading of "power." The best sleep is the deep sleep after the food has passed its first digestion in the upper belly and the quieting down of distention and rumbling, since sleeping on them is harmful in many aspects and is not enjoyable and accompanied by tossing and turning. Therefore, a stroll is beneficial if the food is slow in its movement downward before going to bed.

Sleeping on an empty stomach is bad and weakens the "power." Equally bad is sleeping on a full stomach before the food moves down from the stomach. Both cases will prevent deep sleep and cause tossing and turning, and the latter causes unsettling and indigestion due to the body's engagement in digestion. Daytime sleeping is bad and causes diseases of humidity, catarrhs, corruption of skin color, sleep problems, laziness of nerves, sluggishness, weakness of appetite, swellings, and fevers. The reasons behind its problems are the ease of its interruption and the slowing down of [physiological] functions. Among the benefits of night sleep are its completeness, continuity, and deepness. However, the daytime sleeper should not switch to night sleep suddenly, but rather gradually.

The best **sleeping positions** are by starting on the right then switching to the left—recommended medically and religiously

---

*Boqaileh is cooked leafy vegetables.

[according to the prophet Mohamed]. Starting sleep facedown is very helpful for digestion due to keeping the belly warm. However, sleeping on the back is of low quality and helps induce bad diseases, like sudden death, palsy, and nightmare. This is because wastes gather and are stuck in the back away from the frontal ducts, like the nostrils and mouth. Sleeping on the back is a habit of weak patients due to the weakness of their muscles and organs, and thus cannot tolerate side sleeping since the back is stronger than the sides. Such individuals sleep with mouths open due to the weakness of the jaw muscles. There are two sections on this topic that we mentioned in the books on particulars that complete discussions on the topic.

Topics That Are Mentioned Here But Should Be Delayed

These topics include sexual intercourse, its modifications, and the treatment of its harmful effects (this will be mentioned in the other volumes of the book under the particulars), and the laxative drug and treating their harms (we place this in the article on laxatives), we recommend that the individual who aspires to preserve health practice gentle emesis, diuretics, sweating, and bloodletting (women do it naturally by menstruating).

The Strengthening of Weak Organs, Their Fattening, and Size Increase

Small and weak organs can be strengthened and enlarged. For individuals still in the growing phase, this is done with nutrition; however, in adults it is done with moderate massage and continuous exercise that is special for the organ, then covering with pitch resin.* Also, by holding

---

*Pitch resin is produced by the heating (dry distilling) of the green branches, which causes tar and pitch to drip away from the wood and leave behind charcoal.

the breath inside the organ if it is close to the chest and lungs. An example is in the individual with leg weakness, we apply constriction around the legs and then massage and cover with pitch on the first day. On the second day, we continue with massage and increase the exercise; the same applies for the third day unless there are signs of vessel enlargement and accumulation of material that may cause swelling and the organ's specific disease of fullness. Also, in this particular case, there is fear of developing varicose veins and elephantiasis. When such signs start to appear, exercise and massage are reduced, the individual is laid down, and the organ massaged in the opposite direction, beginning from its end to its origin.

If we want to carry out this process on an organ close to the respiratory organs, the chest, for example, we would wrap with moderate tightness at a position below it with a wide piece of cloth. This is followed with exercising the arms, holding the breath, shouting, talking in a loud voice, and gentle massage. These are details in the particular books; look them up in the Book of Cosmetics (كتاب الزينه).

TWELFTH SECTION

Fatigue That Follows Exercise

Types of fatigue are three and a fourth can be added, and they occur in two ways. The three types are **soreness, expandedness,** and **swollenness.** The additional, fourth one is **dryness** (hardness, brittleness).

The soreness fatigue is felt on the outer surface of the skin, similar to the touch of a sore, or deep in the skin. The most severe is the deepest, and it may be felt by touch or during movement, which may be felt as the pricking of a thorn. Individuals afflicted with it shun movement, even stretching, or they stretch weakly. When it is severe they shiver, and if the severity increases, their shivering becomes stronger and they develop fever. It is caused by excess of thin wastes or the disintegration of flesh and fat by severe movement. In general, they are bad humors that spread in the vessels, and their harm is broken down by good blood, so when they spread to the skin they are harmless.

This type of fatigue is the least harmful. Slight movement causes shivering, and excessive movement causes strong shivering; this may lead to the exit of sharp humors and the settling of the raw humors, which can be in the flesh.

The expandedness fatigue is felt as if the body has been beaten, with a feeling of heat and stretching; the afflicted person dislikes movement and stretching, especially if it is caused by fatigue. This type is produced from wastes that are trapped in the muscle; however, these are good in nature without burning or due to gas. These are distinguished by their lightness or heaviness. These occur after an incomplete sleep; however, if fatigue occurs after a complete sleep then it is of a different type that is worse. The most severe is the one that straightens the muscle parts.

Symptoms of swollenness fatigue are warmer than usual, similar to the swollen in size and color, painful to the touch and movement, and a feeling of distention. The dryness fatigue is a condition that feels as if the body has severe dryness and hardness; this occurs from excessive exercise on food of good chyme and the use of rough massage afterward. It may also occur due to air dryness, insufficiency of food, and fasting.

The cause of fatigue could be exercise, which is the safest and has specific methods of treatment. However, if it happens without a cause, then it is an introduction of a sickness and has its specific methods of treatment. Causes may occur in combination and in sequence, according to their initiation, which is either on their own or by exercise. If you know the treatments of the single fatigues you can apply them to the compound according to the instructions that I will tell you. Treatment should focus on the most important followed by the less important; the focus should be on strength, dominance of function, and integrity. If two or three of these are at hand, it is important that one does not dominate the other two because the latter two will weaken the first. An example of this is swollenness fatigue, which is stronger and dominant, but soreness fatigue is more advanced in its dystemperament and abnormal course, and thus resists the causes of swollenness fatigue and becomes dominant if swollenness fatigue has not already dominated the body.

THIRTEENTH SECTION

Stretching and Yawning

Stretching is due to accumulated wastes in the muscle; this is the reason it occurs often after sleeping. The increase of these humors causes shivering and spasm, and any further increase causes fever. Yawning is a form of stretching due to something in the muscles of the jaws and sternum. Its occurrence in the healthy has no reason, however, its excess is not good. The good type of yawning is that occurring at the last digestion. Yawning may be occurring to push wastes. Yawning and stretching may cause coldness and condensation, slowing of decomposition, and waking up before completing the cycle of sleeping. Their pushing action is the squeezing type. Equally mixed wine [one-to-one with water], unless otherwise contraindicated, is good for yawning and stretching.

FOURTEENTH SECTION

Treatment of Fatigue

Treating fatigue saves a person from many diseases, including fevers. When soreness fatigue starts to appear, exercise should be curtailed if it is the reason behind the fatigue; if it is due to an excess of humors, they should be removed from the diet; if it is due to recent indigestion [fullness], then treatment should include fasting, emesis, and cutaneous decomposition through a lot of massage with soft fat that lacks astringency. On the third day recuperative exercise should be applied. Food on the first day should be of the usual quality but less in quantity. On the second day, feed with moisturizers; however, if the vessels are clean and the humors are in the gut's fat, then massage may get them to mature, especially if warming medications reach them. The following medications are good for such conditions: oil of willow (*Salix babylonica,* شجره الغرب), oils of dill and chamomile and alike, the cooked beet root in oil on a water bath [double pot], oils of the root of marshmallow (*Althaea officinalis,* الخطمـي), squirting cucumber (*Ecballium elaterium*) and white bryony (الفاشرا), and oils of good lichens. All oils with lichens are suitable for this condition.

The aim in treating expandedness fatigue is to relax hardened tissue. This is done with gentle massage using sun-warmed oil, bathing in lukewarm water for long periods, sitting in the bathtub for two to three times, and applying oil after each bathing. If there is a dry area, oil should be applied to it. Food should be moist of a small quantity—less than in the case of soreness fatigue. Humors of expandedness fatigue are decomposed and spread out through exercise; however, if the fatigue is caused by thick waste, it will require emesis. Fatigue caused by expanding gas is decomposed by cumin, caraway, and anise.

The aims in treating swollenness fatigue are to relax the extended tissue, cool the warm tissue, and evacuate waste. These are achieved with long gentle massage, using a lot of lukewarm oil, lengthy lukewarm baths, and rest.

The treatment of dryness fatigue is a hotter than the usual bath. Very hot water condenses the skin and does not harm like cold water, where its hardening effect allows coldness to penetrate, especially in a skinny body (its skinniness may be due to the looseness of the skin). On the next day, the patient should do a gentle light exercise and bathe, as in the first day, then jump in a cold-water bath to condense the skin, reduce decomposition, and preserve moisture. This generates the heat and adaptation to resisting coldness; these two reasons cooperate to prevent the harm of coldness, especially if the individual is thrown in and pulled out instantly, since there is no reason to stay longer in the cold-water bath.

The patient should eat at noon a moist gentle food so that they can undergo another massage late in the afternoon or early evening; thus, the dinner should be delayed while the patient is massaged with sweet oil to assist in waste elimination. The oil massage should not touch the patient's belly unless they feel that something is wrong with belly muscles, then it should be massaged very gently. The patient should enlarge the diet, avoiding very hot food.

Every fatigue is caused by movement; therefore, if one stops at the beginning of the fatigue it prevents its occurrence. This should be followed by recuperative exercise so that the moderate movement pushes the materials to the skin; they are decomposed by massage between the exercises. Proper assessment can be carried out by bathing the patient; if bathing produces shivering, then there is excess of humor, especially if there is fever. In this case, bathing should be stopped and the patient should vomit to fix their dystemperament. On the other hand, if bathing does not cause any side effects, then the patient is benefiting from it.

If the vessels of the intestines contain hardened or raw humors, then the physician should attend first to the fatigue and later work on maturing the humors, softening them, and purging them. If there is an excess of humors, the patient should stop exercising and calm their movement since calm is more helpful for digestion. Venesection should not be applied because it often pushes out the pure and retains the raw. A laxative should not be given before maturation because it does not improve the situation and may cause harm. Induction of urine is fine. Avoid giving the patient warming substances [drink or food] because they will spread the raw humor in the body; their use should be gentle and in moderate amounts.

The diet should include pepper, caper, ginger, caper vinegar, garlic vinegar, assa-foetida vinegar and seeds, and jawarish. After maturation and the appearance of sediment in urine and the maturation of most of the humor, wine should be used to complete maturation and induce urine. The wine should be of the light and gentle quality. Emesis should not be used.

FIFTEENTH SECTION

Other Conditions That Fall under Exercise

These include **hardness, looseness,** and **overhydration.** Looseness is caused by gentle massage and bathing. It is also treated with gentle massage that is slightly hard [includes more pressure] with astringent oil. Hardness is caused by (1) cold, (2) an astringent, (3) an excess of thick or viscous waste that gets trapped in the skin pores, (4) an exercise that brings waste from inside without prior cause, (5) dusty atmosphere, or (6) strong, hard massage.

Hardness caused by cold or astringents gives white skin color, lower temperature, and reduced sweating; redness is regained by exercise. These patients should bathe in warm water and lay down in bath rooms of different moderate temperatures until they sweat, then rub gentle warming oils to help decomposition of wastes. However, if hardness is caused by exercise, then patients lack these symptoms and they have dirty skin. Treatment is by getting the wastes out through decomposing baths and oil rubs.

Hardness due to dusty conditions or the effect of harsh treatments [like hard massage] needs bathing rather than oil rub; patients will need a gentle massage before and after bathing.

Weakness and looseness may develop after excessive exercising that was not followed by massage, excessive sexual intercourse, and successive bathing. Treatment in this case is recuperative exercise and hard massage with astringent oil; the diet should consist of a small quantity of moisturizing food that is moderate in heat or slightly warming. This treatment should also apply to those with weakness, insomnia, depression, or dehydration due to anger; if these symptoms are accompanied by indigestion, then recuperative exercise or any other type of exercise is not suitable for them.

Due to an excess of bathing, food, drink, and excitement, an individual may feel that some of their organs contain moisturizing waste. This is especially felt in the tongue and may harm the functions of the organs. The causes are explained in the latter volumes of book on particular medicines; however, if this is due to that we mentioned above, like excess of drink, pleasures, and moisturizing bathing, then the patient should start hard exercise and rough massage without oil or with just a little warm oil.

Excessive dryness that is felt in the body is considered as a dryness fatigue and should be treated as such.

SIXTEENTH SECTION

Treatment of Spontaneous Fatigue

Soreness fatigue must be identified as to whether it is inside or outside the vessels. Indications of its presence inside are urine stinkiness, quality of consumed food, formation of wastes in the vessels, the speed of their elimination, and the need for treatment, as well as the quality of consumed drinks (pure or turbid). Otherwise, the fatigue is outside of the vessels and their inside is clean, and it can be treated only with recuperative exercise and the treatment mentioned for soreness fatigue due to exercise.

The other type cannot be treated with exercise but rather with rest, sleep, fasting, oil rubs, and bathing with moderately warm water (if the patient can tolerate it according to the condition we mentioned earlier), and food should be a small amount of good-quality chyme, such as watery soups of moderate nutrition like barely, spelt, and light meat of birds, and drinks like honey oxymel, diluted honey, and light white wine, which promote maturation and induce urine. The patient should start with wines that are slightly acidic and move gradually to the gentle white wine. If this measure does not help, it means that there is a dominant humor that should be pushed out. If the dominant humor is blood, venesection is in order; otherwise, give a laxative or other treatment for blood humor. However, you should not carry out any of these actions if the strength declines.

Indicators of the humor type are in the urine or sweat and the state of sleep or insomnia. If the patient cannot sleep despite your treatment, it is a bad sign. Upon concluding that the good blood in the vessels is scarce and the raw humors are the dominant ones, you should rest the patient and give them gentle and ameliorating food and drink that does not induce excessive heating. The drink, such as honey oxymel, should be causing the breakdown [of raw humors]. To increase the strength of the diet, add to the food, or to the barley drink, some pepper. If you deem it necessary, because of the extreme rawness of humors, use the amount of one small spoon of the cuminy or peppery oxymel before and after meals and before sleep. The pennyroyal oxymel is not suitable for these patients because it heats beyond what is required here.

If you conclude that the raw humors are not in the vessels but rather in the original organs, then massage them at noon with loosening viscous oils, give the patient warming drinks, keep them calm, bath them with moderately hot water, and give them the pennyroyal oxymel before meals and exercise without any worries. If a digestive is needed after a meal, do not give a strong transporter like the pennyroyal oxymel but rather ones like the cuminy, peppery (whichever is easier), or quince oxymels. However, you should check that the body of the patient is not hot before giving them these drinks. These patients will benefit from the spread of the oils of chamomile, dill, and oregano, alone or with wax; these also can be strengthened with fennel oil, or fennel oil by itself in one to twelve parts of oil.

If it is evident that the [raw] humors are inside and outside the vessels, then go after the larger of the two without neglecting the smaller one. If they are equal in distribution, then start the digestive action with the peppery oxymel, and you may add to it the seeds of wild celery and an equal amount of anise seeds to make it more diuretic. Also, you may mix it with some of the pennyroyal oxymel, but reduce the cuminy and peppery or gradually increase the pennyroyal oxymel until it becomes the only component; this is done when all the humors in the vessels have been digested and moved out and the only thing left is the raw humors outside of the vessels. The pennyroyal oxymel is beneficial in the second state and harmful in the first, as you have just learned. The patients with the two states [inside and outside raw humors] should not be given whatever pushes [the humors] in or out; therefore, no initial emesis, laxation, or exercise should be done unless it is preceded by amelioration, digestion, and maturation. Once the fatigue has stabilized, skin color improved, and urine matured, follow that with a lot of massage and gentle exercise; if the sickness returns then stop, otherwise continue their gradual return to their normal state of bathing, rubbing, massage, and exercise, and finally try to increase their mental alertness. If the fatigue returns to a recuperating patient with the feeling of sores, then repeat the treatment, but carry the recuperative exercise treatment if it is without the feeling of sores. The case of mixed, confusing signs without strong feeling of fatigue is treated with putting the patient to rest.

Expandedness fatigue is fullness without bad humors, and its treatment in bodies with dystemperament is venesection and amelioration regimen. In this case, the initial treatment should be amelioration and digestion [of the normal humors], then followed by assessment of the follow-up treatment.

Swollenness fatigue is treated by venesection from the vein that is suitable to the organ that is fatigued or in which the fatigue appeared initially. If the organs are equal in their condition, then carry out the venesection from the median cutaneous vein; you may have to repeat the next day and the third day. It is better to do the venesection on the first day when the symptoms appear so that the fatigue does not get hold [in the body] and in the evening of the second and third days. The patient's diet on the first day should be barley water or simple soup of spelt if there is no fever and only barley water if feverish. On the second day, add cold or moderate oil like almond oil. On the third day, add lettuce, cucurbits, mallow and its salad, the *homadhya*, ground fish, and soup. The patient should not be allowed to drink water if possible during these days. However, if they become impatient on the third and cannot digest their food, they may drink honey water or light white wine, pure or diluted. They should not be given a full meal after evacuation so that the undigested food does not rush inside the vessels, for three reasons. First, if the food amount is small it stays longer in the stomach (the retentive faculty of the stomach resists the attractive faculty of the liver); however, when it is plentiful the stomach aids its movement with its expulsive faculty; the same applies for every initial vessel in relation to the one that follows. Second, the excess is hard to digest in the stomach. Third, the excess of food goes to the vessels before it has been fully digested and cannot be fully digested in the vessels.

SEVENTEENTH SECTION

Management of Bodies' Dystemperament

These bodies are of two types: mistreated (acquired) or altered (innate). The mistreated are the ones that used to have good, mountainous temperaments that have become dystemperamental over time due to their mismanagement. The altered are the ones with initial dystemperaments. In the mistreated, the quality and quantity [of dystemperaments] should be determined so that they will be treated with antagonists; however, this is impossible if there is a fever. The altered dystemperament is the one where the dystemperament is a corruption of the initial temperament or a dystemperament of age.

CHAPTER 14

Health Management
of the Elderly

Third Lesson of the Third Art:
Health Management of the Elderly

- First Section: General Description
- Second Section: Diet of the Elderly
- Third Section: Wine of the Elderly
- Fourth Section: Opening Obstruction in the Elderly
- Fifth Section: Massaging the Elderly
- Sixth Section: Exercise of the Elderly

THIRD LESSON OF THE THIRD ART

Health Management
of the Elderly

(6 sections)

FIRST SECTION

General Description

Briefly, health management of the elderly is in the combined use of
moisturizing and warming foods, drinks, and baths; extended sleep by

staying in bed longer than young people; constant induction of urine; evacuation of phlegm from the stomach through the intestines and bladder; preservation of moisture through gentle massage in quantity and quality with oil rubbing; and walking or riding (if possible). The weak should be massaged often, applying a generous amount of moderately warm perfume, and rubbed with oil after sleep to stimulate the animalistic faculty; then use walking and riding.

SECOND SECTION

Diet of the Elderly

Foods should be divided into small portions and served in two or three servings according to their digestive strength and weakness. They should eat at three o'clock in the afternoon, good bread with honey; at seven o'clock in the evening; and after bathing, they should eat something that softens the bowels (as we will mention); and eat at dark good nutritious food. If the individual is strong, then the food portion should be increased slightly. They should avoid every dense food that generates black bile and phlegm and every sharp biting food, like pickles and spices (except when they are applied as medicine); however, if they do eat from the first type [that they should not], such as salty food such as eggplant, dried meat, flesh from the hunt, fish with hard flesh, watermelon, and cucumber, or make the mistake of eating from the second type, such as pickles, sardines, and milk, they should be treated with antagonists [of each food type]. Soothers should be used if it becomes obvious that they have waste, and fed with a moisturizing diet after cleansing and some soothers with the food. Milk benefits those that digest it and do not get distension in the liver or bowels. Milk induces sleep and moisturizes. The best is that of goats and donkeys. Donkey's milk does not curdle [denature] easily and is fast to digest, especially if mixed with salt and honey. The animal should not graze on pungent, hot, acidic, or salty plants.

Leafy vegetables and fruits consumed by the elderly should be like chard, celery, and a little of leek cooked in murri and oil, especially before the main course, to help in digestion. They will benefit from garlic if they are used to it. Ginger jam is a good medication for them, and so are other hot jams; therefore, they should be ingested according to the heat they generate and the digestion they promote and not according to the dryness they incur.

Their diet should be moisturizing, promoting digestion and warming and not dehydrating. Among the fruits that soothe their nature and their bodies are figs and pears (in summer) and figs cooked in honey water (in winter); all of these should be served before the main course to promote digestion; also boiled liblab cooked in salt, water, and oil; and the roots of common polypody (*Polypodium vulgare*, بسفايج) cooked in chicken soup or in the soup of chard or cabbage. If their bowels are soft every other day, then laxatives and softeners should not be used. However, if they are normal one day and constipated for two, then it is sufficient to use liblab, cabbage water, and safflower pith with barley milk, or the amount of one "walnut" or two (no more than three [weight measure = ~18.72 grams]) of pistacia (بطم) resin; this will evacuate the bowels without any harm. Also, they will benefit from the compound drug made of one part of safflower pith and ten parts of dry figs taken in the amount of one "walnut." An oil enema softens the bowels in addition to the evacuation it induces, especially if the oil is sweet. Hot enemas should be avoided because of their drying effect; however, the moist oily enema is the most beneficial if their constipation lasts for a few days. There are other laxative medications that we will mention in the formulary. Evacuation in the elderly must be as possible without venesection since moderate diarrhea is more suitable.

THIRD SECTION

Wine of the Elderly

The best wine for them is aged red wine, which is diuretic and warming together. They should avoid the young and white wine unless they have bathed after eating and felt thirsty; in this case they should drink light wine with little nutritious value; however, this is not a substitute for water. They should avoid the sweet and obstructive drinks.

FOURTH SECTION

Opening Obstruction in the Elderly

The easiest of these [obstructions to open] is the one caused by drinking alcohol. This should be opened with pennyroyal or peppery oxymels, or by sprinkling pepper on wine, or, if they are used to it, by the use of garlic and onion. The antidote (teryaq) is very beneficial in treating obstruction. Similarly, tansy (*Tanacetum vulgare,* أتـانـاسـيـا) and sea ambrosia (*Ambrosia maritima,* أمـبـروسـيـا، دمـسـيـسـه) are beneficial but require moisturizing by bathing and oil rubs afterward and eating meat soups with spelt and barley. Honey drink is good and prevents obstruction and joint pain. After the obstruction has developed and is felt in an organ, or at the feeling of impending obstruction, add the celery seeds and root for treating urinary organs; for stones, cook them with seeds of wild celery; for the lung, cook them with maiden hair fern, hyssop, and cassia.

FIFTH SECTION

Massaging the Elderly

The massage of the elderly should be moderate in quality and quantity without touching weak organs or the bladder. For multiple massages, it should be applied with a rough cloth and bare hands since this will be beneficial to them and prevents the relapse of their organ sicknesses. They also benefit from combining bathing and massage.

SIXTH SECTION

Exercise of the Elderly

Exercise of the elderly varies depending on the state of their bodies, illnesses, and habits of exercise. For the elderly with moderately healthy bodies, they can do moderate exercise. In the presence of a weak organ, its exercise should be connected to the exercise of the other organs; for example, when the elderly suffer from headache, epilepsy, or the pouring of substances in the neck and the frequent ascension of vapors to the head and brain, they should avoid exercise that requires lowering the head; however, they should exercise by walking, riding, and every exercise that affects the lower half of the body. If the illness affects a leg, they should use upper body exercises like weight lifting, throwing stones, and lifting stones. If the illness is in the middle part of the body like the spleen, liver, stomach, and intestines, then exercise of the upper and lower extremities should be fine. If the illness is in the chest, then upper body exercise is the only suitable one. They should gradually include the weak organs in the exercise to strengthen them. These instructions are for the elderly and differ from the other age groups, and also from the very old, that have different tolerance; they should strengthen the weak organs by gradually doing exercises that are suitable to the organs; however, the ill organs may be exercised, but not if they are warm or dry or contain substances that could become putrefied and lack maturation.

CHAPTER 15

Management of the Dystempered Body

FOURTH LESSON OF THE THIRD ART

Management of the Dystempered Body

(5 sections)

FIRST SECTION

Treatment of Hot Dystemperament

Hot dystemperament is either with two other balanced reactants [wetness and dryness] or the dominance of one of them. When the two reactants are balanced, it becomes evident that the increase in heat is moderate and not excessive; otherwise, it would cause dehydration. Hot dystemperament with dryness may increase the duration of the dystemperament; on the other hand, hot dystemperament with wetness does not last for long; they alternate in dominance; sometimes the wetness dominates and extinguishes the excess heat, and other times the heat dominates and dries up the wetness.

A person dominated by wetness will be in a better state in old age when wetness becomes balanced; however, later in old age the wetness and heat decline, and abnormal wetness increases.

In general, management of individuals with hot temperament has two goals: first, to bring them back to balance, and second, to preserve their health. The first goal is best suited to those who are calm, self-sufficient, and patient to tolerate the gradual process of bringing their bodies back to balance over a long period, since trying to do it quickly may cause illness. The second goal is realized through diet that opposes temperament to preserve health.

Those of hot temperament and balanced in the two reactants [wetness and dryness] are healthy in the early stages of life, and their temperament is suitable for the rapid growth of teeth and hair, as well as good speech and speedy walk. However, if their heat becomes excessive and dryness increases, they develop irritant temperament and generate lots of yellow bile. These should be managed as having balanced temperament; however, when they move to the hot category, they should be treated with diuretics and evacuation of bile in the normal direction of their waste (i.e., purgation and emesis). If nature does not help in the elimination, then it should be encouraged by light substances. Emesis can be accomplished with excessive drinking of hot water, alone or mixed with wine, and purgation with viola jam, tamarind, mana (exudate from *Atraphaxis cotoneaster,* المن، شيرخشت), and *Genista purgans* (الترنجبين); additionally, lighter exercise, a diet of good chyme, three baths a day, and avoiding every cause of heating. If bathing does not cause distention or obstruction in the area of the liver and abdomen, they should use it safely; otherwise, they should use openers, such as the infusion of absinth, aloe, anise, bitter almonds, and oxymel, and abstain from bathing after meals. These openers should be drunk after the digestion of the first meal and before taking in the second meal. In the period between the two meals, they should bathe and rub oil, as well as drink light white wine and cold water. All of this is more beneficial to individuals with dry hot temperament.

Individuals with wet hot temperament are susceptible to putrefaction and the movement of substances to their organs. Therefore, they should do a lot of light exercise to break down material, but not to generate heat, and avoid movements that make the humors generate pustules. Those in this category who are not used to exercise should avoid doing it; the most proper for them is to do it after evacuation, to bathe before eating, and to purge all wastes. In the early spring, they should carry out venesection and cleansing.

SECOND SECTION

Treatment of Cold Dystemperament

There are three types of these [cold and wet, cold and dry, and cold and balanced in wetness and dryness]. Individuals with two balanced reactants (wetness and dryness) should increase their heat with hot foods that are moderate in moisture and dryness, warming oils, grand pastes, humidity-specific cleanser, sweat-inducing baths, and suitable exercise. Even though they are balanced in moisture, their wetness may increase if they are in a cold place. Individuals with dry cold dystemperament should be managed like the elderly.

THIRD SECTION

Treatment of Susceptible Bodies

Individuals with bodies that are susceptible to disease are in such condition due to their fullness. Thus, they require balancing of the quantity of humors or, due to the rawness of the humors, require the balancing of their qualities. Their food should be moderate in quantity since the balancing of humors is done by balancing the quantity of food, increased exercise, massage before bathing (if they are used to it, or by the lighter of the two [exercise or massage] if they are not used to it), and by dividing the meals over a period of time to avoid fullness in one session. If their bodies are easy to sweat then they should be made to sweat several times. If delaying food does not bring bile into the stomach, then food should be eaten after the bath, and the best time for this is four o'clock in the afternoon of the equitable day. The drawing of bile into the stomach necessitates early eating; however, if this induces obstruction in the liver, the individual should be treated with the mentioned openers that are compatible with their temperament. If this induces harm to the head, it should be treated by walking. If the food gets corrupted in the stomach and induces diarrhea, then this is a benefit; otherwise, induce diarrhea with cumin, oxymel, and the figs cooked with safflower that we mentioned.

FOURTH SECTION

Fattening of the Skinny

The strongest causes of leanness, as we will describe, are dryness of temperament, dryness of the mesentery, and dryness of the atmosphere. Dryness of the mesentery causes less absorption of food; therefore, it is treated by massage before bathing, where the rubbing is moderate (between soft and rough) until the skin gets reddish, then the rubbing becomes harder, and finished by rubbing pitch resin. The massage is followed by moderate exercise and immediately into the bath. Rough, dry towels should be used for drying, followed by rubbing oil and eating suitable food. If the individual's age, season, and habit can tolerate cold water, then they should pour it on themselves. The massage mentioned above before applying pitch resin should end when tissue engorgement starts to disappear, which is similar to what we mentioned about the enlargement of small organs. The full description is in the Book of Cosmetics of the 4th Book.

FIFTH SECTION

Thinning of the Obese

The treatment involves acceleration of food's exit from the stomach and intestines so that it does not get completely absorbed; using a large quantity of low-nutritious food; bathing frequently before eating; fast exercise; as well as applying disintegrating oils and pastes such as small Arabian pea (bitumen or pitch trefoil, *Psoralea bituminosa*, الاطريفل), massage medicine, and teryaq antidote; also drinking vinegar with murri on an empty stomach in the morning.

CHAPTER 16

Transitions, Seasonal Management, and Travelers

Fifth Lesson of the Third Art: Transitions and Seasonal Management, Traveling

- First Statement: Transitions and Seasonal Management (1 section)
- Second Statement: A Statement on the Management of Travelers (8 sections)

FIRST STATEMENT

Transitions and Seasonal Management

FIRST SECTION

Transitions and/or Seasonal Management

Early in the spring, venesection and purgation should be carried out according to the necessities and habit, and especially to apply emesis. One should abandon warming and moisturizing meats and drinks, simplify the diet, exercise harder than in the summer, not get full on food, and set apart meals, as well as use cooling drinks and extracts and not hot, bitter, acrid, and salty ones.

In the summer, one should reduce food, drinks, and exercise; stay calm; use cooling substances; apply emesis if possible; and stay in the shade and avoid direct exposure to the sun.

In the fall, and especially in a fall of changing weather, one should take the best precautions, such as abandoning all drying substances [dehydrators] and avoiding: sexual intercourse, drinking excessive cold water and pouring it on the head, sleeping in a cold place that causes goosebumps, sleeping on a full stomach, noontime heat, cold mornings, and fruits of the season. One should protect the head at night and in the morning from cold and bathe in warm water only. At the equinox, emesis should be carried out in order to prevent the congestion of waste during the winter. In most bodies, the fall is not the right time to work on their humors and get them moving, and it is better to keep their humors calm. Emesis is not recommended in the fall because it induces fever. As for wine, the heavy varieties should be used, but without excess. Plenty of rain in the fall protects from the season's bad effects.

In the winter, one should do a lot of exercise and consume plenty of food; however, if it is a southerly winter, one should increase the exercise and reduce food consumption. The wheat bread of the winter should be more nutritious and denser than that of the summer, and the same should be applied to meats, kabobs, and alike. Green, leafy vegetables should be like cabbage, chard, and celery, and not white goosefoot, amaranth, purslane, and true endive. It is very rare that healthy bodies become sick in the winter; however, if it occurs, treatment should be carried out promptly and emesis induced (if needed). Disease will not take place unless there is a serious cause, especially if it is a hot disease, because the innate heat, which is the prime force, becomes very strong in the winter from the digested and released food, as well as its accumulation; additionally, all the natural faculties are functioning well. Hippocrates recommends purgation in the winter over venesection, and he dislikes emesis, although he favors it in the summer, because the humors are floating in the summer and sedentary in the winter;

we should follow his opinion. If the air becomes corrupt and epidemical, one should take precaution by drying the body and adjusting the residence with substances that cool and humidify by their action—this is the correct action in an epidemic—or carry out a warming action against the corrupting element. Pleasant perfumes are the most effective in this regard, especially if they are antagonistic to the temperament favoring the epidemic.

In an epidemic, one should reduce excessive intake of air through ventilation and distribution. Very often, the source of air corruption is from the ground; therefore, it is preferred to sit on sofas and seek well-aerated, high locations for residence. Frequently, the air itself is the source of corruption due to its mixing with neighboring contaminated air or an inexplicable atmospheric cause. In this case, it is better to seek shelter in houses that are surrounded by walls and bedrooms. The incenses most suitable for treating corruption of air are galingale, oliban (Boswellia gum), myrtle, roses, and sandalwood. *The use of vinegar during epidemics is protective.* We will mention the rest of this in the particular books.

A Statement on the Management of Travelers

(8 sections)

FIRST SECTION

Management of Early Symptoms of Illness

An individual with constant palpitation should get treatment to avoid sudden death. Excessive nightmares and dizziness should be treated by purging the great humor [the one in excess] so that the patient does not develop epilepsy and apoplexy. Frequent trembling in the body must be treated by removing the phlegm to avoid spasms and apoplexy; similarly, an extended period of dullness of the senses and weakness of movement with [a feeling of] fullness, especially numbness of all senses, must be managed by eliminating phlegm to prevent partial paralysis.

Frequent trembling of the face is treated by cleansing the brain to prevent facial paralysis. Frequent redness of the eye and face with running tears, photophobia [fear of light], and headache should be treated by venesection and purgation and alike to avoid meningitis. An increase of depression or anxiety without a reason and an increase of fear are treated by the elimination of charred humor so that the individual does not get melancholy. Furthermore, if the face becomes red, puffed, and darker in color, and lasts, it is sign of leprosy. If the body feels heavy and tired with fullness of vessels then venesection should be carried out to avoid the rupture of a vessel, apoplexy, or sudden death. The puffiness of the face, eyelids, and extremities indicates that the liver should be treated; otherwise, the individual may develop edema. Very malodorous stools should be managed by removing putrefaction from the vessels to prevent fevers. Also, malodorous urine is a stronger indication of putrefaction. Fatigue and pain are indicative of impending fever. A decreasing or increasing appetite is indicative of illness; in general, every unusual, quantitative, or qualitative change in appetite, stools, urine, sexual desire, sleep, sweat, skin, attention, taste, or dreaming is a forewarning of illness; likewise are abnormal habits such as hemorrhoids, menorrhea, vomiting, nosebleed, or strong desire for something that is corrupt or good. Habits are like nature; therefore, the very bad ones [practiced for a long time] are abandoned gradually.

Some specific signs may be indicators of other specific issues; for example, persistent headache and migraine forewarn of water going into the eye [cataract], and seeing a spot in front of the eye like an insect and alike; if it persists and becomes permanent and the eyesight weakens, it is indicative of cataract. Persistent heaviness and pain in the right side are indicative of illness in the liver. Heaviness and distention in the lower back and waist accompanied by change in urine forewarn of kidney illness. A stool with much less color than usual is a sign of jaundice. A long duration of burning urination is a sign of ulceration of the bladder and urethra. Diarrhea with a burning sensation to the anus is a portent of ulceration. Loss of appetite associated with vomiting, distention, and aching extremities is a sign of approaching colic. Stomach itching [irritation], without small worms in it, is indicative of hemorrhoids. An excess of boils and lipomas is a sign of many cold abscesses. Ringworm will cause black leukoderma, while vitiligo is a sign of white leukoderma.

SECOND SECTION

Comprehensive Statement on the Management of the Traveler

Travelers will not have some of the things that they are used to in their native setting and may get tired and sick; therefore, they should be keen on treating themselves so that they do not develop many diseases. The most important aspects are diet and fatigue.

The traveler should eat good food of good nature, in reasonable but not large quantity, that is easily digestible and does not produce waste in the vessels. The traveler should not ride on a full stomach to avoid putrefaction and should not drink water in excess to avoid shaking that causes vomiting and lying down. Food should be delayed until the end of the ride (unless there is a reason that we explain later); however, if eating is a must, the traveler should eat a small amount for the sake of entertainment that will not induce thirst, whether the travel is during the night or the day.

The traveler should manage their fatigue according to what we describe in the chapter on fatigue. The traveler should not travel with fullness in blood humor or other humors, but rather should cleanse the body, then travel. When having indigestion before travel, the traveler should fast, sleep, and resolve the indigestion before traveling. The traveler should gradually exercise more than usual. If the traveler has to stay up at night during travel, they should gradually build up their tolerance; the same for getting used to hunger, thirst, and other matters.

Also, the traveler needs to get used to the type of food they will be eating during the travel; they need to make their food low in quantity and high in quality and abandon leafy vegetables, fruits, and all that may produce raw humor unless necessary for treatment with certain quantities. The traveler may have to prepare to tolerate hunger and diminish appetite; this can be done by eating a diet of roasted liver and alike that can also be prepared as a kabob and eaten with heavy soups and melted fats mixed with almonds and almond oil. Fats such as beef fat help the individual tolerate hunger for a measured period. It has been said that if a human drinks the amount of one "pound"* of viola's oil, mixed with melted wax to bring it to the consistency of cerate,† they will not have appetite for ten days. Travelers should be prepared for thirst and carry with them thirst-quenching medications, which we have explained in the 3rd book under the chapter on thirst, especially among these are purslane seeds (three drams in vinegar); abandon thirst-inducing

---

*In this case, a "pound" is equal to 373.24 grams.

†Cerate (from the Latin *cera*, "wax") is a soft preparation for external application that is intermediate between that of an ointment and a plaster in consistency. Cerate consists of wax mixed with oil, lard, and various medicinal ingredients. The cerate of the United States pharmacopoeia is a mixture of three parts of paraffin and seven parts of lard. The wax can be substituted with resin or spermaceti.

foods like fish, capers, and salted and sweet foods; reduce talking; walk slowly; drink water mixed with vinegar since a little bit of it silences thirst when water is scarce; and drink the seed mucilage of blond psyllium (*Plantago ovata*).

THIRD SECTION

Precautions for Hot Weather, Especially for Travel and the Management of Travelers

Those who do not take precautions will end up weak without strength and eventually cannot even move and will be dominated by thirst. The sun may harm their brains; therefore, they should cover very well their heads from the sun. The traveler should also protect their chest and rub on it the mucilage of psyllium or purslane juice. Travelers may want to eat or drink something before embarking, such as *suewaiq** of barley, fruit drinks, and others. Hungry travelers will get weaker as they will consume the nutrients in their bodies without replenishment; therefore, they should eat something as we mentioned above and wait until it passes through the stomach so it does shake in their bellies. They should take with them oils of rose and violet to sprinkle them each hour on their heads. Those who are harmed from traveling in hot weather will recover by swimming in cold water; the proper way is not to rush into the water but to gradually get immersed in it. Travelers who are afraid of the very hot and dry wind called *samoum* (Arabic) should cover their nose and mouth with a scarf and tolerate this hardship. Additionally, before traveling in samoum conditions, the traveler should eat an onion cooked or soaked overnight in buttermilk and drink the buttermilk; the onion should be cut into small pieces before soaking it in the buttermilk. To protect from the harmful effects of samoum, the traveler should rub oils of rose and pumpkin. Those affected by the samoum need to pour

---

Suewaiq is an old dish in the Arabian culture made of barley, dates, butter, and cardamom. It is made from the flour of roasted wheat or barley.

cold water on their extremities and wash their faces; eat cooling leafy vegetables; and put cooling oils on their heads, such as rose oil, juice of houseleeks (*Semipervivum*), and oil of willow; then wash and abstain from sex; salty fish is beneficial if symptoms calm down; mixed wine is also good; milk is the best food if there is no fever. Buttermilk is used when the fever is ephemeral and not due to putrefaction. A mouthwash rather than drinking should be used to quench the thirst; however, if it is necessary to drink it should be sip after sip until the discomfort of thirst stops. Before drinking large amounts of water, it is better to mix it with rose water; it is the proper thing to do. Heat-struck individuals should sit in a cool place and wash the feet with cold water, drink cold water, little by little, and eat food that is easy to digest.

FOURTH SECTION

Precautions for Travelers in Cold Weather and Frost

Traveling in cold weather is very dangerous, even when prepared for it, let alone without preparation. Numerous travelers wrapped with everything they could to keep warm were killed by cold and windy snowstorms from spasm, lockjaw, freezing, and apoplexy. Their deaths are similar to those who died from opium or mandrake. If they do not die, they usually reach a state of hunger called bulimia (we have mentioned the treatment in this case and others in the proper place). The first steps to take are to close the skin pores, cover the nose and mouth to prevent cold air from going in, and protect the extremities according to what we will mention. The traveler affected by the cold should gradually warm up and should not get close to the fire source very soon. It is better not to get close to the fire; however, if they have to, they should do it gradually. These steps are for travelers who have not been severely weakened by the cold. However, if the traveler develops frosts in the extremities they should be quickly warmed and rubbed with warming oils, especially those with *teryaq* [antidote] property, such as lily oil.

When cold and hungry travelers eat hot food, they will develop abnormal heat. There are foods that make traveling in the cold easier; these are the ones with lots of garlic, walnuts, mustard, and asafetida. Milk whey can be added to improve the taste of garlic and walnuts. Ghee is also good for travelers, especially if they follow it with undiluted wine. Traveling in cold weather should not be on an empty stomach; the traveler should eat well and drink wine instead of water, wait until it moves out of the stomach, they feel warm, and then depart. Asafetida warms up the frozen in the cold, especially if it is mixed in wine. A complete drink is a dram of asafetida in one "pound" (ratell [Arabic], رطل) of wine.

There are rubs for the traveler in the cold to put on the skin to prevent the effect of the cold; some of these are oils and others. Garlic is the best for traveling in cold wind, even though it is harmful to the brain and mental health.

FIFTH SECTION

On Protecting the Extremities from Harmful Effects of Cold

The Extremities should first be massaged until they become warm, then rubbed with warming oils such as lily oil and frankincense oil. The alcoholic extract of lily makes a good rub; however, when it is unavailable, oil can be used, especially when it is mixed with pepper, pellitory, euphorbia, asafetida, and castoreum. Among the wraps that protect the extremities are the ones containing galbanum and garlic, which is safe, unlike pitch resin. The slippers and gloves should not be tight on the feet and palms such that they cannot move. Movement is important to keep coldness away, and the smothered organ will be severely affected by the cold. It is better to protect the organ by covering with paper and wool cloth made of long or short hair.

If the leg or the hand stops feeling the cold [i.e., has become numb due to frosting] without decrease in coldness or increase in their protection, then the feeling in them is getting destroyed by the coldness, and treatment should start from what you have learned here. If the cold extinguishes the innate heat of the organ and the products of its decomposition are trapped within, putrefaction may develop; the treatment in this case may be similar to that of pustules, especially gangrene. However, if the organ has frosted and is on its way to become putrefied, then the proper action is to place it in ice water specifically or in cooking water of figs, cabbage, basil, dill, or chamomile; all of these are good. A poultice of fatty buttermilk is good. Also, the water of absinthe (wormwood), pennyroyal, mint, or thyme, and wrapping with turnip are good treatments. The patient must avoid getting close to fire and should walk and move the affected extremity by exercising and massaging it, then rub, smear, and rinse with mentioned treatments. It should be known that leaving the extremities still in the cold without movement or exercise is the strongest reason for their frosting. Some people soak the affected extremity in cold water and find benefit that removes the harm, similar to putting frozen fruits in cold water, which removes the freezing, tightens, softens, and ripens them. However, if the fruits are placed near fire they will be ruined. Understanding the mechanism here is not needed for the physician.

If the color of the affected extremity starts to change, it must be slit and allow blood to flow out while the part is immersed in warm water to prevent the blood from freezing at the bleeding slit and allow it to bleed until it stops on its own. Afterward, it should be smeared with Armenian clay* and diluted vinegar to prevent its putrefaction. Tar works at the beginning and the end. If the color becomes black and green and starts to rot, do not do anything else besides cutting out the rotten part quickly to prevent its spread to healthy neighboring parts and to prevent the infection from spreading. Follow what we have mentioned in its chapter.

---

*Armenian bole (bolus armenus, bole armoniac) is an earthy clay, usually red, supposed to be native to Armenia. Its red color is due to the presence of iron oxide; it also contains hydrous silicates of aluminum and possibly magnesium.

SIXTH SECTION

Protecting Skin Color during Travel

The face should be coated with viscous materials such as the mucilage of the seeds of blond psyllium, sap of milk vetch or its extract diluted in water, diluted gum [several species], egg white, a water-soaked cake made of cream of wheat, and a disk made from Criton's* recipe. If the skin cracks from the effect of wind, cold, or the sun, seek treatment in the Book of Cosmetics [a separate book].

SEVENTH SECTION

Protecting the Traveler from the Harms of Various Waters

The variation in water may cause more illnesses than the variation in foods; therefore, precaution should be taken to manage the water issue. Among the precautions are allowing it to settle, filtering it through ceramic, and boiling it. As we have shown, these methods may remove impurities and separate the pure water from its contaminants; the best is distillation. Another method is using a wool wick between two containers, one filled with water and the other empty; the water will start dripping into the empty container; this is a type of settling and is better repeated. Bitter and low-quality water may be improved by boiling it, adding pure clay and strands of wool, then taking the wool out and squeezing the water out, which should be better than the original. Water can be purified by mixing it with pure clay, especially clay burned by the sun, then filtering it. Mixing water and wine reduces the harmful effect of water contamination, especially the type of contamination that has less penetration [i.e., microorganisms]. When water is scarce it should be mixed with vinegar, especially in the summer, to reduce thirst and demand. Salty water must be drunk mixed with vinegar and

---

*Criton of Heraclea was a second-century (ca. 100 CE) Greek chief physician. He wrote a work on cosmetics in four books, which were very popular in Galen's time.

oxymel, as well as with carob, myrtle, and azarole thrown in.

After drinking water contaminated with alum, a laxative or wine should be taken. Bitter water should be followed with fatty and sweet food or the water mixed with *jallab*.* Also, drinking water of chickpeas before drinking bitter water or alike pushes away its harm; similarly, eating chickpeas has the same protective effect. Drinking from stagnant putrid water should not be accompanied by hot food; however, it should be consumed with astringent and cold fruits like quince, apples, and red currants, as well as leafy vegetables like lettuce. Drinking thick turbid water should be followed by eating garlic. It can be purified with Yemeni alum. Onion neutralizes the contamination of various waters; it is an antidote, especially the mixture of onion, vinegar, and garlic.

It is good practice for those who travel between areas with different waters to carry with them water from their hometown and mix it with the water of the first destination, then mix the latter with that of the second destination, and continue to do so until reaching their final destination. Also, one can carry clay from their hometown in order to mix it with water and shake it, and then let it settle before drinking it. A filter must be used when drinking water to prevent leeches from being swallowed. One should not fill up on bad humors. Travelers should carry with them acid concentrates to mix with various waters as a good precaution.

EIGHTH SECTION

Precautions for the Maritime Traveler

During the early days of the voyage, a traveler by sea may develop dizziness or become disoriented, and progress to nausea and vomiting, then calm down and stabilize. The traveler should not try to suppress their nausea and vomiting unless excessive. However, precautions to prevent vomiting are fine to apply, achieved by eating fruits such as quince,

---

*Jallab (Arabic, جلاب) is a popular sweet summer drink in the Middle East made from carob, dates, grape molasses, and rose water.

apples, and pomegranates. A drink of celery seeds prevents nausea from exacerbating and calms it down when it occurs. Absinthe has the same effect. Also preventive are astringents that strengthen the mouth of the stomach and prevent vapors from going upward to the head, such as lentils with vinegar, sour grapes, pennyroyal, and Persian thyme, or bread cooled in a basil drink or cold water (possibly with Persian thyme), and to rub the nostrils with white lead.

ASPECTS OF TREATMENTS ACCORDING TO GENERAL DISEASES

32 Sections

Disease is treated by the opposite and health is preserved by the similar. . . . Usually we treat the disease rather than its symptoms unless the symptoms become more dangerous.

AVICENNA

In this part of the *Canon*, Avicenna deals with thirty-two topics that include aspects of the patient's diet management; basis for selecting medicinal drugs; treatment of abnormal temperaments; purgation through diarrhea, emesis, enema, lotions, douches, venesection, cupping; and use of leeches; stopping of purgation; treatments of obstructions and swellings; incisions; amputation; dislocation of organs; cauterization; pain relief; and priority of treatment. The usage of the term *power* as used by Avicenna throughout his book signifies the metabolic strength and health of an organ or the whole body.

Avicenna elucidates how diet management is part of the patient's treatment (1st Section). He outlines reasoning for selecting the quantity and quality of food and how these two aspects depend on the interplay between preserving the strength of the patient and reducing the severity of the disease. Furthermore, Avicenna deals with aspects of digestion and absorption and the characteristics of the ingested and digested food as its components mix with the blood and affect its consistency and function.

On selecting drugs for treatment, Avicenna clarifies here the rules governing this topic, such as drug temperament, potency, and time of administration, as well as how the choice of a drug depends on the nature of the affected organ, which includes the organ's temperament, structure, position, and "power" of its metabolic health. The latter is related to the importance of the organ to the whole body, its shared functions with other organs, and its drug sensitivity. The choice of the drug also depends on the severity of the disease, its phase, and duration. Avicenna reiterates here the importance of including the six factors (fresh clean air, food and drink, movement and rest, sleep and wakefulness, eating, exercising, and healthy mental state) that are necessary for good health as complementary to a successful treatment. He also outlines the strategy for treating dangerous diseases, dealing with ambiguous illness and its confusing diagnosis, handling an organ's drug sensitivity, and strengthening the psychological and animalistic faculties of the patient.

In the section on treating dystemperament (2nd Section), Avicenna clarifies three ways of dealing with dystemperament; he calls them absolute treatment (allopathic), progressive preservation, and simple progressive preservation (prophylaxis), and cites examples on each. He details the complications related to each dystemperament, offers solutions, warns about harming the innate heat along each step, and gives away some of the "tricks of the trade" for mixing drugs to strengthen the targeted organ and amplify the effect of the drug.

Elimination of waste humors associated with causing disease, by various methods, is an important modality in Unani medicine that is applied to restore or preserve health (3rd Section). In this section, Avicenna enumerates the factors that determine the readiness for elimination and their contraindications, as well as the five goals of elimination. He covers the two strategies for elimination through the distant opposite or the proximate opposite and explains them with examples. He then delves into how venesection is an indiscriminate drainer of all types of humors and the safe approaches of applying venesection. He also compares the actions of diarrhea, emesis, and venesection as to the areas that they cleanse and the direction of elimination. He further explains when to apply each of the methods of elimination or otherwise treat with medications and how the emetic drugs become laxatives and vice versa. Additionally, he specifies how the drug should be compatible with the targeted humor, lists a few scenarios where the process may go unexpectedly awry, and describes who should use these methods of elimination and when.

In the 5th Section, Avicenna follows with the rules of purgation, starting with the preparation for purgation, individuals who should not take laxative drugs, the various conditions of purgation, the drugs' actions and reactions, purgation diet, and dealing with the side effects of purgation (sections 5–7).

Avicenna starts the 11th Section on emesis by listing the individuals who should not undergo emesis and its contraindications, followed by diet for emesis (before and after), times of emesis, the cleansing effect of emesis (its goals, phases of emesis, signs of ineffective emesis), the procedure to apply after emesis (12th Section), benefits of emesis (13th Section), harmful effects of excessive emesis (14th Section), and managing the side effects after emesis (15th and 16th Sections).

In a brief section on enema (18th Section), Avicenna covers the benefits of using enema and its side effects, as well as body position and time of its application. The reasons for the use of lotions and wraps as well as douches in disease treatment are well explained in the 19th and 20th Sections.

On venesection (21st Section), Avicenna describes at length many aspects of venesection. He explains why and when venesection is needed, the types of patients who will benefit, the diseases it preempts, and its contraindications. Avicenna enumerates the veins and arteries that can be venesected, the location and direction of incisions for each vessel, and the specific benefit from the venesection of each vessel. He also addresses a panoply of complications that may arise during venesection.

Following the style of other sections, Avicenna in the section on cupping (22nd Section) explains the mode of action of cupping, its benefits, contraindications, locations on the body, and the characteristics of each location and the effect of its cupping. He also indicates when cupping is done with fire (hot cupping) and with or without scarification of the skin, the age for cupping, and diet for the cupped.

In the section on leeching (23rd Section), Avicenna describes the characteristics of the poisonous leeches, which should not be used in medical treatment, and those that are safe. He further describes the types of water sources that are fine to find leeches and those that are not favorable for this purpose, and the leech's benefit in drawing out blood, preparation of the leech, preparation of the patient's skin, cupping after leeching, removing the leech, and treating the skin after the removal of the leech.

Sometimes it is necessary to stop ongoing *depletions* or those that were started by treatment modalities. Avicenna cites several examples of various types of depletions and prescribes the methods to stop them, divert them, or encourage them in order to stop them (24th section).

The obstruction of vessels and organs is addressed in the 25th Section, where Avicenna explains the nature of humors that may cause the blockage, the methods and strategies to remove the obstruction, and precautions when treating obstructions.

Avicenna has classified swellings in the 2nd Art of his 1st Book (chapter 2 in this book); however, in this 26th Section, he outlines the different treatments of swellings. He explains the use of a combination of drugs and techniques to cause warming, softening, desiccation, resolving, draining, and maturation of all types of swellings, such as solid, unripe, gaseous, internal, and hot and cold swellings. Additionally, he recommends the use of cupping, piercing, and venesection in some situations to treat swellings.

Avicenna briefly covers the basics on making incisions in the 27th Section. He describes the direction of the incision, the qualifications of the practitioner, the preparations for the process, and some precautions on incising an abscess. He follows this with a section on organ degradation and amputation, where he describes removing degraded flesh and the conditions that necessitate amputation of the organ (28th Section). He also describes the steps of the amputation surgery.

The 29th Section covers a number of related topics on the treatments of discontinuity, ulcers, sprain, trauma, and falling. Avicenna discusses the treatment of discontinuity in bone fractures and soft tissues; the principles that should be followed in the case of discontinuity in soft organs; treatment of ulcers by chemicals, cauterization, and manually, and the formation of scabs; treating the dystemperament of the ulcer and its organ; consideration of the strength of the desiccant drugs; and the interplay between drying the ulcer and the diet. He also discusses the treatment of a rip and the probable accompaniment of a nerve split, as well as sprains.

According to Avicenna, there are several good reasons to carry out cauterization (30th Section). He describes how to cauterize hidden locations of the body and the precautions for doing it, stopping bleeding with cauterization, the depth and limit of cauterization, and cauterizing spots on the head.

On the topic of pain relief (31st Section), Avicenna explains briefly the causes of pain and its consequences, as well as its treatment strategies. He clarifies the use of resolvents, laxatives, purgatives, and alike in pain relief, as well as anesthetics and their types. He advocates consideration of the side effects of the anesthetic versus the relief that the patient gets. He also favors the use of the simplest form of the anesthetic and compound forms if antidotes are available to stop them. Avicenna explains the use of several types of fomentation to relieve gaseous pain.

In the last section (the 32nd) on the priority of treatment, Avicenna elucidates the application of the principle of treating the disease rather than its symptoms in the situation when more than one disease occurs at the same time. He lists the three conditions that determine which of the diseases to start with.

Aspects of Treatments according to General Diseases
(32 Sections)

FIRST SECTION

General Discussion of Treatment

We say that treatment can be carried out in three ways: first, management and diet, second, drugs, and third, manual manipulation. By management we mean the administration of the necessary ordinary essentials, which include diet. Qualitative management is suitable to drug administration; however, diet has its specific rules that deal with quantity because food may be held back from the patient, reduced, modified, or increased.

The physician may hold off the **food** from the patient when the purpose is to busy the body system with the digestion of humors or reduce it to preserve the "power" by bringing power from the ingested food and reducing the system's investment in digesting large quantities of food. Attention is always aimed at the more important of two issues, which is the "power" when it is too weak and the disease when it is very strong.

Food is reduced from two aspects: quantity and quality, and a third if you combine the two. The difference between quantity and quality is that the food can be of large quantity but low quality, such as leafy vegetables and fruits. One who takes a large amount of them has a large quantity but not quality. Some food in low quantity has high nutritious value, like eggs and testicles of roosters. Sometimes, we need to decrease the quality and increase the quantity if the appetite is dominant and there are raw humors in the vessels; therefore, we satisfy the appetite by filling up the stomach and protect the vessels from new humors until the existing humors are digested, and also for other reasons. In other situations, we need to increase the quality and decrease the quantity, such as strengthening the "power" when the stomach digestion is weak and cannot digest large amounts of food. Food reduction and stoppage are important in acute diseases. In chronic diseases, food is reduced as well, but less than in acute diseases because we focus more on the strengthening of "power" because we are aware that the patient's healing crisis and recovery are distant; therefore, if the "power" is not preserved it will not last to reach the crisis and digest the humors that take a long time. However, acute diseases have a proximate healing crisis, and we expect that the "power" will not fail before reaching the crisis; if we fear that then we start reducing the amount of food. In the early stages of the disease symptoms, we give food that is strengthening to the "power," but when the disease worsens and symptoms increase, we need to reduce the food quantity according to our confidence in what we mentioned above, thus reducing the burden on the "power" in the height of its engagement, and at the end we have to manage the situation very gently. In case the disease is more acute and the healing crisis is very close, our management is usually very gentle unless there are reasons that prevent it, as we will mention in books on the particulars.

There are two other aspects to the choice of food: these are (1) speed of absorption, fast (as in wine) or slow (such as roasted and fried foods); and (2) the consistency and stickiness of the materials it generates in the blood. Meats of pig (pork) and calves (veal) produce heavy and thick substances that take a long time to break down, while the nutrients of wine and figs produce the opposite. We are in need of quickly digested and absorbed food if we want to prevent the total collapse of the "power" of animalistic faculty and revive it, especially if the time is short and does not allow for slow digestion. We usually avoid following a slow-digested food with a fast-digested one, so that they do not mix, as we have explained before. Also, we avoid eating dense food when sure of the existence of an obstruction. However, we prefer good, nutritious, and slow-digested food when we want to strengthen an individual and prepare them for heavy exercise and choose light food for those whose skin pores get easily blocked.

Treatment with drugs has three rules: first, selecting the drug's qualitative temperament, whether it is hot, cold, wet, or dry; second, selecting its quantity, which is divided into measuring its weight and its temperament (degree of hotness or coolness, etc. [potency]); and third, time of administration. The absolute rule for selecting the drug is by knowing the type of disease; when the temperament of the disease is known it is necessary to select the drug with the opposite temperament since the disease is treated by the opposite and health is preserved by the similar. Determining the quantity of the drug in the two aspects [weight and temperament] together is carried out by estimating the diseased organ temperament and the severity of the disease. The temperament of the organ is estimated by assessing it against gender, age, habit, season, profession, "power," and physique [including skin condition].

The **nature of the affected organ** includes four issues: the organ's temperament, structure, position, and "power." As for the organ's temperament, if its normal temperament is known and its diseased temperament is known, then the departure from the normal temperament can be estimated and the quantity required to bring it back to recovery becomes evident. For example, if the normal temperament is cold and the disease is hot, then it has greatly deviated from the normal and requires a lot of cooling, however, if both are hot then it requires little cooling.

As for the **structure of the organ**, we have listed the different aspects under this term, so look it up there [it is mentioned in the anatomy section, which is not included in this book]. Also, learn that some organs have structures with accessible openings, where their inside and outside are similar; waste can be pushed out of them with gentle moderate drugs, while others are the opposite and require stronger drugs. Some organs are loose and others dense; the loose require gentle drugs, and the dense need strong medication. Organs that are mostly in need of strong drugs are the ones without cavities, not accessible from any side, and without space around them; then there are those accessible on one side, followed by those with two accessible sides, but dense, such as the kidney; these are followed by organs with cavities on both sides, like the loose lung.

As to the **position of the organ**, which as you know requires a location or sharing relationship [relationship of an organ to other organs]. Sharing is beneficial to know because it specifically determines the area of drug target; for example, if the substance of interest is in the convex area of the liver we carry out the evacuation by urination; however, if it is in the concave area of the liver we evacuate with diarrhea because the convex area is shared with urinary organs and the concave area is shared with intestines. As to the **location**, there are three aspects: First is proximity; for example, if it is close to the stomach, the moderate drugs reach it in the shortest time and act on it without losing their power. However, if it is distant, like the lungs, the moderate drugs lose their power before reaching it and will need to be stronger. The drug potency should be equal to the severity of the disease in the near organ receiving the treatment; however, if the organ is far, the drug needs penetrating power and should be stronger than the usual, such as poultices of varicose veins and others. The second aspect is to know which adjuvant to mix with a drug to speed up its arrival to the target, such as mixing diuretics with the medications of urinary organs and saffron with heart drugs. The third aspect is to know the location of the drug delivery; for example, when we know that the ulcer is in the lower part of the intestine, we deliver the drug with enema, and if we think it is in the upper part of the intestine, we deliver the drug with alcohol.

There is also a benefit from **considering the position and sharing together** in regard to the treatment options when the waste product has stopped accumulating in the organ or if it is still pouring into it. In the latter case, we bring out the waste from its location according to four conditions: one, pull it in the opposite direction of its movement, as in from right to left and from top to bottom; two, consider the sharing relationship with other organs, as when stopping menstruation by cupping the breasts (i.e., attracting the waste from the partner); three, consider adjoining organs, such as in liver illnesses where venesection is done on the right basilic vein, while in the case of spleen illnesses it is done on the left basilic vein. The fourth aspect is distancing; the waste should be taken away from the diseased organ to a safe distance. If the waste has completed its accumulation in the organ, taking it out will benefit the diseased organ; or moving it to another organ and then draining it out from there. Examples are venesection of the saphenous vein for treating illnesses of the uterus or venesection of the sublingual vein for treatment of tonsillar swelling [quinsy]. To drain the waste in the opposite direction of its accumulation in the organ, start by relieving the pain and be sure that the drained waste does not go into a principle organ.

There are three aspects to the benefit of the organ's "power." First, consider the **importance of the organ.** The principle organs should not be treated with strong medications, as possible, to avoid harming the rest of the body. For this reason, the brain and liver should not be totally drained of waste in one session or be cooled down severely. Also, when decomposing poultices are applied to the liver, they should not be devoid of good fragrant astringent to preserve "power"; the same applies to oral treatment. The most essential of organs is the heart, followed by the brain and liver. Second, consider the **shared function of the organ,** even if it is not a principle one like the stomach and the lung. For this reason we do not give very cold water in fevers due to the weakness of the stomach. Also note that using softening agents on the principle organs and what follows them is very dangerous in general. Third, consider the **sensitivity and tolerance of the organ.** Sensitive nervous organs should not be treated with drugs of bad temperament, or biting [irritant] and harmful drugs, such as the euphorbiaceous plants* and others. Drugs to be avoided are of three types: resolvents, coolants by action, and those with opposing temperaments, such as verdigris ([copper carbonate], الزنجار), white lead (اسفيداج), burned-copper, and the like. The preceding was a detailed explanation of drug selection according to the nature of the organ.

The **degree of severity of the disease** is similar to a very high temperature that requires a very cold drug to extinguish it, and the person with a very cold temperature requires a drug that warms them up a lot; however, if conditions are not severe, it is sufficient to use less strong drugs.

---

*By euphorbiaceous plants, Avicenna probably means plants with milky poisonous sap.

As for the phase of disease, it is easy to determine that. For example, if the swelling is at the beginning we use something to arrest it only; at its end, we use a resolvent alone; and in between, we mix all the treatments. If the disease is acute at the beginning, we treat it with moderately gentle treatments; however, at the end, we are very gentle in its management. In the case of a chronic disease, we treat gently only at the end. Many of the chronic diseases other than fevers respond well to gentle treatment. A patient with overactive humors is initially treated by purging the humors without waiting for their maturation. However, in a moderate patient, maturation precedes purging.

Knowing the other issues that are suitable for treatment are easy, air among them. It is the most important factor and is supportive to the effect of the drug and the patient's health. [The other five issues were mentioned earlier.]

Dangerous diseases that may lead to the loss of "power" from delaying treatment should be treated first with a strong drug that poses no danger, and gradually apply stronger ones if the lighter does not work. Do not deviate from the proper treatment, because its effect will take a while to appear, and do not build on a mistake, because the damage cannot be fixed. Also, do not rely on one drug for one treatment; change drugs because the familiar drug [to the patient's body] does not produce a reaction. For every body, every organ, and the body and organ together, there is a specific time of reaction to a drug that is different from other drugs.

If the diagnosis of an illness is problematic, then let the body system take care of it and do not rush because the body may defeat the illness or the illness may become more obvious. If the illness is with pain, painlike, or produced by fall or trauma, then start by silencing the pain; when anesthesia is needed, do not surpass poppy seeds since their sedative effect is known and they are edible. When an organ is very sensitive, then the food has to be aimed for enriching the blood with food such as mashes, and if you are confident of your regimen, then feed with coolants such as lettuce and alike.

Note that good successful treatments are those that include something that strengthens the psychological and animalistic faculties, such as happy events, amusements, friends, conservative well-behaved company, and respectful people. The latter prevent the patient from indulging in harmful behavior. Similar types of treatments can be employed, such as in travel between countries and climates. Exercising of physical attributes, and having fun doing it, include asking a cross-eyed boy to focus on an object moved in front of him or having a stern-faced person look at himself in a narrow mirror to relax his face and eyes. Such conscious effort may fix a problem.

One of the rules you need to remember is not to use the strong treatments (like harsh diarrhea, cauterization, incision, and emesis) during the summer and winter in situations of excessive wastes, if you can.

One of the situations that requires careful examination is the presence of two opposing conditions within an illness, such as when the illness treatment requires cooling while its cause requires warming, as in the case of a fever needing cooling and its cause, the obstruction, needing warming; the opposite may occur. Sometimes the disease treatment requires warming while its cause needs cooling, as in colic where it needs warming and the breakdown of its material and its pain needs cooling and anesthesia; the opposite is also possible.

Also note that not every fullness or dystemperament is treated with the opposite or changed to the opposite state, but rather it is sufficient to carry out the necessary management steps in the treatment of fullness and dystemperament.

SECOND SECTION

Treatment of Diseases of Dystemperament

Dystemperament without a bad humor requires only changing of temperament; however, if it is associated with a bad humor then it requires the elimination of the humor. Elimination alone may be sufficient if the dystemperament goes back to the normal state, but if the dystemperament remains after elimination, then it has to be treated separately.

Treatment of dystemperament is of three types. Because dystemperament may be chronic and it is treated with an absolute opposite, which is the **absolute treatment** [allopathy], it can be treated by stopping the progression of dystemperament, fixing it, and halting the cause, which is called **progressive preservation**. The following examples show the difference between absolute treatment and treatment by progressive preservation. Absolute treatment of putrefaction of quartan fever is with the *teryaq* antidote, and drinking water in tertian fever to quench heat, progressive preservation treatment is emesis in the quartan with hellebore, and in the tertian with scammony if you want to prevent an episode from taking place. [The third treatment is by anticipating the dystemperament and preempting it, which is called] **simple progressive preservation** [prophylaxis]; [it can be illustrated by these two examples]: inducing emesis with hellebore to preempt quartan fever due to the dominance of black bile and using scammony to preempt tertian fever due to the dominance of yellow bile.

If you are not sure whether an illness is caused by heat or cold and you want to experiment, then do not experiment by giving a powerful drug and watching for any side effects. Also, note that the durations of heat and cold are equal; however, the danger of cooling is more because heat is supportive of the body. The dangers of moisturizing and drying are the same; however, the duration of moisturizing is longer. Moisturizing and drying are preserved by strengthening their causes and are replaced by removing their causes. Heat is strengthened by the causes that we mentioned, then by refreshers such as expunging dregs and fullness, clearing an obstruction, and by that which preserves it, such as moderate moisture. Coldness is strengthened by fortifying its causes; it is extinguished by heat or by excessive decomposition, such as dryness specifically, and accidental heat.

When treating excessive heat by unblocking an obstruction one should be cautious not to cause excessive coldness to avoid solidifying the obstruction, thus increasing hot dystemperament. But rather to slowly treat with cleansers, such as barley water and juice of true endive. If this does not work, then use something moderate in strength; otherwise use a drug with moderate heat, without worrying, because the benefit from its cold unclogging is much more than its warming effect, which is easy to treat after unclogging. Also, excessive cooling may prevent the maturation of sharp humors. Some physicians are against this opinion without knowing that strong cooling extinguishes the "power," especially if it is weakened by illness; even though the treatment may fix the problem, later it will cause other illnesses, such as single cold dystemperament, or generate other substances that are antagonistic to the ones that the treatment fixes.

Heating cold dystemperament is easy at the beginning but difficult if it has become chronic. In general, heating the cold at the beginning is easier than cooling the hot at the beginning; however, cooling the hot later, although difficult, is still easier than heating the cold later. This is because excessive cooling indicates the extinction of the innate nature. Also, be aware that cooling may be accompanied with dryness or moisture, or it may be without them. Dryness is a better fixative to the coldness when it takes place, and moisture is a better inducer of fresh coldness. Dryness will progress by all causes of heat when in excess, and wetness is increased by all the excesses of coldness. The buildup of moisture is strongly aided by rest, light regular bathing, bathing in a tub (we have mentioned this before), and drinking wine mixed with water.

Also, be aware that when an elderly person needs cooling and moisturizing it is not sufficient to bring them back to [normal] equitability, but rather to that which surpasses the normal cold and wet temperaments, because although it is accidental, it is close to their normal.

It is often necessary when altering a temperament to add something to the mixture that will strengthen the temperament, such as using vinegar with warming drugs to strengthen the organ, or the use of saffron in the cooling drugs of the heart to get the drugs to the heart. Frequently, the drug initially has a strong effect on temperament, but later becomes gentler when it starts its action; therefore, it will require another substance mixed with it to concentrate and confine it, even if the latter substance is antagonistic in its action to the primary drug, such as mixing wax with balsam of Mecca (*Commiphora gileadensis,* syn., *C. opobalsamum*)* and others to keep it confined to the organ and carry out its action.

---

*Balsam of Mecca, also called balsam or balm of Gilead, is a resinous gum of the tree *Commiphora gileadensis* (syn., *C. opobalsamum*), native to southern Arabia.

THIRD SECTION

How and When to Carry Out Elimination

There are ten factors that determine the aptness of elimination:

- Fullness
- "Power"
- Temperament
- Suitable symptoms (such as the targeted material for elimination has not been depleted before, since two successive eliminations are dangerous)
- Body condition (physique)
- Age
- Season
- Weather
- Familiarity with elimination
- Profession.

If there are contraindications to elimination, then the elimination should not be carried out. For example, an empty stomach prevents elimination, so does weakness of any of the three faculties; however, we may prefer to weaken one faculty, the perceptive and responsive, if the elimination is more beneficial in a dangerous situation, and this applies to all faculties. Elimination is contraindicated in the hot and dry temperament, in the cold and wet temperament, and due to lack of heat or its weakness; however, it is highly recommended in the hot and wet temperament.

As for the body condition, excessive thinness and looseness are against elimination for the fear of weakening respiration and "power"; therefore, the weak and skinny, with an excess of yellow bile in the blood, should be treated and not purged, and should be given food that generates good blood, which tends to be cold and moist. This may fix their humors' dystemperament or strengthen the individual to tolerate elimination. A scarce eater should not be purged unless it is a must. Very obese individuals should not be purged for fear of becoming cold and causing the flesh to press against the vessels and collapse them, thus confining the heat and squeezing dregs into the viscera.

Bad signs that prevent elimination include propensity to diarrhea, spasm, incomplete growth (childhood), wilting of old age, very hot and very cold weathers, and hot southern country. Most laxatives are harsh; therefore, combining two harsh effects is intolerable since the faculties are weak and relaxed. External heat attracts substances to the outside, and the drug attracts them to the inside, thus antagonism occurs. Elimination is contraindicated in the following: cold northern climate, unfamiliarity with elimination, and tiring professions like bathhouse workers and porters.

There are **five goals for elimination: First**, eliminating what should be purged out of the body; this produces relief and comfort unless it is followed by problems in the vessels, abnormal heat or ephemeral fever, or other illness that may accompany elimination, such as loose stools and bladder sores. These effects may mask the benefit of elimination and cause immediate harm until the effect disappears. **Second**, elimination is applied in its natural direction. For example, nausea is cleansed with emesis, and gastrointestinal cramp with purgation. **Third**, elimination from an organ should be in the direction of the waste flow. For example, the right basilic vein is drained in liver illnesses, and not the right cephalic vein; such a mistake may cause danger. Additionally, the collecting and outlet organ should be of less significance than the drained organ, and with a natural exit, like the urinary organs to the convex side of the liver and the intestine to the concave part of the liver. The collecting organ may have a problem such as an illness or may not tolerate the passing through of humors; therefore, elimination should be diverted to another proper organ. Treat carefully if it is feared that the humors will adversely affect the organ, as when the material moves from the eye to the throat, which may induce pharyngitis. The body's nature may carry out such elimination by exiting the waste material from an unusual direction to protect the organ when it is weak or keeping the waste in an opposite distant area, which is confusing, such as when the waste comes from the head and moves down to the bottom, leg, or foot, because in this case it is unknown whether the source is the brain as a whole or one of its ventricles. **Fourth**, time of elimination. Galen asserts that in chronic diseases it is important to wait for maturation, and you have learned what maturation is. After maturation and before elimination, the patient has to drink soothers like the water of hyssop herb, Persian thyme, and seeds [such as anise, celery, and fennel]. In acute diseases, waiting for maturation is also the right thing to do, especially if the bad humors are calm; however, if they are on the move, then elimination should be carried out first because the harm from their circulation is more than the harm of their elimination before their maturation, especially if the humors are light in the vessels and outside the organs. When the bad humor is confined to an organ, it should not be moved at all until its maturation and turning into moderate texture [density]—as you have learned in its chapter. **Fifth**, if the instability of the "power" is feared while waiting for maturation, then elimination is carried out with precautions as to the bad humors' cycle and density. If these are dense and meaty, they should not be moved before thinning them; their thickness is inferred from early indigestions, distending pain in the epigastrium, and swelling in the viscera. In this case, one should be sure that exits are unblocked. After all these steps, diarrhea should be induced before* maturation.

There are two **ways to eliminate a substance** and remove it from its location. One of them is by bringing it to the **distant opposite** side, and the other to the **proximate opposite** side. The best time to carry out elimination is when there is not fullness in the body and the substance is not on the verge of moving. Let us assume that a man is profusely bleeding from the mouth and a woman has excessive bleeding from hemorrhoids. In the first case, the proximate opposite is by bringing the matter out through a nosebleed, and in the second, by inducing menorrhea. However, to carry out the treatment by the distant opposite in the first case, venesection should be carried out in the lower vessels, and in the second case, venesection through upper body vessels and locations.

In the distant opposite, one should not do the elimination by

---

*The Rome 1593 copy says "after."

selecting an exit that is two regions far from the location of the waste substance; it should not be more than one region. If the substance is in the upper right side of the body, it should not be pulled to the lower left, but rather to the lower right, which is the proper side; alternatively, it can be brought to the left from an upper location if it was distant from the waste location by a distance that is equal to the shoulder girdle. This does not apply to the head's sides; if the substance is in the right side of the head, it is brought down and not to the left. When bringing the substance to a distant location, sedate the original locality first to stop the pain and weaken its retentive power over the substance since pain is an attractant. Do not force a substance out because force may move and thin it and make it go to the painful location. Sometimes, it is sufficient to draw it out without elimination since diverting it prevents it from accumulating in the organ, even though it does not get out of the body. Thus, the pulling away by itself performs the goal, even though without elimination but transferring the waste substance to the opposite organs by applying pressure, cupping, or the application of rubefacient* drugs—in general with something that causes pain.

The easiest materials to eliminate are those in the vessels. Those in the organs and joints are difficult to extract and eliminate and have to come out with other substances. The individual who has undergone elimination should not rush to eating too much food or raw food that gets absorbed without full digestion; however, if it is a must, eat in a small quantity that increases gradually and gets fully digested when absorbed inside the body.

Venesection is a special elimination that equally removes excesses of all humors. Venesection cannot be applied to eliminate the excess in quantity or quality of one particular humor. Excessive elimination often causes fever. If elimination causes the cessation of a habitual diarrhea, it can be restored by repeating the elimination that caused its cessation. For example, with the cessation of discharge of the ear or nose by the formation of an obstruction, whatever caused the cessation will

---

*A rubefacient drug is a substance for external application that produces redness of the skin.

also bring back the discharge. Be aware that retaining some of the substance that needs elimination is better than overelimination that may lead to weakness of "power"; most of the time the system takes care of what is left over. As long as the eliminated substance is the proper one to eliminate and the patient can tolerate the process, then there should not be a fear of excessive elimination; elimination can be continued until the patient faints. In the case of individuals of strong "power" but with excessive bad humors, carry out the elimination little by little. Similarly, if the substance is very sticky or well mixed with the blood, elimination cannot be carried out in one session; this is the case in varicose veins, chronic arthritis, cancer, chronic scabies, and chronic pustules.

Diarrhea attracts substances from above and eliminates from below. Therefore, diarrhea has two types for gathering substances: the active and the passive pulls. It is also good when the substances have settled; if they are in the lower part of the body, it pulls them to the opposite direction and extracts them. **Emesis** pulls and extracts in opposite directions to diarrhea; it attracts from below and eliminates from above. **Venesection** varies in its pulls according to its location, as you have learned. Individuals who are least in need of elimination are those who eat and digest well. People in warm countries are less in need of elimination.

FOURTH SECTION

Common Rules between Emesis and Purgation, and Mention of the Method of Directing the Laxative and Vomiting Drugs

Individuals who are to undergo purgation or emesis should divide up their daily food ration into allotments to be consumed in small portions over several meals and diversify food and drink because the stomach craves what it loses, whether pushed up or down. The stomach tends to strongly retain homogenous food, especially if it is in small amounts. However, in loose bowels none of this occurs. Be aware that emesis and purgation are not suitable for a person who manages their body well; they need lighter treatment such as exercise, massage, and bath; however, if they develop fullness, especially of good humors like blood humors, then venesection is needed for cleansing without purgation.

When it is necessary to carry out venesection or elimination with hellebore or strong drugs, then treatment should start with venesection; this is from the instructions of Hippocrates in his book on *Iblimia* [epilepsy],* and he is right. The same treatment should be followed when the phlegmatic humors are mixed with the blood. However, if the humors are cold and viscous, venesection will increase their thickness; therefore, purgation should be the first step. In general, if the humors are equal in quantity, then start with venesection, and if one humor becomes dominant, then treat with elimination. Unequal humors require the reduction of the excessive humor by emesis to bring all humors to equality; this is followed by venesection. If medications were given first, then venesection should be delayed for a few days.

An individual who needs elimination but has undergone venesection recently should be treated with medications. Often, the treatment with drugs in a situation that requires venesection causes fever and imbalance; if this is not resolved with demulcents, then it becomes obvious that venesection should have been done first. Elimination is not required for every type of excessive fullness, but rather its need is based on the graveness of the disease and the quality and quantity of fullness. Very often, better management is a good alternative to venesection when needed. Frequently the physician calls for elimination, but when delayed, the alternative is fasting, sleeping, and treating the dystemperament caused by the fullness.

Elimination is sometimes carried out as a prophylaxis in cases of gout, epilepsy, and other illnesses at a specific time, usually the spring. The prophylaxis should be done before the time of the attack episodes by carrying out the elimination that is specific for the disease, whether it is venesection or purgation.

Drying agents (desiccants) can be used externally with internal dry drugs for elimination, as is done in patients with edema. A drug that is

---

*Known in the West by the title "On the Sacred Disease."

compatible with the targeted humor for quantitative elimination should be used, as in the case of eliminating yellow bile with scammony. In this case, scammony is mixed with a substance that is opposite in quality but compatible with its purgation action or does not prevent diarrhea, such as black myrobalan, and is used to treat any dystemperament that may develop due to its use. Patients with visceral swellings have weak diarrhea and vomiting; therefore, the use of the following drugs may be needed: *Dolichos lablab*, common polypody, and Indian laburnum.

According to Hippocrates, emesis is easier for thin individuals and should be their first choice for cleansing in the summer, spring, or fall, but not winter. Diarrhea should be the choice of those of moderate body size; however, if emesis is recommended, they should wait until the summer and not do it at any other time unless needed. Before commencing with emesis or purgation, the targeted humor should be softened and the ducts enlarged and cleared since this makes the process less laborious. It is a good practice to soften the system to get the most out of purgation and emesis before the use of strong medicine. Purgation and emesis are difficult, tiring, and may be dangerous for individuals with a skinny belly.

Emetic drugs may become laxatives if the stomach is strong, if taken on an empty stomach, when the patient has been having loose or soft bowels, if the patient is unaccustomed to emesis, or if the drug is dense and passes through quickly. A laxative becomes an emetic due to weakness of the stomach, excessive hardness of stools, repulsiveness of the drug, or the patient's indigestion. If the laxative does not induce diarrhea or induces it without maturation of the targeted humor, then the laxative moves the humor throughout the body; thus it dominates the body and converts other humors to its kind, which increases its quantity in the body. Some humors are often responsive to emesis, like yellow bile, others are not, like black bile, and others vary, like phlegm.

It is more proper for a patient with fever to induce diarrhea rather than emesis. It is impossible to induce emesis for those with loose bowels—lienteric diarrhea.

The worst of the laxative drugs are those composed of a very diverse mixture of ingredients that vary in their time of induction, thus disrupting the diarrhea. One of the components will induce diarrhea before the other and one may push out the other.

Inducing diarrhea and emesis in a healthy individual causes headache, colic, distress, and difficulty in completing the emesis. In general, as long as emesis pushes out wastes, it does not cause disturbances; however, if disturbances develop, then the emesis does not contain waste. When the expelled humor, by emesis or diarrhea, changes to a different humor it is an indication the body has been cleansed from the targeted humor. However, it is a bad sign if it changes to shavings and malodorous black material.

Deep sleep after emesis and purgation is an indication that the body has been cleansed very well. Be aware that a severe thirst after purgation and emesis is a sign of a good cleansing.

A laxative drug carries out its action by active pulling of the humor itself. It may pull out the thick humor and retain the thin one, as the laxative does to black bile. This is contrary to the saying that the laxative produces that humor or that it pulls out the thin humor first. Galen is of the opinion that a nonpoisonous laxative, when it does not induce diarrhea and continues, generates the type of humor that it pulls out. This is not correct. It appears from what Galen explains that the laxative pulls because there is a similarity in substance between the pharmacological pulling and the pulled humor; this is not correct. If this were correct, then the larger of two iron pieces would pull the smaller, and the same with gold pieces; however, the proof of this should be done by nonphysicians. The pulling mechanism of humors in the laxative and emetic drinks is the way they react in the intestines to produce the action where the body will push the humors to the outside. It is very rare that the laxative drug moves up from the intestine to the stomach; however, when it happens, it tends to induce vomiting. A laxative does not move up to the stomach for two reasons: one, the laxative drug moves fast to the intestines, and two, the body will push the laxative drug into the vessels of the mesentery in the lower direction, and not the upper direction, because it is easier for the body to push in that direction and closer to the exit. If the drug has a pulling power specific to the humor, and the body of healthy individuals may oppose the drug, the drug may still pull in the proper direction. The action of the laxative drug becomes contrary to this if it stands in the stomach because it then pulls the waste humor to itself from the intestine by its action and against the body's will. Be aware that most of the pulling of humors by the drugs is from the vessels, except in the areas next to the stomach, where the humor is drained from the vessels and nonvessels, such as when draining humors from the lung, where the humors move to the stomach and intestine through tissue and not through vessels. Drying drugs cause the draining of humors from the body, similar to elimination.

FIFTH SECTION

Description of Purgation and Its Rules

We talked earlier about the necessity of preparing the body to accept the laxative, enlarge the pores, and soften the bowels, especially in cold illnesses. In general, softening the bowels before purgation is a good safe rule except for individuals with a tendency to loose bowels because this should not be done to them for fear of causing excess purgation. The laxative for such people should be mixed with an emetic to keep the laxative in the stomach longer and prevent it from moving on before carrying out its action. The mixing of the two drugs, the laxative and the emetic, moderates the action of the two; thus the laxative carries out its action and the emetic works in the opposite direction. Lispers with a tendency for loose bowels do not tolerate a strong drug, and most of their diarrhea is caused by their head catarrhs. It is risky to give the laxative while there is dense waste; it should be moved out, even by an enema or an emollient soup.

Bathing for a few days before taking the laxative softens the waste humor; it is a good preparation unless there is a reason to abstain from bathing. There should be some time between bathing and taking the drug; do not go into the bathhouse after taking the drug because it pushes the drug out. Bathing is good to prevent diarrhea, except in winter, where it is fine to go into a first room of low heat in the bathhouse; its temperature is incapable of pulling at all, but rather softens the bowels.

In general, when taking the laxative drug, the temperature should be moderate and not induce sweat or fatigue; this is a factor in the preparation of the body. Other preparatory steps are massage and rubbing with oil. The physician should not give strong laxatives to individuals who are not used to them. Individuals with indigestion, thick humors, distention of the epigastrium, and inflammations and obstructions in the viscera should not be given laxatives until these problems are fixed with soft foods, bathing, rest, and abandoning all that moves their humors or causes inflammation.

Individuals drinking old water and those with spleen problems should be given strong drugs. It is better to sleep after taking the strong laxative before the drug starts acting; this ensures a better result. However, if the laxative is weak, the patient should not sleep because the drug may get digested. When the laxative starts to work, the patient should not sleep, no matter what the situation, and should not move, but stay calm and let the body work on the drug, *because if the body does not work on the drug, the drug will not work on the body.* The patient, in the meantime, should smell antinausea fragrances such as mint, common rue, celery, quince, and Khrasani clay* mixed with rose water and a little red wine. If the smell of the laxative drug is revolting, the patient should close their nostrils. For those who cannot stand the taste of the drug, they should chew some tarragon until the mouth becomes numb. If the patient fears that they may vomit the drug, their limbs should be tightly wrapped before taking it, and follow the drug with some astringent.

The physician may mix the tablets with honey or coat them with thick honey or sugar to form an outer crust; another trick is to coat them with cerate. An effective way to take the drug is by filling the mouth with water or other liquid, then swallowing the tablets as they are or prepared with some of these tricks; these will prevent the aftertaste of the drug. The decoction should be drunk warm, and the tablets should be taken with warm water. The stomach and the feet

---

*Khrasani clay is a type of clay eaten cold and dry. It is hot in action due to salinity, which strengthens the mouth of the stomach. It acts as an antinausea agent.

of the patient taking the medication should be warmed up. After the nausea goes away, the patient should get up and move little by little since movement is helpful. The patient should take sips of warm water in amounts that will not drain the drug, bring it out, or reduce its effect, except when stopping diarrhea is needed. Drinking warm water diminishes the normalcy of the drug. An individual planning on taking the drug while with hot temperament, weak build, and weak stomach should take barley water, pomegranate juice, and light food before ingesting the drug. It is better for a person without these issues to drink the drug first thing in the morning [on an empty stomach]. Purgation during hot weather causes fever. No food or drink should be taken until the drug effect is over. Sleep should be delayed as well until the drug action is over unless the patient resorts to stopping the purgation. If the patient cannot tolerate fasting because the stomach is bilious due to the continued rapid pouring of bile into it or from prolonged fasting, the patient should eat a little wine-soaked bread after the ingestion of the drug and before the start of the diarrhea; this should help the process of purgation. Warm, not cold, water should be used to wash the anus.

It has been said that when the tablets are prepared in a decoction, the decoction should be compatible with the nature of the tablets; for example, tablets that target yellow bile for elimination should be drunk in a decoction of fumitory (*Fumaria officinallis*), the drug targeting black bile should be cooked in absinth, common polypody, and alike, and for phlegm, in branching centaury (*Erythraea pulchella*).

If you need to carry out purgation on a dry and muscular body with a strong drug like hellebore and alike, then you should first moisturize the body with fatty food. In general, strong drugs are dangerous, I mean like hellebore, because they cause spasms in the healthy body, and in a body full of moistures they induce the movement of wet humors in a suffocating way and bring bad humors in the viscera that are hard to push out. The actions of euphorbiaceous plants like alpine daphne and euphorbia (*Euphorbia pithyusa*) are stopped, when their effect becomes excessive, with yogurt.

Very often the smell of a drug remains in the stomach as if it is still there; in this case suewaiq of barley should wash it away, since it is the most compatible of the flours.

If, after a long period, the drug has not induced diarrhea, the patient should sit still; however, when there is a fear of danger, the patient should drink diluted honey, honey syrup, or water with natron dissolved in it. Alternatively, the patient may use a suppository or enema if it can be tolerated. Among the reasons for the failure of a drug to act are congenital narrowness of ducts, dystemperament, or the close presence of an illness. For example, patients with palsy or apoplexy have narrow ducts that prevent the exit of waste humors in the same vessels that brought in the drug, thus they cannot be purged. Doing two purgations on the same day is dangerous and incorrect.

A humor-specific drug will cause disturbances and difficult diarrhea if it does not find its target humor, similarly, if the humor is covered by its opposites. Every drug works first on its specific humor, then on the one that follows it in quantity, scarcity, or thinness, according to this order, except for the blood humor, which is delayed and held tightly by the system. Pulling out the distant humor is difficult. For those that fear distress and nausea after drinking the drug, it is better to vomit two or three days before taking the drug by taking the leaves or root of radish. The food of an individual who will undergo purgation should not be excessively salty.

Very often the drug causes distress, nausea, fainting, palpitation, and colic, especially if it does not induce diarrhea or its action is delayed, which then requires the induction of emesis; however, very often it is sufficient to take astringents. Drinking barley water after the diarrhea prevents the side effects of the drug and washes away the remains of the diarrhea by mixing with it. A person with a cold temperament dominated by phlegm should, after the conclusion of purgation, take watercress seeds washed in hot water with oil; those with a hot temperament should use the seeds of blond psyllium (*Plantago ovata*) with cold water, violet oil, rock sugar, and jallab. The patient should take Armenian clay mixed with pomegranate juice after diarrhea if ulceration is feared; otherwise the purgation should be stopped. Barley water is best when fever develops after the ingestion of the drug. Oxymel should not be taken if the purgation causes ulceration for two to three days until the intestines regain their health.

On the day after purgation, the patient should go to the bathhouse; if any of the humors are still within the body, the patient will enjoy the bath because it will cleanse the remaining waste humor. However, if the patient does not enjoy it and becomes restless, then they should leave the bath.

An individual with weak intestines may develop persistent diarrhea after purgation with laxatives and require treatment to harden the intestines. Likewise, the elderly are prone to the risks of purgation. Drinking wine after purgation drugs causes fevers and problems. Frequently, purgation and venesection cause pain in the liver; this should dissipate by drinking hot water.

The appearance of the dog star (Sirius), snowfall, and very cold weather are not the time to start purgation; the treatment should be done in the spring or fall. Spring is followed by the summer, so its purgation drug should only be gentle. The fall is followed by the winter, thus a strong drug can be tolerated. The body should not get accustomed to using drugs for purgation every time it needs softening because it becomes a habit with bad consequences.

Every person with a dry temperament is weakened by a strong purgative and should minimize movement when taking a weak drug to avoid the disintegration of their "power." A good weak purgative drug is violet mixed with sugar. If purgation is needed in the winter, the time should be when the southerly wind occurs, and in the summer, it is the opposite direction [i.e., northerly winds]. There is a detailed explanation for this. When the patient takes a weak purgative and it does not work, no further action should be taken, but rather left alone. Purgation may revive an illness and cause fever; in this case, venesection is preferred.

SIXTH SECTION

Excessive Purgation and When to Stop It

Thirst is one of the signs that should dictate stopping purgation. However, if purgation persists without thirst, it should not be feared that an excess may have occurred. Thirst may happen not due to purgation or its excesses, but rather due to the condition of the stomach; the stomach induces thirst quickly when it is hot or dry, or both. Also, thirst occurs when the drug is sharp, is an irritant, or the waste humor itself is hot like yellow bile. With these reasons, the thirst appears early, and their opposites push it back. If you see excessive thirst and little purgation, then stop the process, especially if the causes of thirst are absent. In such a situation, stopping purgation should not be delayed until the appearance of thirst, and the exiting material should be the indication of the stopping point. When purging yellow bile is followed by phlegm, this is indicative of excess; imagine if this goes on to drain black bile! The exiting of blood humor is a greater danger. The treatment of colic after taking the drug is detailed in the books on particulars under the chapter on colic.

SEVENTH SECTION

Treatment of the Patient with Excessive Purgation

Purgation becomes excessive either due to the weakness or wideness of vessels or irritation of their openings, and dystemperament and related problems are caused by purgation itself. If purgation becomes excessive, wrap tightly the extremities, starting at the armpits and groin, and continue downward. Give the patient a little of *teryaq* to drink or a decoction of felty germander (*Teucrium polium*). Make the patient sweat by a bath or running steam under the clothes while the head is out; if the patient sweats profusely, they should be given astringents, fruit juices, and massage with good-smelling rubs like basil, sandalwood, and camphor. Also, all outside body parts should be massaged and warmed up, even with fire cupping placed under the rib cage and between the shoulders. If needed, place plaster wraps of suewaiq and astringent water on the stomach and intestines, as well as oils of quince and mastic. Patients should avoid cold wind because it causes squeezing that leads to diarrhea; they should also avoid hot wind as well because it weakens their strength. Patients should be strengthened with good perfumes and astringent drinks and dip bagels in warm basil-flavored wine after eating a piece of bread soaked in pomegranate juice. Suewaiq with powdered poppy peelings may also be used. A formula that has been tried: frying three drams of watercress seeds, cooked in buttermilk until it becomes thick, and then given to the patient to drink. The patient's food should be astringent and cooled down with ice, like the juice of sour unripe grapes and alike.

Purgation arrest is aided by exciting emesis with hot water. Extremities should also be placed in hot water and not allowed to cool, even if fainting occurs. Patients should not drink alcohol. If all of the above does not work, then eventually resort to narcotics and strong treatment, as described in the chapter on preventing diarrhea. It is better if the physician is ready beforehand with pills and astringent powders as well as the enema and its instruments.

EIGHTH SECTION

Treatment of the Patient Who Has Taken an Ineffective Purgative

If the drug does not induce purgation and causes colic, disturbance, headache, stretching, and yawning, then the patient should be treated with an enema and known suppositories and drink mastic in warm water. The purgative may act if the patient drinks astringents and eats things like quinces and apples because they squeeze [shrink] the mouth of the stomach and the parts below it, stop nausea, turn the drug movement downward, and strengthen the body.

If the enema fails and bad side effects appear, such as distension of the body, bulging of the eyes, and upper movements, then venesection should be applied. Also, if the drug does not cause diarrhea and is not followed by bad side effects, then the proper action is venesection as well, even if it is two or three days afterward, because the waste humors may move into some vital organs.

NINTH SECTION

States of Purgative Drugs

Some of the purgative drugs are dangerous and bad, like black hellebore, turpeth* when it is not white and good but yellow, white agaric mushroom that is not pure white but tilting to black, and alpine daphne. If any of these is ingested, the proper thing to do is to push it out as much as possible by emesis or purgation followed by teriac. Very often, the danger of these drugs such as yellow and moldy turpeth is neutralized by drinking very cold water or sitting in it, also, by the use of substances that break down the danger of the drug by their gluing, softening, and fatty (with gluing) actions. Some drugs are suitable for only particular temperaments and unsuitable for others; for example, scammony (*Convolvulus scammonia*) is ineffective in people of cold climates unless it is used in large amounts, as in Turkey. In some countries and some people, it is necessary to use the extract strength of the drug rather than its parts by weight. Laxative drugs should be mixed with aromatic drugs to preserve the strength of the organs; similarly, beneficent drugs may be used here to strengthen the animalistic "spirit" in every organ, and most of them are beneficial by ameliorating and liquefying.

It is possible to use two laxatives, one fast-acting on its humor type and the other slow-acting on its humor type. When the first drug is done acting, it may compete with the second drug and lessen its action. If the second drug starts after the first, it is usually not strong enough to move the waste humor; therefore, an adjuvant accelerator should be added to it, such as ginger to the turpeth, which prevents its latency for a while, similarly, if both drugs work on the same humor.

The facts that we have outlined about the strengths of laxative drugs

---

*Turpeth is also known as *fue vao* and St. Thomas lidpod.

should be studied. We have elucidated there the facts about single-drug laxatives. A laxative drug may work through its properties (specific nature) by breaking down, such as turpeth; squeezing [inducing contractions, peristalsis], like black myrobalan (*Terminalia chebula*); softening, like manna (exudate from *Atraphaxis cotoneaster*); or lubrication, like the mucilage of blond psyllium (*Plantago ovata*) and pears. Most strong drugs have some toxicity that forces diarrhea, despite the will of the body; thus they should be managed with something that contains an antidote. Bitterness, tanginess, astringency, pungency, and acidity may greatly enhance the action of the drug if these are congruent with the drug's specific nature. Bitterness and tanginess aid in decomposition, pungency promotes contraction, and acidity acts on the decomposition for lubrication. Lubricant drugs should not be combined with those promoting contraction in equal strengths. Rather, one should be slower than the other, so that one softens by its action (before the action of the contractor), then is followed by the contractor and expels what has been softened, and draw on this principle.

TENTH SECTION

Issues That Should Be in This Book That Are Listed in Others

Find in the *aqrabadhin* (formulary or pharmacopoeia) laxative and emollient drugs that can be taken as drinks or used as rubs according to the age of the patient. In the single formulary are the drugs that counter the effect of every single drug, its management, and its method of use, either as a drink or tablet. For example, the drug can be used if it has not hardened like a stone or if it is not so soft that it causes ulcers and irritation; it should have started to dry but still feel soft between the fingers.

ELEVENTH SECTION

On Emesis

There are people in whom the physician should not induce emesis because of the nature of their bodies, such as those with tight chests and very weak breath who are prone to hemoptysis; all individuals with thin necks, a tendency to form swellings in their throats (pharynx), and weak stomachs; and the very obese (they should rather undergo purgation, while emesis is more suitable to thin individuals because of their excessive yellow bile). Also, because of habit, individuals who have difficulty vomiting or are not used to strong emetics or those whose lung vessels would be burst by emesis and may develop tuberculosis. When the status of an individual is ambiguous, try on them the light emetics; if these do not cause any problem, then the physician may try stronger ones like hellebore and alike.

A patient who does not like undergoing emesis, but should, has to prepare by getting accustomed to it through reducing their food amount and increasing their food's fat and sugar, stopping exercise, and eating fats and oils with wine.

Before emesis, the patient should be fed good-quality food, especially if they are not easy vomiters; it is better they vomit good food. If the patient vomits after eating food that is specific for emesis, they should refrain from eating until they feel very hungry; meanwhile quench thirst with apple juice and no jallab or oxymel because they will cause nausea. The suitable food in this case is roasted chicken followed by three glasses of wine. If the patient's vomit is acidic, which is unusual for them, and their pulse is showing a slight fever, then eating should be delayed until the middle of the day and should be preceded by a drink of hot rose water.

If emesis produces black bile, the patient should then place a sponge soaked in warm vinegar on their stomach. It is best that emesis food differs from the regular one in case the patient develops diarrhea due to laxation induced by coldness. After a moist vomit, the patient will benefit from eating sparrows, young birds, without eating the bones of extremities because they are heavy on the stomach and slow to digest. After eating, the patient should be taken to the bathhouse.

Once the patient drinks the emetic, they should get ready, exercise until they get tired, and then vomit around midday. During emesis, the eyes should be covered with a piece of cloth and the belly wrapped with soft cloth at moderate pressure. Among the emetics that are preparatory for emesis are arugula, radish, citron, pennyroyal, onion, leek, barley water with crushed seeds sweetened with honey, sweetened soup of cod (*baccala*), sweet wine, almonds with honey, unleavened fried bread kneaded with butter, watermelon, cucumber and its seeds (or its roots soaked in water, grinded, and mixed with sweetener), and radish broth.

A person trying to vomit using a little alcoholic drink should drink more if it does not work with only a little. Drinking *fouka'a** beer mixed with honey after bathing will induce vomiting and diarrhea. To induce vomiting, the food should not be masticated well.

A strong emetic like hellebore should be taken on an empty stomach in the morning (if there is no contraindication), two hours after sunrise and after evacuating the intestine. Afterward, a feather is used to induce vomiting. If this does not work, use slight movement or take the patient to the bathhouse. The feather used in emesis should be coated with oil of henna.

If the induction process causes pain and distress, give the patient hot water or oil; this may cause vomiting or diarrhea. Warming up the belly and extremities aids in emesis. When the effect of the emetic drug starts taking place quickly, the patient should sit still, smell some good perfumes, finger massage the extremities, drink some vinegar, and chase that with apple and quince with some mastic.

Be aware that movement maximizes the volume of vomit and stillness reduces it. The summer is the best time for carrying out emesis. The summer is also good for patients with a nature unsuitable for emesis to have the procedure.

The ultimate **goal of emesis** is primarily to cleanse the stomach alone and not the intestine, and secondarily to cleanse the head and the rest of the body as well as pulling and extracting from the bottom.

**Fouka'a* is a beer made of oatmeal and herbs.

Beneficial emesis is distinguished from ineffective by subsequent improvements in feeling lighter, appetite, pulse, and breathing, as well as all other faculties.

Emesis begins with nausea, and most of emesis is associated with pain and burning in the stomach if the emetic drug is strong like hellebore; this is followed by runny saliva and vomiting in many throws, and ending in a clear runny substance. The biting and pain should be steady without other complications except nausea and its associated distress, and they may let the bowels loose. After four hours, the pain should ease and the patient feels restful.

Ineffective emesis does not induce vomiting and increases the patient's distress; it causes enlargement and bulging of the eyes and their redness, excessive sweating, and dysphonia (difficulty in speaking). If these symptoms are not treated they may cause death. Their treatment involves an enema, drinking honey in warm water, smearing of teriac oils such as lily oil, and continued effort to vomit. Precaution should be taken to prevent choking during vomiting, and be ready with a stomach enema.

Emesis is indicated primarily in difficult chronic diseases such as edema, epilepsy, melancholy, leprosy, gout, and sciatica. Despite its benefits, emesis may bring about some diseases like hearing loss. Emesis should not be followed directly by venesection. The latter should be delayed for three days, especially if there are humors at the mouth of the stomach. Very often, emesis becomes difficult due to the thinness of the humors. In such case, the humors should be thickened by eating suewaiq of pomegranate seeds. Be aware that a malodorous stench after emesis is a sign of a downward movement of indigestion, and throwing up after such a malodorous smell is also a sign of it.

The **best time to carry out emesis** that is prescribed for pain is midday in the summer. Emesis is beneficial in the case of eyelid swelling or sores on the internal side, but harmful to the eyesight. A pregnant woman should not undergo emesis because it does not bring out the waste of her menses [as is the case in normal time] and fatigue may cause her some trouble; therefore, her tendency to vomit should be quieted; otherwise, a woman who wants to vomit should be assisted.

TWELFTH SECTION

Procedure for After Emesis

After the patient is done vomiting, they should wash their mouth and face with diluted vinegar to alleviate any heaviness of the head; also, drink mastic in apple juice, abstain from eating and drinking, rest, oil the epigastrium (the upper middle section of the belly), and quickly bathe and wash. If it is necessary to eat, then it should be a nutritious and delicious food that is easy to digest.

THIRTEENTH SECTION

Benefits of Emesis

Hippocrates instructs to apply emesis once a month on two successive days to bring out on the next day the remainder of what stayed behind on the first day and to bring out from the stomach what has solidified in it from the first day. Hippocrates guarantees health preservation with such a regimen. Excessive use of emesis is harmful because it evacuates phlegm, yellow bile, and cleanses the stomach. There is no better cleanser for the intestines from the bile that is always pouring into them. It removes heaviness from the head, clears the eyesight, and pushes out indigestion. It also benefits those with bile backed up into the stomach, which corrupts food. Thus, emesis removes corrupt food and returns the stomach to normal digestion of fat, brings back normal appetite, and stops the desire for hot, acidic, and pungent foods. Furthermore, it is good for preventing the sagging of the body and heals the kidneys and bladder sores. It is a good treatment for leprosy, bad skin color, epilepsy (the digestion-related type), jaundice, orthopnea (shortness of breath when lying flat), tremors, and palsy. It is a good treatment for ringworm.

Emesis should be used once or twice a month* on fullness without keeping track of periodicity or the number of days. It is most

---

*Whether to use emesis once a month or twice a month—as advised by Hippocrates—is a choice made at the discretion of the Unani physician.

agreeable to skinny individuals whose normal temperament is choleric.

FOURTEENTH SECTION

Harmful Effects of Excessive Use of Emesis

Excessive emesis is harmful and weakening to the stomach and makes it vulnerable to the accumulation of waste humors. It is also harmful to the chest, eyesight, and teeth, and causes chronic head pains (except those shared with the stomach) and headache not caused by the lower organs. Additionally, excessive emesis is harmful to the liver, lungs, and eyes, and may burst some vessels.

Some people like to eat and get full quickly, and when unable to tolerate the fullness, they resort to vomiting. This leads to terrible chronic diseases, and they should refrain from filling up, but rather eat and drink moderately.

FIFTEENTH SECTION

Managing Conditions That Happen at Emesis

As to the inability to carry out emesis, we have discussed what is needed. Distention and pain that occur under the epigastrium can be treated with hot water pads, emollient oils, and fire cupping (hot cupping). However, the severe burning that remains in the stomach should be treated with fatty soup that is easy to digest and by rubbing the spot with oil of violet mixed with oil of wallflower, also known as gillyflower (*Erysimum cheiri*), and some wax. When the condition is accompanied by persistent hiccups, it should be stopped with thirst and sipping of hot water, little by little.

As to its effects on blood, we have mentioned that in the section on the effects of emesis. If trismus, cold diseases, sleepiness, or loss of voice appear after emesis, then the extremities should be tied and wrapped and the stomach should be fomented with oil in which common rue and squirting cucumber have been cooked, and drink honey mixed into hot water. For the patient who has been overcome by sleepiness, the same oil should be dropped into the ear.

Managing the Patient with Excessive Emesis

The patient should sleep or be put to sleep by any means, their extremities tied as done in arresting diarrhea, and their belly treated with wraps loaded with tonics and astringents. If the emesis is strong and the patient throws up blood (hematemesis), then give them four *cowtools** (قوطولات) of milk mixed with wine to weaken the emetic drug, stop the bleeding, and relax the body.

To cleanse the areas of the chest and stomach from blood in order to prevent its clotting, give the patient ice-cooled oxymel to drink slowly. It may also be beneficial to give the patient the juice of purslane mixed with Armenian clay, which causes the vomiting to stop, in case of drug overdose.

Issues That Should Be Sought in Other Locations

Emetic drugs should be used according to their degrees of strength and the method of administration, as written in the books of compound drugs and single drugs.

Enema

An enema is a good treatment for expelling waste from the intestines, calming pain and swelling of the kidneys and bladder, in colon diseases,

---

*A *cowtool* is 340 grams, which equals nine okas.

and in pulling down the waste humors from the upper organs. However, a strong enema weakens the liver and causes fever. An enema is used to bring out the leftovers from emesis.

The shape of the enema device and its instructions for use have been described in the chapter on colic. The best position for the patient receiving the enema is to be lying on the back, then later to shift to the side of the pain. The best time for the enema is when the air has cooled down in order to minimize distress, disturbance, and loss of consciousness. Bathing excites the humors and disperses them, while the goal of the enema is to attract the congested humors. Therefore, bathing should not precede the enema. The patient with intestinal injury [or perforation] who requires an enema due to a fever or other disease and fears the arrest of the enema inside, should place a pad with hot *jawarish* (a set of compound herbal preparations) on the anus and navel and around the navel.

NINETEENTH SECTION

Lotions and Liquid Rubs

Lotions and liquid rubs are treatments that reach the core of the disease. The drug may have two powers: light (gentle, thin) and heavy (harsh, thick), and the need for the gentle is stronger than that of the harsh. Therefore, if the two powers are equal, then using liquid rubs allows the gentle and arrests the harsh; thus, benefit comes from the penetrating lotions, as in the use of coriander in suewaiq to treat scrofula.

Wraps are like liquid rubs; however, they differ in that they are solid and rubs are liquid. Liquid rubs are usually applied by loading them on a piece of cloth, and sometimes are perfumed with the smoke of agarwood, which is beneficial to the main organs.

TWENTIETH SECTION

Douches

These are good treatments to change the temperament of the head and other organs. To change the temperament by applying hot or cold douches to the organs when there is no accumulation of humors, one should start with a hot douche and follow it with cold water to firm it up. If the situation is in reverse, start with the cold water.

TWENTY-FIRST SECTION

On Venesection

Venesection is a general cleansing method to drain out the excess. The excess here is the overabundance of humors in vessels in equal amounts. Venesection should be applied to two types of patients. The first type includes those that are susceptible to disease if their blood becomes excessive, and the second is those that are already diseased. Venesection is carried out due to the excess of blood, low quality of blood, or both. Those susceptible may develop one of the following diseases: sciatica, gout, joint pain due to blood humor [rheumatism], coughing up blood due to bursting of vessels in the skinny individuals when the amount of blood increases, epilepsy, apoplexy, melancholy when there is plenty of blood, shortness of breath [suffocation], internal swellings, hot conjunctivitis, cessation of regularly bleeding hemorrhoids [in this case it signifies a change has taken place in the blood], women who may develop amenorrhea (in the latter two groups, their skin color does not indicate their need for venesection due to their darkness, whiteness, or greenness), and those with weak internal organs and hot temperament. All these individuals should be bled in the spring if they have not yet developed any of these diseases.

Patients with physical trauma (from falling or beating) should be venesected so that they do not develop swelling, and the individual with swelling who fears its bursting before maturation should be venesected even if it is not needed and there is no excess of humors.

When diseases are feared but have not yet occurred, it is widely permissible to carry out venesection. However, when these diseases occur, venesection should not be applied in the early stages of disease because it causes the thinning of waste humors, distributes them in the body, and mixes them with the proper blood. Thus, ineffective evacuation may require tougher repeats.

The appearance of maturation when the disease has surpassed the early and final stages dictates venesection if there are no contraindications. Neither venesection nor emesis should be carried out on a day when the disease is active because it is a day of rest and sleep and it is at the height of the disease. In a case of a disease with several crises, bleeding too much blood should not be done in the first place; rather the disease should be calmed down. However, if venesection is carried out, it should be done with little blood and the rest left for several later venesections, if possible, in order to preserve the patient's strength to fight the crises. If during the winter following venesection, the patient complains of pain (breaking-like pain), then they should be venesected again with little blood so they can cope with the winter.

Venesection pulls out the blood and very often causes constipation. Weakness due to excessive venesection will generate a lot of bad humors. A patient who is not used to venesection may lose consciousness at the beginning of venesection and may vomit; when this happens venesection should be stopped. This also applies to vomiting during venesection.

Venesection activates the humors until calm is reached. Venesection should not be carried out during colic. Pregnant and menstruating women should not undergo venesection unless there is a great necessity, such as to arrest menstrual bleeding when it is successive and strong. Venesecting a pregnant woman would kill her fetus.

Signs of fullness do not always necessitate venesection since they could be due to raw humors; in this case, venesection is harmful and does not induce maturation and may cause the death of the patient. Individuals with dominant black bile should be venesected if diarrhea does not evacuate it [in other versions of the book: to follow venesection with purgation], and take into consideration the color [or complexion] according to the condition that we will mention. Furthermore, attention should be paid to distention since its occurrence in the body is a sign of necessity of venesection. Venesection carried out on an individual with little good blood but an excess of bad humors will result in the loss of the good fraction and the retention of bad humors. Only a little amount of blood should be drained from an individual who should be venesected but whose blood is of low quality and quantity or is dominated by an organ that causes harm. Additionally, they should be fed with good-quality food, undergo venesection once more, and then venesected again after a few days to draw out the bad blood and retain the good fraction.

If the bad humors are choleric, they should be evacuated through gentle diarrhea, emesis, or by calming them down and working on calming the patient. When the humors are thick, ancient physicians used to order patients to bathe and walk and perhaps drink oxymel with hyssop herb and Persian thyme, before and after venesection, as well as before a second venesection. If you are obliged to do venesection on a patient weakened by a fever or due to bad humors, then venesection should be carried out in steps.

Restricted venesection preserves strength; however, it may drain the gentle and pure and retain the turbid thick humors. Liberal venesection causes loss of consciousness, purifies well, and slows recovery; it should be applied for prophylaxis in obese individuals and in the winter to prevent blood gelation. Restricted venesection is more appropriate in the summer for those in need of it.

The patient should be venesected lying down in order to preserve strength and prevent fainting. Venesection should be avoided in the case of inflammatory fevers and all nonacute fevers and during their initial steps and days of dizziness, and reduced in fevers accompanied by spasms. If venesection is needed for fear that a spasm will prevent the patient from sleeping, make them sweat profusely and diminish their strength, then a fraction of blood should be retained [for the patient to function]. Similarly, when venesecting a nonputrefactive, feverish patient, the amount of drained blood should be reduced to allow the remaining fraction to break down the fever. If the fever is not inflammatory but putrefactive, then look up the ten laws,* then examine [the urine] in the a glass jar. If the water fraction is thick and reddish, the pulse is great, and the face is puffy without the harmful effects of the fever, then it is safe to venesect the patient when their stomach is empty. However, if the urine is thin and fiery in color and the body signs show the effect of the disease since it started, then do not venesect.

If the fever is intermittent, then venesection can be done, and take into consideration the presence of shivering. If shivering is strong, then venesection should not be done. Examine the color of the blood that is coming out; if it is thin and tilting to white, then stop venesection and be cautious that one of two things does not happen to the patient: exciting choleric humors or exciting cold humors. If venesection is a must in a fever, then do not pay attention to what is said that venesection cannot be done after the fourth day; it can be done even after the fortieth day; this is Galen's opinion. However, early or late, venesection should be carried out according to the proper signs; if not clear, then do it when necessary according to the ten laws. More often, venesection in fevers, even when it is necessary, is strengthening to the body system over the matter by reducing it; that is, if the physique, age, strength, and alike permit venesection. Venesection is a must in sanguineous fevers. It should be started with gentle venesection followed by an excessive one at maturation. Very often, this type of fever disappears after venesection.

Venesection is contraindicated in very cold temperatures, countries of very cold weather, during severe pain, after a decomposing bath [a bath that breaks down and disperses raw humors], after sexual intercourse, and in individuals under the age of fourteen years old, if possible, unless you are sure of their body strength, full musculature, wide, full vessels, and redness of their skin. The elderly and youth who have these characteristics are fine to undergo venesection. Youth should be venesected in small amounts. One should be very careful when venesecting the following individuals: very skinny, very obese, loose [body has a

---

*The ten laws refer to considering the following: (1) strength, (2) age, (3) original temperament, (4) dystemperament, (5) habits, (6) physique, (7) profession, (8) previous treatment, (9) season, and (10) geographic location.

lax appearance], white and pale and flabby, and yellowish with scarcity of blood; venesecting them should be avoided if possible. Venesecting patients with a prolonged state of illness should be avoided unless the severity of their blood corruption dictates it. If, upon draining blood, it looks black, then continue venesecting; however, if the blood is white [meaning not red] and thin, then stop venesection because this signifies a great danger. Venesection should be avoided when there is fullness of food so that it does not attract raw substances to the vessels instead of evacuating them. Also, venesection should be avoided on a full stomach or intestines and when anticipating fullness or nearness of fullness. In this case, the stomach should be evacuated by emesis, and the intestines by enema. Avoid venesecting a person with indigestion, and wait until their indigestion has been resolved through digestion.

People with digestive issues such as sensitive or weak stomach mouth [cardia] or generating yellow bile [through regurgitation] should be carefully venesected, especially if it is done on an empty stomach in the morning. A sign of sensitive cardia is sensitivity to biting [spicy] food, weakness of cardia manifests in weak appetite and pain, and excessive bile occurrence and persistence causes constant nausea, vomiting of bile, and bitterness of the mouth. Those people if venesected without the proper preparation of their stomachs will be in grave danger, and some of them may die. Therefore, those with a sensitive and weak cardia should be given pieces of bread soaked in the concentrate of an aromatic acid. If the weakness is due to cold temperament, the bread should be soaked in sugary water of aromatics, constipating mint drink, or constipating styrax, then they should be venesected. The patient with bile should be vomited by drinking an excess of hot water with oxymel, fed a few bites, rest for a short time, then venesected.

The good blood lost during venesection should be quickly replaced by eating *kabob*, which is very nutritious once it has been digested; however, the quantity should be as minimal as possible because the stomach has been weakened by venesection.

Venesection may be done to stop the bleeding in cases of nosebleed, menorrhagia, anal bleeding (hematochezia), internal chest bleeding (hemoptysis), or bleeding sores by pulling the blood to the opposite direction from the bleeding spot. This is a strong and effective treatment. The incision should be very small and bleeding should be done many times over successive days, but not in one day unless necessary, where the amount of drawn blood gets reduced day after day.

In general, it is better to do several sessions of venesection over one session of large quantity. Unnecessary venesection excites the bilious humors and is followed with dryness of the tongue and alike. The latter can be fixed with a drink of barley water and sugar. If a second venesection is needed and there were no adverse effects from the first (such as palsy), then the vein should be slit longitudinally and widely to prevent the muscle from closing the slit. Keeping the slit open can be assisted by placing a piece of cloth soaked in oil with some salt on top of the incision. Rubbing the incision area with oil before slitting prevents its fast closing and reduces pain. This can be done by gentle rubbing with an oil-wet cloth or by dipping the area in oil and then rubbing with a piece of cloth. Sleeping between two successive venesections speeds up the healing of the incision. Remember that we have mentioned that emesis should be carried out on a southerly wind day; it is the same for venesection.

The venesection slit should be small to prevent excessive bleeding in individuals who have been cauterized, in the insane, and in those who do not require a second venesection. A second venesection is delayed according to the weakness of the patient; if there is no weakness, then the second venesection can take place after an hour. When the goal of venesection is to attract the waste humor, then the second venesection should take place after a day. The incision should be diagonal to the direction of the vein if the patient will undergo a second venesection within the same day, across the vein for a second immediately following the first, and lengthwise for those who will undergo more than a second venesection. The more painful the slit, the slower its recovery. Bleeding of a large quantity in the second venesection causes fainting unless the patient eats something before it. Sleeping between the first and second venesection prevents waste from exiting with blood because sleeping pulls humors to the inner parts of the body.

The benefits of a second venesection are the preservation of strength while continuing the cleansing process. The most beneficial second venesection is the one that has been delayed two or three days after the first. Sleeping after venesection may cause aching of organs. Bathing before venesection may make it difficult because it thickens and softens the skin and makes it slippery, except in the case where the patient has very thick blood. After venesection, the patient should not fill up with food but rather eat gradually the things they like. Similarly, the patient should not exercise after venesection but rather lay down and should not do a decomposing bath. If during venesection the bled arm becomes swollen, venesection should be switched to the other arm as tolerable. The arm should be treated with Venetian ceruse ointment (white lead) and covered with strong cooling lotions.

The venesection of a body dominated by an excess of humors causes their excitement, movement throughout the body, and mixing with other body fluids. This situation requires successive venesections. The domination of black bile requires successive venesections, which will immediately improve the health status. In the elderly, venesection may cause apoplexy. Venesection may bring on fevers, and these fevers break down the putrefactive substances. Every healthy individual who undergoes venesection should follow our instructions on what to drink in the chapter on alcohol.

Be aware that the venesected vessels are either veins or arteries. The arteries are less often venesected, and one has to be careful to avoid the danger of hemorrhage, which in its least serious situation forms an aneurysm, especially if the slit is very small. However, if venesecting an artery can be performed safely, its benefit is great, particularly in a disease that requires arterial venesection. The most beneficial is the venesection of an artery that is in close proximity to an organ with abnormal symptoms. If the symptoms are due to a light and active blood humor, the organ will get great benefits from a safe venesection of the closest artery.

Arm vessels subjected to venesection include six veins: (1) **cephalic** (القيفال), (2) **median cubital** (median cutaneous, الاكحل), (3) **basilic** (الباسليق), (4) **funis brachii** (accessory cephalic or vena mediana cephalica, حبل الذراع), (5) **salvatella** (third dorsal metacarpal vein, الأسيلم), and

(6) **axillary vein** (الأبطي), which branches into the basilic and where the cephalic originates. In the last three, the incision should be done above the wrist, not below or next to it, so the blood will come out easily; also care should be taken to avoid damaging the nerve or artery. Longitudinal slitting of the cephalic vein at the joint delays its healing, and it is the opposite for nonjoint areas of the veins; for example, in the salvatella and other veins, it is more appropriate to slit longitudinally. When selecting a region to venesect in the cephalic vein, it is better to move away from the tip of the muscle and find a softer spot and open it widely without doing repeated cuts. A large slit in the cephalic vein does not damage the vein, as repeated cuts do, since they slow down the healing of the vein. The slit in the cephalic vein should be large if a second venesection is planned. If the cephalic vein cannot be located, then its branches in the outer side of the forearm should be used.

Venesecting the median cubital, or median cutaneous vein may damage the nerve below it. The vein may be positioned between two nerves; therefore, an effort should be made to slit longitudinally while holding onto it. Also, there may be a thin nerve lying on top of it like a tendon; this should be investigated lest it gets hurt by the incision and causes permanent loss of sensation. When the median cutaneous vein is thick, this nerve branch is easier to detect, but it is terrible to slit it by mistake and cause damage. However, if by mistake the nerve is nicked during venesection, do not close the wound, and place on it substances that prevent it from closing, and treat the nerve with the remedies that are specific for the nerves; we have mentioned them in the 4th Book. Do not place any coolants on it, such as European black nightshade (*Solanum nigrum*) and red sandalwood (*Pterocarpus santalinus*), but rather rub around it, and the whole body, with warm oil.

It is more appropriate to venesect the accessory cephalic vein in an oblique direction, except when difficult; then it should be slit longitudinally. Venesecting the basilic vein is very dangerous because the artery is located below it; therefore, you should be careful when venesecting it because bleeding from the artery may not stop or become difficult to stop. In some people, the basilic vein is located between two arteries; if one finds such a case and thinks it is safe to venesect, they may inadvertently damage the other. Therefore, you should check for this condition. Strapping the arm area will make either the artery or basilic vein bulge; therefore, the strap should be released and the bulge massaged gently, and then strap again and see if the vein appears. If it does not, then you have to abandon the basilic and venesect the axillary vein, which is located on the lower, inner side of the forearm. Very often inflation increases the thickness (diameter) of the vessel and strapping flattens it. Inflation in the pulse of the artery [ballooning] brings the artery higher [in the skin] and makes it look bigger, and thus it is mistaken for a vein and is venesected. If you strap any vein it will cause it to bulge, like a lentil or chickpea; therefore, carry out what we mentioned for the basilic vein. The deeper the basilic vein, the safer it is to venesect in the upper arm area. Slitting the vein with the scalpel should be done in the opposite direction of the artery. The artery is not the only site where a mistake could happen when venesecting the basilic vein, since there are also a nerve and a muscle below the vein, and the damage may occur to either one of them as well, which we have already mentioned. Signs of a mistake in venesecting the basilic vein and the slitting of the artery are the gushing out of light blondish blood and the vessel's softness and movement downward when touched. When this happens, treat the wound by wrapping the scalpel with the threads of rabbit hair and load it with the powder of oliban (*Boswellia* gum), Socotra dragon tree (*Dracaena cinnabari*), aloe, and myrrh (*Commiphora myrrha*); also place on the wound red iron oxide, sprinkle with cold water as possible, and bandage tightly to stop the bleeding. If the bleeding stops, keep the bandage for three days, and after that, take all necessary precautions and apply astringents to the wound. Some people resort to cutting the artery to make it shrink and collapse and stop bleeding. Many people have died because of bleeding, and others because of tying the organ and the excessive pain it generated when the organ started to die.

Be aware that bleeding occurs in the veins as well. Also be aware that the cephalic vein drains more blood from the neck and above, and little from below the neck, but it does not exceed the liver area or the epigastrium, and it does not significantly cleanse the lower parts.

The median cutaneous vein has a function that is midway between the cephalic and the basilic veins. The basilic vein drains the trunk and below. The accessory cephalic vein is similar to the cephalic. The right third dorsal metacarpal vein is beneficial in liver pain, and the left one in spleen pain. Either side is drained until the blood stops flowing. It is necessary to place the venesected hand in warm water to prevent the blood from clotting as well as maintain the flow and ease of flowing, especially if the blood flow is weak, as is usually the case when venesecting the third dorsal metacarpal vein, which is usually slit longitudinally. Venesecting the axillary vein follows that of the basilic.

The artery to venesect in the right hand is the one on the back of the hand between the thumb and the index finger [radial artery]. It is strangely beneficial in the chronic pains of the liver and diaphragm. It is told that Galen had a vision in his dream that a person told him to venesect the artery to cure his liver problem, which he did, and recovered. Alternatively, another artery closer to the middle of the hand may be venesected for the same benefit.

When venesecting the vessels of the arm does not bring out blood, do not rush to cauterize; strap the arm, then repeat the incision, or leave for a day or two, and if necessary to make a new incision, make it above the old one and not below it. A strong constricting strap causes swelling; therefore, it is better to wet the cloth with rose water or clean cold water. The strap should not displace the skin before and after venesection.

In skinny bodies, strapping causes the emptying of vessels and prevents blood flow. In very obese people, their flabby skin does not show the vessel unless the skin is pulled. A venesecting practitioner may behave gently and try to minimize pain by tightly strapping the arm for an hour, thus causing it to sleep; some of them may rub oil on the edge of the scalpel, which reduces the pain but delays healing.

If the above mentioned vessels do not appear on the arm but their branches do, then massage them with some pressure; if the blood comes back quickly after removing the pressure, then venesect them; otherwise do not venesect. To wash the venesected area, pull the skin above the incision of the vessel and wash, then pull it back to its original place.

When fat covers the incision area move it gently but do not cut it out; in this case, a second venesection requires another incision.

Be aware that there is a limited time for stopping blood flow and bandaging the incision that may vary. Some people can tolerate the loss of five to six "pounds" (one "pound," or ratell, equals 373.24 grams), even when they have a fever, and other healthy ones cannot tolerate the loss of one pound. There are three conditions that should be watched when venesecting: first, blood pressure; second, blood color (in some situations the color could be misleading, such as when the blood is too thick and it comes out initially as thin and white, when there is full-ness, or the presence of swelling and inflammation where the swelling attracts blood); and third, pulse (when the pulse becomes weak and small and the blood color changes, then venesection should be stopped). Similarly, venesection should be stopped if the venesected patient starts yawning, stretching, or becomes nauseated. Additionally, if the blood color changes quickly, check the pulse health to determine whether to continue or cease venesection. The fastest people to faint are the skinny with loose bodies and hot temperaments, and the least affected are those with moderately well-built bodies.

It has been said that the practitioner of venesection should have plenty of scalpels with and without fine tips, the latter is used for slippery vessels like the **jugular vein** (وداج); a ball of wool and silk thread; a wooden stick or feather to induce vomit; rabbit wool; aloe; oliban (*Boswellia* gum); and musk pod of the deer musk; musk drug;* and musk tablets. Fainting is one of the accidents that are feared in venesection. When a patient undergoing venesection faints, the wool or silk ball should be placed in the mouth, vomiting induced with the instrument, and give the patient the musk pod to smell and a dosage of the musk drug or its tablets to revive strength. If blood squirts out, stop it with the rabbit's wool loaded with oliban. Fainting rarely happens when the blood is coming out, but more often after it has stopped unless excess was taken. However, fainting is not an issue in incessant fevers, initial phases of apoplexy, suffocating afflictions,

---

*Used for heart weakness and fainting.

large dense tumors, and severe pains, only if the body is strong.

We have simplified the discussion about the vessels of the arm and not mentioned those of the leg and other vessels; therefore, we need to connect to them. Among the leg vessels is the **sciatic vein** (inferior gluteal), which can be venesected at the outer side of the heel or below, or above, between the hip and the heel. It should be wrapped or strapped with strong bandages. It is better to bathe before venesecting the sciatic vein. Its incision should be longitudinal. If the vein is hidden, then the branch between the two smallest toes (the fourth and the small toe) is the one to venesect. There is a great benefit in venesecting the sciatic vein in cases of sciatica, as well as in gout, varicose veins, and elephantiasis. It is difficult to carry out a second venesection on the sciatic vein.

Among the veins is the **great saphenous vein*** (GSV), which is on the inner side of the heel. It is more obvious than the sciatic vein. It is venesected to drain the blood from the organs below the liver and to bring the blood from the upper parts to the lower parts; for this reason, its venesection brings on menstruation and opens the tips of hemorrhoids. By analogy, the venesection of the sciatic vein and the GSV should have similar effects; however, experience has shown that the sciatic vein is much more effective in treating the pain of sciatica, which may be due to proximity. The best way to venesect the GSV is to use oblique to cross incisions.

Also among the veins is the **popliteal vein** [which carries blood from the knee joint and muscles in the thigh and calf back to the heart; its origin is defined by the junction of the posterior tibial vein and anterior tibial vein]. It is similar to the GSV in its effect; however, it is better than the GSV in inducing menorrhea, as well as relieving anal and hemorrhoidal pains. There is also the vein behind the Achilles' heel, which appears to be a branch of the saphenous vein and has its own characteristics in venesection.

---

*The great saphenous vein (GSV), also greater saphenous vein, is the large (subcutaneous) superficial vein of the leg and thigh. The terms *safaina* (Greek, meaning "manifest," "to be clearly seen") and *el safin* (Arabic, meaning "hidden or concealed") paradoxically have both been claimed as the origin for the word *saphenous* (Caggiati and Bergan, "Saphenous Vein").

In general, venesecting the leg's veins is beneficial in diseases caused by the accumulation of waste humors in the head and black bile diseases. Venesecting the leg's veins strongly weakens more than does venesecting the arm's veins.

Except for the jugular vein, all the venesected vessels of the head region should be slit obliquely. These vessels include veins and arteries. Among the veins is the **frontal vein** (supratrochlear vein), running vertically between the two eyebrows. Its venesection is beneficial in heaviness of the head, especially the back of the head, heaviness of the eyes, and chronic lasting headache. The **parietal branch** of the superficial temporal vein is venesected in the case of migraines and head sores.

The **temporal veins** that clasp the temples and the **vena angularis*** become visible only after choking the neck. In these veins, the incision should not be deep in order to prevent it from becoming a fistula. They will bleed a good amount of blood. Venesection of these veins is beneficial in headache, migraine, chronic conjunctivitis, epiphora,† leucoma,‡ trachoma,§ styes,¶ and night blindness.

There are three small veins (posterior auricular veins) located behind the ear where it meets the hair. One of the three veins is more visible and is venesected at the start of water and vapor accumulation in the head coming from the stomach; for this reason it is beneficial in the case of ear and back-of-the-head sores, as well as in head disease. Galen rebuffs the notion that venesecting the veins behind the ears causes sterility as sought by reclusive individuals.‖

Among the head veins are the **jugulars,** which are venesected at

---

*The vena angularis is a short vein formed by the supraorbital vein and the supratrochlear vein and continuing as the facial vein.
†Epiphora is the overflow of tears onto the face.
‡Leucoma is an eye disease consisting of an opaque white spot on the cornea.
§Trachoma is a bacterial infection of the eye.
¶External styes form on the outside of the eyelids and can be seen as small red bumps due to the infection of the sebaceous glands of Zeis at the base of the eyelashes. Internal styes are infections of the meibomian sebaceous glands lining the inside of the eyelids.
‖Avicenna uses "reclusive individuals" to indicate those who sought to suppress their sexual desire. Some had resorted to venesecting the veins behind the ears to achieve low libido and sterility.

the beginning of leprosy, severe pharyngitis, shortness of breath, severe asthma, voice hoarseness, and vitiligo due to an excess of hot blood, as well as diseases of the spleen and the sides of the body [such as pleurisy]. As we have explained before, the vein should be punctured with a very fine blade. As to the method of restricting the vein, the head should be tilted to the opposite side of the venesected side, and select an area of the vein that is stable. As in the saphenous and sciatic veins, the clamping should be horizontal, while the incision should be longitudinal.

There is also the vein in the nose tip, the **nasal branch of the anterior facial vein.** Its venesected spot is usually where it branches into two upon pushing on it. It produces only a little amount of blood upon bleeding. Its venesection is useful in cases of freckles, unhealthy facial color, hemorrhoids, nose boils, and itchy nose. However, its venesection produces permanent redness of the face that looks similar to favus,* which spreads over the face; therefore, its harmful effect outweighs it benefit.

Venesection of the **veins below the mastoid process of the temporal bone** is beneficial in cases of dizziness caused by light blood and advanced pains of the head. The **labial veins** are four, two for each lip. Their venesection is beneficial in cases of mouth sores, stomatitis, and painful, swollen, and receding gums, as well as hemorrhoids and their cracks. The **sublingual vein,** which is below the tongue and above the interior of the chin, is usually venesected in breathing problems and swelling of tonsils. Another sublingual vein below the tongue itself is venesected in cases of speech heaviness due to blood humor; this should be venesected longitudinally since a crosswise incision may not help in blood clotting later. The area between the lower lip and chin is venesected in cases of foul mouth smell. Additionally, a **gum vein** is venesected to treat problems of the stomach mouth.

Among the arteries of the head that may be venesected is the **temporal artery.** In addition to venesection, it may be cut, drained, or cauterized; this is done sometimes to stop the acute catarrh of light humors

---

*Favus, Latin for "honeycomb," is a disease affecting the scalp, but occurring occasionally on any part of the skin.

that pours into the eyes and at the early stages of a condition called pupil dilation. The arteries behind the ears, the **posterior auricular arteries**, are venesected in cases of conjunctivitis, beginning of glaucoma, leucoma, night blindness, and chronic headache. Their venesection is not free of risk, and the incision is slow to heal.

Galen has told the story of a person who was injured in the throat's artery and lost a large amount of blood. Galen treated the bleeding wound with oliban, aloe, Socotra dragon tree, and myrrh, and stopped the bleeding and cured the patient of a chronic pain in the hip.

Among the vessels that are venesected in the body are two on the abdomen. One connects to the liver, and the other to the spleen. The one on the right is venesected in edema, and the other in diseases of the spleen.

There are two times to carry out venesection, one of choice and the other of necessity. The preferable time of choice is midday after completion of digestion and evacuation. However, the time of necessity is when venesection has to be done without delay or regard to any contraindication. Be aware that the dull scalpel causes a lot of harm; it is a source of mistakes, does not reach, and induces swelling and pain. When working the scalpel, do not push it, but rather move it gently to get its tip to the tissue of the vessels. Roughness with the scalpel may cause small, invisible nicks in the tip of the blade; thus, it becomes slippery and causes injuries to the vessels. If you insist on using this damaged blade, you will cause more problems. For this reason, the blade's action on the skin should be tested first before venesection and when recutting—if you prefer. Also, you should make an effort to fill up the vessels with blood because this minimizes slipping and the movement of the vessel. If the vein is difficult and does not appear after strapping, then untie the strap and retie it several times, massage the area, and pressure the vein up and down until it appears. While doing this, use two fingers to try to catch the vein along its known path; sometimes stop its blood flow, and other times release one finger until you clearly feel the vein. Thus, pull it up to raise it, or let it go to release it. The head of the scalpel should not go deep to avoid harming an artery or nerve. The thinnest areas of the vein should be filled the most. The scalpel should be held by the thumb and the middle finger, while the index finger is used for feeling around the tissue. The scalpel should be held from the lower half of its handle, and nothing above that, because holding it from above the middle makes it unsteady. If the vein moves to one side, then tie it and hold it from the opposite side; however, if it moves to either side, then avoid venesecting it longitudinally. Strapping and pressuring should be according to the condition of the skin in hardness and thickness, as well as the amount of flesh. Strapping should be close to the venesection spot. If the strapping makes the vein disappear, then mark the spot and be careful that the vein does not move away from the marked spot of strapping. If the vein moves after strapping, then venesection should be canceled. If it is hard to locate the vein and to bring it up, then slit the flesh above it in people with skinny bodies, use a hook, and tie the vein. Strapping during venesection prevents the fullness of the vein. The individual who sweats a lot due to fullness is in need of venesection. Very often, the patient with fever and headache who is ready to undergo venesection gets a natural diarrhea that makes venesection unnecessary.

TWENTY-SECOND SECTION

On Cupping

Cupping cleanses the areas of the skin more than does venesection. It extracts more of the thin blood than thick blood. Its benefit is small in bulky, large bodies because it does not efficiently pull and extract their blood, but rather draws the thin fraction with difficulty and causes weakness in the cupped organ.

Cupping should not be prescribed at the beginning of the lunar month because the humors have not yet moved or gotten agitated, nor at the end of the month, when they have diminished, but rather at the middle of the month, when the humors are excited by the increase of the lunar brightness, which also increases in the brain within the skull and in the waters in tidal rivers. Know that the best time of day for cupping is between two and three o'clock. Cupping should be avoided after a bath, except for those with thick blood; they should bathe, rest for an hour, and then undergo cupping.

Most people [i.e., physicians] despise cupping on the forehead and warn about its harmful effect on the senses and the mind. Cupping on the mastoid process [back of the neck] is second in benefit to the venesection of the median cubital vein. It is beneficial in heaviness of the forehead, lightening the eyelids, trachoma, malodor of the mouth, and hardening of the eye. Cupping on the back [between the shoulders] is second in effectiveness to venesecting the basilic vein. It is beneficial in relieving shoulder and throat pain. Cupping on the two veins along the neck is second to venesection of the cephalic vein. Their cupping is beneficial in cases of head trembling and to the organs of the head, such as the face, teeth, ears, eyes, throat, and nose. However, cupping on the mastoid process actually causes loss of memory, as has been said, since the back of the brain is the site of memory and is weakened by cupping. Also, cupping on the upper back weakens the mouth of the stomach. Cupping the veins of the neck may cause head trembling. Therefore, to avoid side effects, cupping on the mastoid process should be done slightly lower, and cupping on the upper back should be done slightly higher, unless the reason is to treat the bleeding and coughing, then it should be moved lower and not higher. Cupping on the upper back and the inner sides of the thighs is beneficial in bloody chest disease (hemoptysis) and bloody asthma; however, it weakens the stomach and causes heart palpitations.

Cupping on the leg is similar to venesection in its effectiveness. It cleanses the blood and induces menstruation. For white women with loose bodies and thin blood, it is better to cup the legs than venesect the GSV. Cupping on the occiput* and the top of the head is beneficial in mental confusion and dizziness, and it has been said that it slows down the advancement of hair graying; however, it should be checked because it varies among different bodies and in most cases it accelerates it. It is also beneficial in eye diseases, which is where it is most effective

---

*Occiput is the anatomical term for the back of the head.

since it helps in the recovery from trachoma and pustules; however, its side effects include senility, loss of memory, mental confusion, and some chronic diseases, and it is harmful to people with glaucoma unless used at the proper time. Cupping under the chin is good for the teeth, face, and throat, and cleanses the head and the jaws.

Cupping on the loins helps in cases of boils, scabies, and pustules of the thigh; gout; hemorrhoids; elephantiasis; gas of the bladder and uterus; and itching of the back. The cupping would have the same effect whether the cupping was with heat or without, or with slitting (scarification) or without. The cupping with slitting is more effective in non-gaseous situations, and the one with slitting is better in disintegrating the cold gas and removing it from the loins and from any other location.

Cupping on the front side of the thighs is beneficial in swelling of the testicles and abscesses of the thighs and legs, and cupping on the back of the thighs is beneficial in the swellings and abscesses of the buttocks. Cupping below the knee is beneficial when the pain in the knee is caused by sharp humors, bad abscesses, and old sores in the shank and the foot. Cupping on the heels is good in cases of amenorrhea, sciatica, and gout.

Cupping without slitting (scarification) may be used to attract the waste matter against the direction of its movement, as when cupping the breast to stop menorrhagia, bringing up a deep tumor for treatment, translocating a tumor from one organ to a less significant organ, warming up the organ by bringing blood to it and disintegrating its gas, bringing an organ back to its original location, as in a hydrocele, and calming the pain, as in cupping the navel in severe colic, intestinal gas, and uterine pain, especially during menorrhea in young women.

Cupping on the hip can be used to treat sciatica and possible joint dislocation. Cupping between the hips is beneficial for the hips, thighs, hemorrhoids, hydrocele, and gout. Cupping the anus brings fluids from all over the body, including the head. It is good for the intestines, corruption of menstruation, and lightness of the body.

We assert that cupping with slitting has three benefits: first, the evacuation from that particular organ where the cupping takes place; second, retention of the organ's strength without getting affected by the elimination of humors; and third, it does not evacuate from the main organs. The incision should be made deep to bring the waste fluids from the lower tissue. If the tissue around the cup swells up and the cup is stuck and difficult to remove, then apply a piece of warm-to-hot, wet cloth or sponge around the cup mouth at first. This happens often when cupping around the breast to prevent menorrhagia or nosebleed; for this reason, the cup should not be placed on the breast itself. Once the location of the cupping has been rubbed with oil, make the slit quickly, and place the cup gently without excessive pressure so that it can be quickly removed the first time. Later, the cup can be left gradually for a longer time. The cupped person should be fed after one hour. The boy can be cupped in the second year of age. After the age of sixty, cupping should not be used at all. Cupping the upper parts of the body is safer than bringing the waste matter to the lower parts. After cupping a person with yellow bile, they should be given pomegranate seeds and juice, juice of true endive with sugar, and lettuce with vinegar.

TWENTY-THIRD SECTION

On Leeching

In India, it is known that some of the leeches are poisonous. Therefore, leeches with the following characteristics should be avoided: those with very large heads, dark blue to black or green color, hirsute bodies, eel-like, with azure striations, and with coloration similar to chameleons. The use of these poisonous leeches causes swelling, fainting, bleeding, fever, muscle relaxation, and bad ulcers. Catching leeches from dirty, muddy water should be avoided. It is better to fish them out of algal water (water with algae growing in it) or water with frogs living in it (disregard any contrary advice). Among the leeches to use are the ones of mixed colors and greenish tops with two arsenic lines,* blondish color [i.e., light brown] with rounded sides, dark brown (like liver

---

*Elemental arsenic is dark bluish gray. In some translations, the color is given as yellow (Michalsen, Roth, and Dobos, *Medicinal Leech Therapy*).

color), looking like small grasshoppers, similar to the mouse tail, and the thin and small-headed; however, do not use the ones that have red bellies and green backs, especially from running water.

Leeches draw out blood more deeply than does cupping. The leeches should be brought in one day before their intended use and hung upside down to empty the contents of the belly, if possible. Then, they are fed on the blood of a lamb or alike before using them. Thereafter, their slime and skin is cleaned with a sponge. The location on the patient's skin should be cleaned with borax and massaged until it becomes red. When needed, the leech should be sent in clean, fresh water. Leeches are encouraged to attach by rubbing the location with clay or blood. Leeches that become fully engorged can be released by sprinkling on them salt, ash, borax, linen ash, sponge ash, or wool ash. The most proper thing to do after the fall of the leech is to apply cupping; this will ameliorate the harmful effect of the leech bite. If bleeding continues from the bite location, then sprinkle some burned astringent, ash, powdered pottery, or alike to stop the bleeding. These bleeding treatments should be available at the leech applicator. Leech application is useful in skin diseases such as ringworm, freckles, and others.

TWENTY-FOURTH SECTION

On Stopping Depletions

Depletions are stopped by diverting the matter without letting it go out; diverting and elimination; supporting the elimination; using drugs that are cooling, agglutinant, astringent, or caustic drugs; or strapping (tourniquet). An example of diversion without depletion is breast cupping to stop bleeding from the uterus. The best application of diversion is that which involves the relief of pain of the depleted organ. Example of a diversion with depletion are venesection of the basilic vein, arresting vomiting by inducing diarrhea, arresting diarrhea by emesis, and arresting both by sweating. Examples of stopping depletion by aiding depletion are the cleansing of the stomach and intestines from the diarrhea-inducing slippery viscous humors, inducing emesis to cleanse the stomach mouth from the humors that cause vomiting, applying cold medications to solidify (coagulate) liquid and constrict openings, using astringent drugs to bind matter and constrict openings, and using glutinous drugs to clog openings. When these drugs are hot and desiccant their effect is stronger. Caustic drugs form a scab on the surface of the opening that blocks the flow and caps it; this may cause an expected harm when the scab is removed and leaves a bigger opening. Some of the caustic drugs have astringent (styptic*) effects, like white vitriol; some do not have astringent effects, like quicklime. The astringents are used for a temporary scab, the noncaustic astringents for a temporary scab that falls off quickly, and the caustic astringents for a stable, strong scab.

Stopping depletion can be done with compression. Compressing the opening and forcing it to close, such as when there is a mistake in venesecting the basilic vein that injures the artery; in this case, a plug is used, such as the hair of a rabbit. We advise that if bleeding is due to an opening, it be treated with astringent to bring its edges closer; if it is due to a burn, treat with glutinous astringent like Lemnian earth [clay from the Greek island of Lemnos; its tablets had the seal of the priestess of Hephaestus, hence the Arabic name, "sealed clay"]; and if it is due to a mixture of growth and scabs, this treatment is described elsewhere [and consists of a dual treatment for growth and cleansing].

TWENTY-FIFTH SECTION

Treatment of Obstruction

Obstruction may be caused by thick humors, viscous humors, or an excess of many humors. If there is no other cause of obstruction, the effect of the humors can be removed by eliminating through venesection and diarrhea. If the humors are thick, then they should be loosened by resolving (liquefying) drugs, and viscous humors (especially thin ones) require decomposing drugs. You are aware of the difference between the thick and the viscous; it is like the difference between clay

---

*Styptic effects slow down bleeding or stop it by causing blood vessels to contract.

and glue. The thick needs thinning to induce its movement, and the viscous needs the decomposer to break down the adhesive property of its components. There are two paradoxical precautions when resolving the thick humor: The first, weak resolving, increases the volume of the humor without reaching a desired liquefaction to undo the obstruction, thus increasing the obstruction. The second is an excessive resolving that liquefies the thin part and solidifies the thick part. When strong resolution is required, it should be followed by a gentle resolvent without thickness in it and with the application of moderate heat to help in resolving all of the obstruction.

The most difficult obstruction is that of the vessels, and the worse of these is the obstruction of arteries, especially in the main organs. If the openers of obstruction combine astringency and amelioration, they would be better since the astringent reduces the harsh effect of attenuation on the organ.

TWENTY-SIXTH SECTION

Treatment of Swellings

Swellings are warm or cold, soft or solid, and we have listed them earlier [see the 2nd Art]. Their causes are either external or predisposed. An example of predisposed causes is fullness, and the external are traumas such as falling, blow, or bite. External causes may be associated with humoral fullness, imbalance, or neither. Swellings caused by external or predisposed reasons associated with humoral fullness may sometimes be in organs that are close to main organs, such as the emunctories that remove waste products from the body [e.g., kidneys, skin]. When the swellings are not close to important organs, none of the resolvents should be initially applied to them, but rather the repelling organ should be treated. The whole body should be treated if the swelling is not due to the malfunction of a single organ. The deterrents, divergents, and astringents should be applied to the swelling, or very close to it. Divergence from the organ to the opposite side [of the matter that contributes to the swelling] can be achieved by exercising the opposite side or carrying a heavy weight. Very often, the matter is attracted away from the swollen arm by carrying a weight in the other hand for a while.

As to astringents, the deterring astringents used in the treatment of hot swellings should be exclusively of cold temperament, while in the cold swellings the astringents should be mixed with a substance that has a hot effect, like lemongrass and oyster shell. An increase in the size of either hot or cold swellings requires decreasing the amount of the astringent and increasing the resolvent until the swelling reaches its maturity, then the two substances are mixed in equal amounts, and at the decline of the swelling, the treatment should include only the resolvent and softening. Cold and soft swellings need a more drying and hardening resolvent than in the hot swellings. Swellings from external causes without humoral fullness are first treated with softeners and resolvents, or as the above treatment of the first type.

If the swollen organ is the emunctory of an important organ, such as the glands of the neck and around the ears for the brain, axilla for the heart, and groin for the liver; it should not be treated with deterrents. Although that is the right treatment for the swellings, in this case it is not the method of choice because we want to attract more of the humors to the swellings, away from the important organ, to avoid worse complications in this organ. We allow more material to accumulate in the swelling of the subservient lower organ than in the higher organ, and we apply cupping and sever attractant wraps to bring the matter to the swollen organ.

The accumulation of these swellings, or alike, in the empty areas may lead to their bursting or they may be given assistance to burst, and they may need maturation and piercing. Maturation is done with local heat that is confined with a gluey substance. When trying to induce maturation, one should examine whether the innate heat is weak and the organ is dying; in this case, gluey and confining substances should be removed and openers and deep incisions should be applied. This is followed with drugs that are resolvents and desiccants. We cover this topic in the books on particulars. Frequently, the swelling is deep and needs to be pulled to the surface, even with fire cupping.

Solid swellings that have surpassed their initial stage should be softened with drugs that have less heating and drying, so that their thick part does not harden by excessive decomposition, but rather prepares all of it for decomposition; then follow with stronger decomposition. In case there is a possibility that the remaining portion may harden, soften it again, and follow this routine until all vanishes between softening and decomposition.

Unripe swellings are treated with substances that warm and soften. Gaseous swellings are treated with warming and softening substances to disintegrate the gas and enlarge the pores since their cause is the condensation of gas [accumulation] and occlusion of pores. The causal substance of gas accumulation should be treated. Some swellings develop into ulcers, such as herpes, which should be cooled down like the phlegmon hot swelling; however, they should not be moistened. If the swelling requires moistening it should not be done because the goal here is to avoid ulceration, and rather, it should be dried since the treatment of an ulcer is drying, and moistening is the most harmful for it.

Internal swellings should be drained by venesection or diarrhea, and the patient should avoid bathing, alcohol, and excessive physical and emotional reactions like anger and alike. Initially, the patient should use mild deterrents, especially if the swelling is in the stomach or liver. When the time to treat with resolvents arrives, the treatment should include resolvents and pleasant smells, as we have mentioned earlier. The liver and stomach are more in need of such treatment than the lungs. The emollients [such as laxatives] used here should have a maturation effect on the swellings and be compatible with the swellings, such as European black nightshade (*Solanum nigrum*, عنب الثعلب) and **golden shower tree** (Indian laburnum [*Cassia fistula*], الخيار شنبر). European black nightshade is very good for resolving internal hot swellings.

The patient with hot swellings should not be fed a large amount of food or at the time of a [fever] episode unless there is a severe loss of strength. A patient with hot swelling and loss of strength will die. Strength flourishes with food, and food in this case is most harmful. If the swelling resolves itself, this is the best outcome, and if it bursts, then there is a need to drink something to wash it away, such as honey water or sugary water, followed with a substance that does gentle maturation, and finally, the desiccant. This is further explained in the book on the particular diseases.

Sometimes, there is a misdiagnosis of swellings below the belly since it is sometimes a hernia, not a swelling, and there is danger in cutting it open, and it may be an internal swelling, not in the peritoneum, but in the intestine itself; there is danger in slitting it, so beware.

TWENTY-SEVENTH SECTION

General Description of Incisions

Incisions in the skin should be made along the lines and wrinkles, but not in the forehead, since an incision along the forehead lines and creases will cut its muscle and the eyebrow will fall. The same applies to the organs whose lines are not in the same direction. The practitioner should be knowledgeable in anatomy, the anatomy of nerves, veins, and arteries, so that they do not make a mistake and cut some of them and cause the patient's death. The practitioner should make available to themselves a few of the drugs that stop bleeding, painkillers, and instruments that are suitable for the process. For example, the practitioner should have Galen's drug*, rabbit hair, spider's cobweb (which has obvious benefit), egg white, and cautery; all of this to prevent bleeding if a mistake occurs, or for a necessity. Additionally, the practitioner should have the single drugs as we have described in the book on single drugs. You are aware that when slitting an abscess and its contents are released, not to approach it with oil or water or an ointment containing fat or a majority of oil, like Basilicon ointment,† but rather an ointment like that of red iron oxide. The latter should be used as needed, and a sponge soaked in an astringent should be placed on top of the open abscess.

---

*Composed of one half part each of wax, pine resin, Euphorbia (*Euphorbia serrate*), and thick pitch resin, and one part of oil and balsam of Mecca.

†Basilicon, or basilicum, is an ointment used as an unguent and is composed of resin, wax, pitch, and oil.

TWENTY-EIGHTH SECTION

Treatment of Organ Degradation and Amputation

If the organ degrades due to dystemperament, with substance or without, and is not recovering after incision and application of creams that are proper for treatment, as in the books on the particulars, then the degraded flesh should be removed. First, the removal should be without using cauterizing instruments, since cauterizing may harm parts of the muscles, nerves, and vessels very badly. However, if this treatment is not healing the problem and the degradation has reached the blood, then the organ has to be amputated. The cutting surface has to be cauterized by dipping it into hot boiled oil to prevent the spread of degradation to other parts and to stop bleeding. On the cutting surface, there will be growth of unsuitable blood and skin that resembles blood in its consistency.

If the decision is made to amputate, then a probe should be inserted in the degraded flesh and moved around the bone until it reaches a properly adhering tissue; this is where pain is felt when the probe goes in, and it is the limit of safety. The area where the tissue is hanging and poorly attached is part of what should be amputated. The bone may be drilled with several holes to make it easy to break, or it may be sawed off. To do this, the tissue should be pulled back to avoid extra pain. If the piece of bone that should be cut is sticking out or a splinter of an arm that may not heal and may degrade and spoil more parts, then the healthy flesh surrounding it should be freed from the bone and pulled back, or by using other tricks that may be arrived at when examining the case at hand. When a sound organ is close to the site of cutting, the organ should be wrapped with cloth to keep it at a safe distance from the saw, and then start the cutting. If the bone is like that of the thigh and the bad part is large and close to the nerves, arteries, and veins, the physician should then find an alternative way.

TWENTY-NINTH SECTION

Treatment of Discontinuity, Types of Ulcers, Sprains, Traumas, and Falling

Discontinuity in the large organs, which can be treated by alignment, proper effective bandaging, as in the bone-setting profession (discussed in its specific chapter), then by resting and by eating proper gelatinous food (like animal feet) that will transform into cartilaginous food, which helps ligate the ends of the fracture. Otherwise, it is impossible to heal fractures, especially in mature bodies, except according to this description. We will describe bone setting in detail in the book on particulars. As to the discontinuity in soft organs, there are three principles that should be followed. First, the initial thing to do if the cause is ongoing: stop the flowing of the material [be it blood, urine, gastric juice and so forth] and cut off its adjacent supply. Second, heal the split with medications and suitable food. Third, prevent sepsis if possible. If you achieve one of the three, then you can pay attention to the other two.

As to stopping bleeding, you have already been exposed to it, and we have finished explaining it. Fusing the parts of the split is done by bringing the two edges of the wound together and applying desiccant ointments and eating gelatinous food.

The goal of treating ulcers is to dry them. Ulcers that are free of putrefaction can be dried; however, others with putrefaction need strong caustic applications such as red iron oxide, white vitriol, arsenic, and quicklime; if these are not effective, then cauterization should be used. The compound medication (containing verdigris, wax, and oil) cleanses by verdigris and prevents by the wax and oil the excess action of the caustic; it is a moderate medication in this regard, as mentioned in the pharmacopoeia (*aqrabadhin*). Every ulcer is either single or compound. The edges of the single small ulcer, if its tissue is intact, can be pulled together and wrapped with caution to prevent the presence of oil or dust, and they will fuse together. Similarly, the edges of a large ulcer with intact structure can be pulled together as mentioned. However, large ulcers, such that their edges cannot be pulled together, with pus within their lumen, or having lost some of their tissue, should be treated by desiccation. If the ulcer has lost some skin, then there is the need for a seal [i.e., a scab], which can be formed by applying an astringent or caustic, like white vitriol and red iron oxide, that induces dryness and scab formation. However, the latter two drugs may increase the size of the ulcer if applied in excess.

If the ulceration has caused the loss of some tissue, as in deep ulcers, then forming a scab should not be the priority. In this case, we should encourage the formation of tissue. The drugs used here to stimulate the formation of flesh should not have a drying effect beyond the first degree [on the Unani scale].

There are some other conditions that have to be followed. Among these are the original temperament of the organ and the temperament of the ulcer. If the organ's original temperament is very moist and the ulcer is not very moist, then a slight drying of the ulcer is sufficient because the illness has not surpassed the original temperament by much. However, if the organ's temperament is dry and the ulcer is very moist, then second- and third-degree desiccants are needed to bring it back to its original temperament. The temperament of the ulcer should be brought to equitability in the equitable organs. Among these conditions also is consideration of the temperament of the body as a whole. If the body is very dry, then its excessively moist organ is equitable in moisture according to the equitable body; therefore, it should be dried according to the equitable body. Similarly, if the body has excessive moisture and the organ is dry. If both are increased in their states, such as both became more moist, then drying should be greater, and if both became more dry, then drying should be lesser.

Additionally, the strength of the desiccants should be considered. For example, desiccants that promote tissue growth, although they do not cause severe drying (as do those that do not promote growth), but scabbing, obstruct the flow of growth materials. Therefore, these regeneration-promoting desiccants are more cleansing of pus than are those that scab and seal. All desiccant drugs without caustic effect have regeneration properties on the flesh, and all ulcers in nonfleshy locations, as well as round ones, are slow to heal. To treat deep or internal ulcers, the desiccant drugs and astringents should be mixed with penetrating drugs, like honey, and location-specific drugs, like diuretics in the treatment of urinary ulcers. Also, to heal the ulcer, the astringent drug should be made viscous, like Lemnian earth.

Be aware that there are inhibitors to the healing of ulcers, such as unhealthiness of the organ (i.e., the organ's temperament); therefore, we need to fix it as you have learned. There is also the low quality of the blood supplying the organ, so you need to follow up with the diet that produces good chyme. Excessive blood supply to the ulcer increases its moisture and should be reduced by depletion, diet, and exercise. Disintegration of the underlying bone and discharge of pus has no drug that can fix that, except scraping or trimming. In treating ulcers, ointments are often needed to bring out the bits of bones and their sharp debris (spicules); otherwise, they will prevent the healing of the ulcer.

Healing ulcers requires a good diet for strengthening the body, but at the same time needs to reduce the ulcer in order to minimize the pus. Therefore, to deal with such opposing needs, the reduction of pus should be followed by an ample diet, and the increase in pus should be followed by reducing the diet; the physician should manage this. In the initial stage of ulcers or during their growth, the patient should not go into the bathhouse or pour hot water in order to prevent attracting material to the ulcers. However, if the ulcer matures and becomes open then it is fine to bathe. An ulcer that begins to heal but keeps reverting back will become a sinus. The color of the pus and the edge of the opening should always be examined. If the pus increases without an increase in diet, it is a sign of maturation.

A rip (فسخ) is deep discontinuity below the skin; therefore, it is obvious that its medications should be stronger than those for surface injuries. Because it causes blood accumulation, it is necessary to use resolvents that are not excessive desiccants to avoid breaking down the light portion and hardening the thick portion. Once the resolvents' action is finished, a cicatrizant is applied to speed up the healing and prevent any foreign residue from going in between the fusing parts, causing putrefaction and reseparation of the parts. If the rip is deep, the location should be scarified to allow the medication to go through deeper. However, it may be sufficient to treat a light rip and light trauma through venesection. If the rip is accompanied by a longitudinal split* (شدخ) that may have split a nerve, the split should be treated first with the medication specific for the split in order to treat the rip later. When the split is large it is treated with desiccants, and if it is small, like the prick of a needle, it is left to nature to take care of it; however, if it is poisonous, twisted, severely disconnected, or injured a nerve, then there is the fear that it will swell and cause throbbing. For a sprain, it is sufficient to bandage it and apply the specific medications for a sprain. A fall or trauma requires venesection at the opposite side, light diet without meat and alike, use of lotions, and specific drinks, as described in the books on particulars. The discussion on the discontinuity of nervous organs and bones is delayed until later.

THIRTIETH SECTION

On Cauterization

Cauterization is carried out to prevent the spread of corruption, to strengthen the organ when its temperament becomes cold, to break down the bad humors attached to the organ, and to stop bleeding. The best material to use for cauterization is gold. The location of cauterization may be obvious and can be seen or may be embedded inside an organ, like the nose, mouth, or anus. The latter situation requires a speculum coated with a baked layer of talcum powder or Armenian clay mixed with vinegar, then wrapped with a cloth and cooled down substantially in rose water or other juices. The speculum is sent into the desired body cavity until it meets the location to be cauterized; the hot cautery is then sent to the location through the speculum. With this setup, the cautery should not harm other body parts, especially if the cautery is thinner than the walls of the speculum and does not touch its walls. The practitioner of cauterization should be careful not to harm neighboring tissues, like nerves, tendons, and ligaments. When

---

*A longitudinal split is a longitudinal opening in a nerve that is deep and large (Avicenna, 2nd Art, 1st Lesson, 4th Section).

cauterization is done to stop bleeding, it should be very effective at a depth that creates a deep and thick scab that does not fall off quickly, since the fall of a cauterization scab brings more trouble than before. The proper limit of cauterizing to remove corrupt flesh is its induction of pain. Sometimes, it is necessary to cauterize all the way to the bone beneath the bad flesh to stop all of its corrupting effect. If this situation exists on the skull, you have to reduce the heat so that the brain does not boil from the heat and the eyebrows do not spasm; in other situations, you should be worry free.

THIRTY-FIRST SECTION

On Relieving Pain

You have learned that the causes of pain fall into two types: discontinuity and sudden dystemperament, which in its later stages becomes hot, cold, or dry dystemperament, with or without humor, gas, or swelling. Therefore, relief of pain takes place by treating the causes. You are aware of the treatments of each type and how to recognize and treat dystemperament, swelling, and gas.

Every pain that becomes severe may kill; initially, it causes coldness and shivering of the body, then decrease of pulse, followed by its cessation and death. In general, the pain is relieved by changing the dystemperament, resolving the humor, or applying anesthesia. Anesthetics relieve pain by stopping the sensation in the organ in one of two ways: by excessive cooling or by the toxicity to the metabolism of the organ.

Resolvents in general are gentle decomposers, such as linseeds, dill, yellow melilot, chamomile, celery seeds, and bitter almonds, and all are hot in the first degree, especially if there is some stickiness, like the gum of pear, starch, soups, saffron, labdanum, marshmallow, cardamom, turnip and its stew, fat, green hyssop, and oil, as we have mentioned. Laxatives, purgatives, and alike have similar resolving properties. Resolvents should be used after evacuation, if evacuation is needed to stop the supply of matter to the organ, in addition to using whatever matures swellings and bursts them.

The strongest anesthetic is opium. Other anesthetics include mandrake (and its seeds and bark of its root), poppy plants, henbane, black nightshade, and lettuce seeds. Ice and cold water are also considered anesthetics. Often the causes of pains are external matters, like exposure to hot or cold conditions, uncomfortable sleeping position, or an injury during drunkenness. Therefore, it is a mistake when seeking an internal cause in the body. Furthermore, it should be explored whether there is fullness and seek the signs of fullness. Also, the cause may be external, but giving hot internally. For example, an individual who drinks cold water that causes severe pain in the stomach and liver does not need a difficult treatment like evacuation or alike, but rather bathing and long sleep. An individual who develops a severe headache after drinking hot drinks needs only to drink cold water.

The drug to use for pain relief may be slow acting but the pain cannot be tolerated (such as expelling the trapped substance in the intestinal fibers, causing colic) or fast acting but with severe side effects (such as anesthetizing in colic). The physician here has to apply their medical sense to figure out which is longer, the duration of strength or the duration of pain, and whether the pain or the drug is more harmful, thus selecting the right treatment. Perhaps the persisting pain could kill by its intensity and severity, and the anesthetic may also kill or harm in other aspects. Sometimes the side effects of the anesthetic can be avoided and another treatment be applied. However, you should examine the composition of the anesthetic and its characteristics, and use its simplest forms or use its compound form with its antidote, unless it is a critical condition that requires a strong anesthetic. Some organs are not very affected by the use of anesthesia, and it does not produce severe side effects, such as the teeth. [For some organs] taking the anesthetic in a drink is safe, as for relieving eye pain, and it is less harmful than putting it on a mascara. However, the harm of drinking anesthetics may be avoided in other organs.

In the case of colic, anesthetics increase the danger because the waste matter becomes colder, thicker, and insulated. Anesthetics relieve pain by inducing sleep, which is one of the methods for pain cessation, especially when combined with hunger in a physical pain condition.

Compound anesthetics that can be stopped with antidotes are safer, such as philonium* and the triangular tablets,† but they are weaker anesthetics. The fresh and soft of these compound mixtures is the strongest; the old [and dry] has no effect, and the one in the middle has moderate strength.

Some of the severe pains are easy to treat, like the gaseous pains. These can simply be treated by pouring warm water on them; however, there may be a danger if the cause is actually a swelling thought to be gas, thus causing greater harm. Additionally, if the hot water treatment does not resolve the gas issue, it will cause its expansion. Hot water fomentation is another treatment for gas, especially if it is mixed with proso millet, except in an organ that can not tolerate it, such as the eye, which is usually fomented with a piece of cloth. Fomentation sometimes is applied with warm oils. Among the strong foments is the cooked flour of ervil in vinegar, dried, and made into a poultice; similarly, you may use the bran for a milder version. Salt fomentation is used for steam burn; the proso millet is better but weaker. Water in a bladder is used as fomentation; it is safe and soft, however, care should be taken as mentioned above.

Fire cupping is similar in its effect to fomentation. It is effective in silencing gaseous pain, and repeating a few times takes away the pain. However, its side effects as similar to the resolvents. Among the relievers of pain is a long, gentle walk because it produces relaxation. Additionally, light known fats, oils as mentioned, nice singing, especially to induce sleep, and distraction with entertainment are strong relievers of pain.

---

*According to Galen, philonium is a compound drug that was invented by Philon of Tarsus. The drug is composed of white pepper, henbane, opium, saffron, euphorbia, pellitory, Spikenard (*Nardostachys jatamansi*), and honey.
†Triangular tablets are a type of compound drug whose pills are shaped as a triangle.

THIRTY-SECOND SECTION

Advice on Which Treatment to Start

If a number of diseases fall together, then we should start treating the one that has one of the three following characteristics. First, healing the second cannot be done without healing the first. For example, if a swelling and a sore occur together, first treat the swelling in order to remove the accompanying dystemperament (that also would prevent the healing of the sore), then treat the sore. Second, when one is the cause of the other, such as the co-occurrence of obstruction and fever, the obstruction should be treated first [because it is the cause of the fever], then the fever. When a warmer or desiccant is needed to open the obstruction, use them without worrying about the fever because it is impossible to treat the fever while its cause remains, and the treatment of its cause is desiccant drugs, which are bad in a fever. Third, treat the one that is more serious than the other. For example, when a continuous fever (synochus) is co-occurring with palsy, treat the fever with coolants and venesection and ignore the palsy.

Usually we treat the disease rather than its symptoms unless the symptoms become more dangerous. In this case, the symptom should be venesected without worrying about the disease, like giving anesthetics in severe colic when the colic becomes difficult, even though it may hurt the colon. Venesection may be delayed due to weakness in the stomach, existing diarrhea, or nausea; or the venesection should not be delayed, but done partially, as in spasmodic episodes where venesection leaves some of the humor so that the spasmodic movement breaks it down without affecting the innate heat.

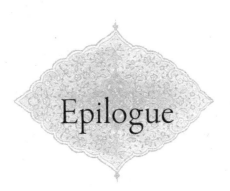

Epilogue

Throughout this book, we have attempted to connect the Unani concepts with the modern scientific knowledge; we explained our interpretation for the scientific basis of Unani and showed areas of agreement and conflict between the two. However, in this epilogue, we are aiming to elucidate how some Unani concepts can provide theoretical and practical solutions to several intractable problems in current biomedical sciences. As scientists in touch with current global biomedical research efforts and working on several of these aspects to provide solutions, we feel confident that our ideas that we offer here provide some directions and may be viable solutions. The reader will realize that our ideas and explanations are just links on the continuum of scientific knowledge that spans millennia; we are simply connecting the forgotten scientific past with that of the present to make progress possible. In so doing, we are paying tribute to those scientists who dedicated their lives and work to keep medicine objective and beneficial to humanity.

For a long period of time starting in the nineteenth century, Unani knowledge has become increasingly marginalized and its contributions to the current Western medical system unacknowledged; the reasons are numerous but mainly due to the lack of good understanding of its principles and concepts, as well as prejudice for its association with Arabic and Islamic cultures. Unani medicine, like other traditional medical systems, is also undergoing a revival that may bring its concepts and modalities to the forefront of medical theory and practice and rewrite them in a modern format that makes Unani better understood, widely accepted, and effectively applied. Most recently, the interest in Unani has been expanding; books, articles, and websites on its various topics have been appearing, and more people are seeking to apply its modalities. We cannot end this book on Unani medicine without speculating on its future, its place in the modern health system, its future influence on Western medicine, and also its own future transformations.

During the process of writing this book, we have found Avicenna's writing to be mostly compatible with our current scientific knowledge and to have some predictive aspects whose accuracy and usefulness we have only recently come to realize. Of course, Avicenna did not invent Unani medicine; however, he was part of the continuum of scientists and physicians who documented the knowledge of their time and added to it their new data and experience. Like great teachers before him, such as Hippocrates, Galen, and Rhazes, Avicenna excelled in writing and teaching; he understood the sciences of his time and expanded on them and left us a voluminous body of writings. Reading the *Canon* shows us how truly fascinating is the amount of the ancient knowledge that was passed on through several cultures and their languages and reached us in a readable and logical format.

There are many fascinating concepts and ideas in Avicenna's *Canon* that have been forgotten by modern Western medicine, and their reintroduction will without a doubt change the latter in a meaningful manner if and when they are incorporated in it. From the preventive aspect of Unani we can point out the six essential requirements for health (fresh clean air, food and drink, movement and rest, sleep and wakefulness, eating and exercising, and healthy mental state), its emphasis on proper healthy digestion, the cumulative nature of intermediate compounds (incompletely digested or assimilated nutrients) and their effect on health, its understanding of the various ranges of homeostasis (i.e., temperaments) of organs and human races within and between populations that are adapted to certain geographical areas, its superb disease concept, and its most impressive insistence on the individualized nonharming nature of applying medicine.

If we have to choose one topic that signifies the strength and sophistication of Unani medicine, which also is important for modern medicine, it is its disease concept. Despite all the latest developments in biomedical research that have taken place during the last fifty years, modern medicine lacks a clear, well-defined disease concept such as that of Unani medicine (for a discussion of the disease concept in Unani see the introduction of the 2nd Art, "Disease, Causes, and General Symptoms"). The disease concept is the bedrock of any medical system because of its deep implications on defining the disease origin (the affected organ tissues and their cellular components), its related symptoms, boundaries (i.e., events marking its starting, peak, and ending phases), and treatment modalities. In Unani, the disease concept centers on the health status of energy production within the tissues of the organs as measured by temperaments; thus disease begins in Unani when normal energy production is disrupted—dystemperament. Although our current scientific knowledge points out the centrality of cellular energy production (as ATP) for cell differentiation and function, this energy-centered concept of disease does not exist in modern medicine, where the search for causation goes beyond this to genetics and epigenetics. Since the Unani energy concept of disease fits well with our current knowledge and the larger evolutionary framework of biology, it should be explored as a disease concept for our current Western medical paradigm. Except for exclusive genetic disorders, a well-defined disease concept is needed for our current biomedical paradigm to make progress on the main issues of modern medicine, such as the search for molecular biomarkers for early detection, progression monitoring, and assessment of response to treatment; subtyping of disease into its natural classes; personalized treatment and adverse drug reactions; and modeling of disease and its biological pathways (systems biology).

The lack of a clear disease concept in Western medicine has created several intractable issues that remain unresolved, and progress on their status remains elusive. One of these main issues is disease definition through its molecular boundaries (molecular events that are associated with producing the disease phenotype). Thus far, modern medicine cannot define the early molecular events of a disease. Take cancer, for example; up until now and after tens of years of research and hundreds of billions of dollars spent worldwide there is no agreement on what constitutes early oncogenic transformations that lead to cancerous growth! This means that we still do not know when the disease starts, and we do not have any biomarker for early detection of the disease. Similarly, modern medicine cannot predict if a patient will develop severe adverse reactions to a drug. Thus far, there are no predictive methods to classify the population according to the individuals' susceptibility to adverse reactions of various classes of pharmaceutical drugs or predict the success or failure of a drug treatment, especially in cancer treatments. The best indicator of a lack of a disease concept in Western medicine, at least within the pharmaceutical industry, is the piled-up list of drugs that have been withdrawn from the market due to their harmful and life-threatening effects. The lack of solutions for these issues make one realize the quandary of the new molecular paradigm and the urgent need for a disease concept that focuses the efforts on the correct mechanisms of disease.

As we have been discovering lately, many of the diseases are composed of multiple molecular subtypes (i.e., a disease phenotype encompasses several genotypes with molecular profiles that are dissimilar). Since the mid-1990s, advances in molecular biology and instrumentation allowed the fast acquisition of high-throughput biochemical data from blood serum or tissue specimens. These data are collectively referred to as "omics," which encompass gene-expression data from microarray technology, genetic data, such as nucleotide polymorphism (difference in DNA sequence) and copy number variation of a gene, and mass spectrometry data, such as metabolomics and proteomics. The omics data have shown that the diseased specimens are heterogeneous in their gene expression, metabolomics, and proteomic profiles, which is also an indication that the disease process itself is heterogeneous (i.e., a disease phenotype may develop by several interwoven genetic events and developmental pathways).

The heterogeneity of the disease process as reflected in the omics data has proven to be a very difficult issue to deal with. Mining heterogeneous data by conventional statistical methods is almost useless, and meaningful conclusions based on such data can only be reached by using the proper analytical paradigms and tools that can deal with such heterogeneity, since eliminating or reducing heterogeneity produces different results. Many researchers have ruined their good careers by proclaiming to have found a biomarker for early detection of a type of cancer that later proved to be useless. Without the proper study design and the right analytical tools the omics data can turn into a "too much of a good thing is not good for us" situation. The current opinion is that single-molecule indicators have not been proven to be the answer for early detection of disease. Prostate-specific antigen (PSA) and cancer antigen 125 (CA 125) are examples of problematic biomarkers that enjoyed wide popularity for a long time until studies proved their inaccuracies and contribution to overdiagnosis. This brings us back to the good old method of Unani profiling for health assessment and diagnosis. Unani physicians have practiced profiling by using the humors as their classes of biochemical molecules for monitoring the health status and for prevention. Because long-term humoral imbalance is the cause of susceptibility to disease and its subsequent development, detecting the imbalance is the responsibility of the physician. Fortunately, profiling and detecting humoral imbalance can also be carried out by using omics data. Two of the authors here (M. S. A.-A. and H. A.) have shown through a series of published research papers that the application of an analytical paradigm termed parsimony phylogenetics is more suitable for the mining of omics data and that profiling can be carried out by producing phylogenetic trees called cladograms. Thus, Unani teaches us that when early events cannot be ascertained by individual biomarkers, then monitoring the health status by tracking a few classes of molecules, quantitatively and qualitatively, is a working alternative to the futile search for single biomarkers.

However, Unani's energy-centric concept of disease may help narrow the search for biomarkers to particular pathways and their aberrations that are the real culprits in disease initiation. Concentrating on the health status of cellular energy and its machines (the mitochondria) narrows the study to fewer events and may allow the determination of predictive biomarkers.

The discussion also brings out the compatibility of Unani's disease concept with the modern theory of evolution. The modern synthesis of the evolutionary theory is approximately less than one hundred years old, and with its latter updates serves as the conceptual framework of modern biology; however, the organic evolution of life on Earth, and probably the universe, as a concept is very old and is described in ancient Chinese, Greek, and Indian writings. The centrality of evolutionary thinking is well stated in the famous statement of Theodosius Dobzhansky: "Nothing in biology makes sense except in the light of evolution."* His insistence on the use of the evolutionary framework to understand biological phenomena has proven to be the right dogma for the field of biology and related subjects, such as medicine. Not surprisingly, the Unani concept of disease is compatible with the theory of evolution. The human body is made up of single units called cells, and these types of cells are termed eukaryotic cells. There are only two types of cells in living organisms: prokaryotic (exist mostly in bacteria) and eukaryotic (all other organisms). Evidence suggests that the prokaryotic cells gave rise to the eukaryotic cells through a symbiotic event where one prokaryote entered the other and remained there (a guest and a host). The guest's specialty was energy production, and it is known to us now as the mitochondria, and the host represents the rest of the eukaryotic system—the nucleus, cytoplasm, ribosomes, and alike. This symbiotic event allowed the new cell to have an internal large source of energy to carry out its functions and to differentiate itself within a multicellular organism and to specialize in functions. Without the mitochondria, the eukaryotic cells, our building blocks, can not function. The Unani energy-centric disease concept teaches us that the disruption of the mitochondrial energy production is the first event in illness.

Unfortunately, evolution is not the conceptual framework within biomedical research or modern medicine. Except for a few lone scientists advocating the need for applying evolutionary reasoning to medical sciences, the evolutionary concept is almost absent within the modern medical establishment. However, the concept of temperament within Unani is evolution compatible (see "Primer: Concepts of Unani

---

*Dobzhansky, "Nothing in Biology Makes Sense."

Medicine" on page 17 and "The Essentials of Life: Heat and Water" on page 41) because it is in agreement with the symbiotic theory of the eukaryotic cell evolution where the symbiotic event permitted the existence of differentiated cells with narrow parameters of function— homeostasis or temperament in Unani terminology. In such a situation, the Unani concept of temperament fulfills, without a doubt, its prediction that health is based on the organ's ability to maintain normal energy production and its failure to do so is the root of malfunction and disease.

Modern biomedicine needs to examine the concepts of Unani because high-resolution and high-throughput instruments are not substitutes for good concepts that are within the right biological framework. The strength of Unani stems from its compatibility and harmony with the modern theory of biological evolution, where its energy-centric concept of disease offers the basis for progress in modern medicine.

It remains to be seen whether modern medicine will make the leap into the realm of Unani concepts to move itself from the logjam that it drove itself into by trying to find the magic bullets of biomarkers and treatments. On the other hand, Unani physicians are using modern technology to update their medicine and expand the power of their practice.* Without a doubt, Unani medicine will stay with humanity because of the strength of its concepts, its adaptability, its emphasis on prevention and personalized treatment, and the cost-effectiveness of its practice. We hope this book serves as an objective tool to understand Unani medicine in the twenty-first century.

---

*Mamtimin, "Plasma Metabonomic Analysis with ¹H" and "Plasma Metabonomics Analysis of Tumor Patients."

Arabic–English Glossary
of the *Canon*

These are the translations we chose for the following words
in Avicenna's *Canon*.

ا

Myrtle (*Myrtus communis*)	آس
Lichens	آشنه
Gangrene	الأكله
Bathtub	أبزن
Axillary vein	الإبطي
Savin (*Juniperus sabina*)	أبهل
Chameleon	أبي قلمون
Epilepsy	إبيليميا، صرع
Female donkey, she-ass	أتان
Tansy (*Tanacetum vulgare*)	أتاناسيا، حشيشه الدود
Citron (*Citrus medica*)	أترج، أطرنج
Citron-yellow	أترجي
Irritation	إثاره
Death	أجل
Congealing, thickening	إجماد
Woods, wetland	أجمه
Conversion	إحاله
States of the body*	أحوال البدن

---

*There are three states of the body: health, disease, and in-between.

Retention	إحتباس
Urinary retention, ischuria	إحتباس البول
Amenorrhea	إحتباس الطمث
Oxygen deprivation, congestion, retention, hyperemia	إحتقان
Burning, charring	إحراق، الإحراق
Running and lifting the feet up high	احضار
Rules, characteristics	أحكام
Dark red	أحمر قاني
Cross-eyed, strabismus	أحول
Trembling	إختلاج
Trembling of lips	إختلاج الشفه
Variable, variability	إختلاف
Hemorrhagic diarrhea	إختلاف الدم
Burning and/or irritating diarrhea	إختلاف لاذع
A vein on the side of the neck	أخدع (أخدعين)
Humors (*akhlāt*)	أخلاط
Flow	إدرار
Skin color, complexion	أدم
To heal	إدمال
Lemongrass (*Cymbopogon schoenanthus*)	إذخر
Purple	أرجواني
Followed with, followed by	أردف
Termites	أرضه
Vibration	إرعاد
Four elements (earth, water, air, and fire), the basics, the origins (*arkan*)	أركان
Groin	إربيه
Nose tip	أرنبه الانف
"Spirits," breaths (*arwah*)	أرواح
External causes	أسباب باديه
Functional causes	أسباب تماميه
Formative causes	أسباب صوريه
Active causes	اسباب فاعليه
Physical causes	أسباب ماديه

Retentive causes	أسـبـاب مـاسـكـه
Transformation	إستحـالـه
Thickness	إستحصـاف
Muscle weakness, relaxation	إسـترخـاء
Recuperative, regain	أسـترداد
Edema	إستسقاء
Ascites	إستسقاء زقي
Tympanites	إستسقاء طبـلـي
Prophylaxis	إستظهـار
Elimination, evacuation, depletion, loss	إستفراغ
Evacuation crisis	الاستفراغ البـحرانـي
Assimilation	إستمراء
Wetting of breath (e.g., by vomiting)	إستنقاع الروح
Constancy	إستـواء
Caused dizziness	أسـدر
Lines on the surface of the skin	أسره
Spinach	إسفانـاخ
Soup	إسفيدبـاج
Ceruse, white lead, zinc oxide*	إسفيداج
Sky-green	أسمانجونـي
Purgation or diarrhea	إسهـال
Salvatella vein	أسيلـم (الوريد الخنصري)
To raise, to carry	إشـالـه
Hand span	أشبـار
Inflammation	إشتعـال
Higher position	إشراف
Confusion	إشكـال
Reddish brown	أصهـب
Imbalance, disturbance	إضطراب
Bandages	أضمده
Citron, sweet lemon (*Citrus medica*)	أطرنـج، أترج
Infants	أطفـال

---

*Venetian ceruse, also known as spirits of Saturn, was a sixteenth-century cosmetic used as a skin whitener. It contained white lead, which causes lead poisoning that would eventually damage the user's skin complexion and cause hair loss.

English	Arabic
Liquid rubs, lotions	أطـلـيـه
Oyster shell	أظفار الطيب
Constipation	إعتقـال الـطـبـيـعـه
Symptoms	أعراض
Organs, also could mean parts of the body (*aʿdhaʾ*)	أعـضـاء
Food potential (the calculated energy of food)	أغذيه بالـقوه
Aromatics	افاويـه
Dodder (*Cuscuta epithymum*)	أفتيـمـون، أفثيـمـون
Recovery	إفراق
Absinth, wormwood (*Artemisia absinthium*)	أفسـنـتـين
Functions (*afʾal*)	أفعـال
Imaginary actions	أفعـال وهـميـه
Gum arabic's fruit juice (*Acacia arabica*)	أقاقيـا
Cranium, skull	قـحف، (ج:أقـحـاف)
Pharmacopoeia (*aqrabadhin*)	أقرابـاذين
Region	إقليـم
Trotters (the feet of any cattle)	اكـارع
Median cubital or median cutaneous vein	اكـحـل
Yellow sweet clover, yellow melilot (*Melilotus officinalis*)	إكليل الـملك
Causes of disease	الاسـبـاب
External or initial causes	الاسباب البـاديه
Distant causes	الاسـبـاب الـبـعـيـده
Predisposition causes	الاسـبـاب الـسـابـقـه
Proximate causes	الاسـبـاب الـمـلاصـقـه
Connecting causes	الاسـبـاب الـواصـلـه
Evacuation crisis	الاستفـراغ البـحـرانـي
Heavy lead	الأسـرب
Cecum	الاعـور
Buttocks	الألـيـتـين
External	البـاديه
Phlegm (*balgham*)	البـلـغم

Simple warming	التسخين الساذج
Inflammation	إلتهاب
Blood, blood humor* (*dam*)	الدم
Quartan fever	الربع
Black bile (*sauda'*)	السوداء
Dog star (Sirius)	الشعري
Yellow bile (*safra'*)	الصفراء
Alzheimer's disease	العته
Orbital nodes (ascending and descending)	العقدتين
Faculties (*quwa*)	القوى
Tropics (Cancer and Capricorn)	المنقلبين
Mastoid process	النقره
Fever	إلهاب
Supernumerary pulse	الواقع في الوسط
Sea ambrosia (*Ambrosia maritima*)	أمبروسياء، دمسيسه
Fullness, repletion	إمتلاء
Diseases of discontinuity and/or separation	امراض تفرق الاتصال
Diseases of organs' surfaces	أمراض صفائح الأعضاء
Diseases of vasculature and cavities	أمراض الاوعيه والتجاويف
Structural diseases	أمراض التركيب
Diseases of form	أمراض الخلقه
Diseases of appearance	أمراض الشكل
Diseases of number	أمراض العدد
Squeezing diseases	أمراض العصر
Diseases of ducts, canals, and tracts	أمراض المجاري
Dystemperament	أمراض المزاج
Diseases of quantity and/or size	أمراض المقدار
Diseases of position	أمراض الوضع
Compound diseases	امراض مركبه
Secondary diseases	أمراض مشتركه
Double pot, cooking on water bath and not direct flame	إناء مضاعف
Dilation of pupil	انتشار العين

---

*Blood and blood humor are not the same, although they have the same name.

Wetting	إنتشاف
Orthopnea, shortness of breath when lying flat	إنتصاب النفس
Swelling, flatulence	إنتفاخ
Coagulation, condensation, thickening	أنجماد
Internal, inner side	انسي
Ruptured vessels	إنصداع العروق
Coagulation, condensation, formation, fusion, thickening	أنعقاد
Explosion, rupture	إنفجار
Lamb rennet	انفحه الجدي
Slitting of vessel	انفرار عرق
Aneurysm	أنورسما
Aching, breaking	إنكسار
Grease	إهاله
Greasy	إهالي
Black myrobalan (*Terminalia chebula*)	أهليلج
Veins	أورده
Partial phases	أوقات جزئيه
General phases	أوقات كليه
Oka, a weight measure (forty drams)	أوقيه
Ileus	إيلاؤس

ب

Chamomile	بابونج
Basil (Persian)	بادروج
External causes	البادیه، الاسباب-
Cut	بتر
Emerald-green	بتلنجي
Boils, pustules, pimples	بثور
Healing crisis	بحارين، بحران
Voice hoarseness	بحه الصوت
Smoky moisture*	بخار دخاني

---

*Ancient authors associated a "smoky" nature with ammonia, and we interpret it as referring to protein; however, in other areas it refers to carbon dioxide.

Foul odor of the mouth, ozostomia	بخر الفم
Persian cyclamen (*Cyclamen persicum*)	بخور مريم
Skin	بدن
Stools	براز
Maidenhair fern, Venushair fern (*Adiantum capillus-veneris*)	برشاوشان، كزبره البئر
Leukoderma	برص
False black pepper (*Embelia ribes*)	برنج كابلي
Has seeds in it, such as seedy oxymel	بزوري
Common polypody (*Polypodium vulgare*)	بسبايج، بسفايج، ثاقب الحجر
Incision	بضع
Incise, incision	بط
Bubbling	بقبقه، بقابق
Purslane (*Portulaca oleracea*)	بقله حمقاء، فرفحين، فرفج
Leafy vegetables	بقول
Cooked leafy vegetables	بقيله
Dullness	بلاده
Acorns	بلاليط (من بلوط)
Balsam of Mecca (*Commiphora opobalsamum*)	بلسان، دهن البلسان
Phlegm (*balgham* [*bālghām*])	بلغم
Vitreous and/or glassy phlegm	بلغم زجاجي
Silliness, senility	بَلَه
Henbane (*Hyoscyamus niger*)	بنج، سكران
Ring finger	بنصر
Violets, pansies (*Viola* spp.)	بنفسج
Vitiligo	بهق
Vitiligo nigra	بهق أسود
Hemorrhoids	بواصير
Borax	بورقيه
Urine	بول
Bulimia	بوليموس
Aconite (*Aconitum napellus*)	بيش

ت

Side effect	تأثير بالعرض
Yawning	تثاؤب
Hardening of the eye	تحجر العين
Breakdown, decomposition, digestion, dispersion, dissolution, evaporation	تحلل، إنحلال
Sore throat	تخشن الحلق
Expansion, looseness	تخلخل
Dyspepsia, indigestion	تخمه
To treat	تداري
Management, handling, precaution, regimen, treatment	تدبير
Turpeth (*Operculina turpethum*)	تربد
Soft swelling	التربل
Fatty buttermilk	تردوغ
Tremor	ترعش
Clavicle, collarbone	ترقوه
Flabbiness	ترهل
Aeration, ventilation	ترويح تهويه
Teriac, antidote, antitoxic*	ترياق، ترياقي
Strain	تزحر
Simple warming	تسخين الساذج
Convulsion, spasm	تشنج
To bandage, to poultice, to paste, to plaster	تضميد
Extinguishing, cooling	تطفئه
Correction, adjustment	تعديل
To glue	تغريه
Irregular	تفاوت
Tasteless	تفهه
Dry skin	تقحل جلود
Progressive preservation	تقدم بالحفظ
Distillation	تقطير
Strangury, slow painful urination	تقطير البول

*An antitoxic compound formula.

Swaddling	تقميط
Pus formation, suppuration	تقيح
Hardness, stiffness, condensation	تكاثف
Condensing, thickening	تكثيف
Mustiness, wetness	تكرج
Fomentation	تكميد
Riding the sea in high waves	تلجيج
Sticky, to stick	تلجج، تلحيج
Burns, stings	تلذغ
Compactness	تلزز
Softness of bowels	تلين الطبع
Functional	تماميه
Distension	تمدد
Rubbing	تمرخ
Depilation	تمرط
Rolling	تمرغ
Stretching	تمطي
Falling	تناثر
Disperse, become less dense	تنفيش، نفش
Cleansing	تنقيه
Body's trunk*	تنور
Nausea	تهوع
Excitation, excite, puffiness	تهييج
Frequency	تواتر

ث

Warts	ثآليل
Density	ثخن
Dense	ثخين
Porridge of bread or pasta in meat soup (*thereadeh* or *treadeh*)	ثريده، تريده، فته
Dregs, residues, sediment	ثفل
Perforation	ثقب
Incisors	ثنايا

---

*A body's trunk corresponds to the Chinese concept of "triple burner" or "*san jiao*."

ج

Galen*	جـالينوس
Miliaria	الـجـاورسيه
Proso millet (*Panicum miliaceum*)	جـاورس
Mesentric vessels	جداول
Smallpox	جدري
Chicken pox	جدري الماء، العنقز، العنكز، الحمقاء
Benign smallpox	جدري سليمـات
Young goat (first year)	جـدي (أجـداء)
Leprosy	جـذام
Active pull	جذب مـخـالف
Passive pull	جذب مـوافق
Active and passive pulls	جـذبين
Scabies	جرب
Trachoma	جرب الاجفـان او الـعـين
Excoriating scabies (*scabies crustosa*)	جرب متقشر
Arugula	جـرجـير
Wound	جـرح
Cut	جز
Palpation, feeling the pulse, touch	جس
Hardness, solid	جسـاوه، جسأه
Belching	جشـاء
Curliness	جعـوده
Acorn's soft peel	جفت البلـوط
Jallab†	جلاب
Pomegranate flower	جلـنار:زهرالرمـان
Carbuncle (*jamra*)	جمـره
Aggregate	جمـع، يَجـمَع
Side	جنـب (ج:جنـوب)
Both sides of the body	جنـبين

---

*Aelius Galenus or Claudius Galenus (129 CE–199 [or 217] CE; Greek: Galēnos), known as Galen of Pergamon (Bergama, Turkey), was a prominent physician, surgeon, and philosopher.
†*Jallab* is a popular sweet summer drink in the Middle East made from carob, dates, grape molasses, and rose water.

Castoreum, European beaver (*Castor fiber*)	جندبيدستر
Jawarish (a set of compound herbal preparations)	جواريش، جوارشنـات
Nutmeg	جوزبوا، جوزالطـيب
Mangosteen (*Garcinia mangostana*)	جوز كندم
Integrity, essence, substance, composition	جوهر

ح

Acute (has great effect), harsh	حـاد
Innate heat, cellular respiration and associated heat	حـارغريزي
Persian thyme (*Thymus capitatus*)	حـاشـا
True myrtle (*Myrtus communis*)	حـب الآس
Hemp seeds	حب السمنـه
Funis brachii (*vena mediana cephalica*)	حبـل الـذراع
Diaphragm	الـحجـاب
Cupping	حجـامـه
Border, limit	حد
Age of youth and renewal	حداثـه
Swelling of skin	حـدر
Sore in the internal side of the eyelid	حَدْرَةٌ: قَرْحَةٌ تَخْرُجُ ببياضِ الجَفْنِ
Seeds of watercress (*Nasturtium officinale*)	حرف (بذور حب الرشـاد)
Eye pupil	حدقه
Innate heat	الـحراره الـغريزيه
Abnormal heat	حراره غريبه
Latent heat	حراره كامنـه
Urethritis	حرقه البـول
Activity, movement	حركـه، حركـات
Hot, burns the tongue	حريف
Sensation	حس
Measles	حصبه
Boxthorn (*Lycium afrum*)	حضض، عوسج
Congestion, retention, trapping	حقن

Enema, clyster, injection	حقنه
Loin	حَقو
Asafetida (*Ferula assafoetida*)	حلتیت (ومنها صمغ الانجدان)
Pharynx, throat	حلق، حلقوم
Homadhya (from *hamedh,* which means "acid"), a salad made with garden mallow	حماضیه
Cardamom (*Elettaria cardamomum*)	حماما، حب هان
Putrid mud	حمأه
Muddy	حمائی، حمئیه
Hyperpyrexia	حمی حاده
Sanguineous fever	حمی دمویه
Quartan fever, tetrataus	حمی الربع
Tertian fever	حمی الغب
Hectic fever	حمی المدقوق
Incessant fevers, synochus, typhoid fever	حمی مطبقه
Ephemeral fever	حمی یوم
Erysipelas	حمره
Lamb, baby lamb	حمل
Warm up	حمم
Irregular fevers	حمیات مختلطه
Blue fenugreek seeds (*Trigonella caerulea*)	حندقوقی
Houseleeks (*Semipervivum*)	حي علم

خ

Scratch	خدش
Abscess (*kharaj*)	خراج
Khrasani clay*	خراسانی، طین
Shaving	خراطه
Flaky, scaly	خراطی
Earthworms	خراطین
Hellebore	خربق

*Khrasani clay is a type of clay eaten cold and dry. It is hot in action due to salinity, which strengthens the mouth of the stomach. It acts as an antinausea agent.

Mustard	خردل
Snoring	خرخره
Cervical vertebra	خرز القفا
Carob	خرنوب، خروب
Wool	خز
Mastoid process	الخشائي، العظم الصدغي
Poppy (*Papaver somniferum*)	خشخاش
Wound scab, slough, crust of a wound	خشكريشه
Frost, frostbite	خصر، خصرين
Shake	خض
Marshmallow (*Althaea officinalis*)	خطمي
Slipper made of leather	خُف
Palpitation of the heart, tachycardia	خفقان
Lightness of symptoms, recovery, recuperation	خفه
Loosen	خلخل، يخلخل
Humor (*khalt*)	خلط
Superfluous humor	خلط فضلي
Form, structure	خلقه
Scrofula (*khanazeer*)	خنازير
Diphtheria, pharyngitis	خناق
Spelt, *Triticum romanum/spelta*	خندروس
Smallest finger	خنصر
Suffocating afflictions	خوانيق قاتله
Galangal (*Alpinia galanga*)	خولنجان
Golden shower tree, Indian laburnum (*Cassia fistula*)	خيار شنبر، خروب الهند
Wallflower, gillyflower (*Erysimum cheiri*)	خيري
Moles	خيلان

د

Lionitis, lion's disease	داء الاسد
Minim, one-sixth of a dram	دانقِ
Cold abscess	دبيله
Filling up of vessels	درت العروق

Dram, dirham, 3.125 grams	درهم
Glove	دستبانج، دستنان
Porridge (a dish of boiled oats [rolled, crushed, or steel cut] or other cereals in water, milk, or both)	دشيش
Rubbing	دعك
Repose, rest	دعه
Suddenly	دفعه
Hectic fever	الدق
Lightness	دقه
Signs	دلائل
Massage	دلك
Restorative massage, calming massage	دلك الاسترداد
Prepping massage	دلك الاستعداد
Blood, blood humor (*dam*)	دم
Socotra dragon tree (*Dracaena cinnabari*)	دم الأخوين
Moaning	دمدمه
Epiphora, the overflow of tears onto the face	الدمعه
Windy snowstorm	دمق
Boil, furunculus, furuncle	دمل (ج:دماميل)
Oil	دهن
Livestock	دواب
Dizziness	دوار
Varicose veins	دوالي
Buttermilk, churned sour milk	دُوغ، لبن مخيض
Threadworms, pinworms (*Oxyuris vermicularis*)	ديدان صغار
Giant roundworms (*Ascaris lumbricoides*)	ديدان طوال
Tapeworms (*Taenia solium*)	ديدان عرائض
Custom, habit	ديدن
Diluted in water	ديف "بمعنى حل في الماء"

ذ

Pleurisy, side disease	ذات الجنب
Tuberculosis	ذات الرئه

Angina	ذبحه
Diarrhea	ذرب
Intermittent pulse	ذوالفتره
Disintegration	ذوبان

ر

Fennel (*Foeniculum vulgare*) [Persian]	رازیانج، رزیانج
Common inula (*Inula helenium*)	راسن
Extracts, concentrates	رُب، ربوب
Asthma	ربو
Trembling	رجرجه
Soft, diffused tumors (*rakhu*)	رخو
Soften	رخی، یرخی
Contusion	رض
"Pound" (373.24 grams)	رطل
Nosebleed	رُعاف
Tremor, shaking	رعشه
Piece of cloth	رفاده
Small intestine	رقاق
To stop the flow of blood from a wound	رقوه الدم
Gentle, soft	رقیق
Ophthalmia conjunctivitis	رمد
Breath, physiological functions, respiration, "spirit"*	روح
Red currant (*Ribes rubrum*)	ریباس
Gas, wind	ریح
Infantile convulsions	ریح الصبیان، أم الصبیان
Basil	ریحان
Fragrant herbs	ریحانی
Gaseous (*reehia*)	ریحیه

ز

White vitriol (zinc sulfate, $ZnSO_4$)	زاج

---

*For an explanation for the multiple meanings of "spirit," see the discussion on this in the chapter "Primer: Concepts of Unani Medicine."

Dysentery, enteritis	زحير
Verdigris, copper carbonate (CuCO₃),* basic copper acetate	زنجار
Verdigris, a type of green color like that of copper carbonate	زنجاري
Foam, froth	زبد
Azarole, mosphilla, and Mediterranean medlar (*Crataegus azarolus*)	زعرور
Pitch resin[†]	زفت
Cold, nasal catarrh, coryza	زكام
Lienteric diarrhea	زلق الامعاء
Zeerbaj[‡]	زيرباج
Hyssop (*Hyssopus officinalis*)	زوفا

س

Predisposition	السابقه، الاسباب-
Forearm	ساعد
Shank, the lower part of the leg	ساق
Dill (*Anethum graveolens*)	شبث، شبت
Pannus, vascular keratitis	سبل
Excessive straightness	سبوطه
Ulceration, abrasion	سحج
Physique, including skin condition	سحنه
Blockage, obstruction[§]	سدد
Dizziness	سدَرُ
Common rue (*Ruta graveolens*)	سَذاب (فَيجَن)
Meningitis	سرسام
Phrenitis	سرسام حار
Lethargia	سرسام بارد

---

*Karpenko and Norris, "Vitriol in the History of Chemistry."

†Pitch resin is produced by the heating (dry distilling) of wood, which causes tar and pitch to drip away from the wood and leave behind charcoal.

‡*Zeerbaj* is a meat stew cooked with cinnamon, chickpeas, salt, sesame oil, vinegar, sugar, ground almonds in rose water, dry coriander, pepper, mastic, and saffron.

§This term most likely means the deposition of large molecules into the arteries, such as atherosclerosis.

Cypress (*Cupressus sempervirens*)	سرو
Galingale (*Cyperus longus*)	سعد
Favus, porrigo	سعفه
Powder, flour	سفوف
Scammony (*Convolvulus scammonia*)	سقمونيا
Fall, collapse, drop	سقوط، سقطه
Powder made from the fruit of Indian gooseberry (*Phyllanthus emblica* [syn. *Emblica officinalis*])	سك من الأملج
Apoplexy, sudden death*	سكته
Rock sugar	سكر طبرزد
Oxymel†	سكنجبين
Seedy oxymel‡	سكنجبين بزوري
Stillness, rest, inactivity	سكون
Tuberculosis	سل
Sharp debris or spines, spicules	سلاءه (ج:سلاء)
Blepharitis, tarsitis	سلاق
Lipoma (*sal' layen*)	سلع لين
Swiss chard	سلق
Cassia, or Chinese cinnamon (*Cinnamomum aromaticum*)	سليخه
Celestial	سماويه
Zenith	سمت الرأس
Roughness	سمج
Ghee, fat (soft fat)	سمن
Age of senility	سن الشيوخ
Middle age	سن المكتهلين
Insomnia	سهر

---

*For apoplexy, modern usage differs from that in ancient times. It was used to describe any sudden death that began with a sudden loss of consciousness, especially one in which the victim died within a matter of seconds after losing consciousness. Sudden cardiac deaths, ruptured cerebral aneurysms, certain ruptured aortic aneurysms, and even heart attacks may have been described as apoplexy in the past.

†A drink made of water, honey, wine, and vinegar.

‡Seedy oxymel is usually made of sugar, vinegar, wine, and water and cooked with the seeds of dodder, celery, fennel, endive, and anise.

Fetidness, offensive smell	سهوكه
Anemia, cacochymia*	سوء القنيه
Melancholic	سوداوي
Lily (*Lilium candidum*)	سوسن
Orrisroot (*Iris florentina*)	سوسن اسمانجوني
Synochus, continuous fever	سوناخس
Suewaiq†	سويق

ش

Fumitory (*Fumaria officinallis*)	شاه أترج، شاهترج
Chestnut	شاهبلوط، كستناء، ابوفروه
Alum†	شَبُّ
Age of strength	شباب
Dill	شبت
Euphorbia (*Euphorbia pithyusa*)	شبرم
Willow (*Salix babylonica*)	شجره الغرب، الخلاف، الصفصاف
Fat (solid fat)	شحم، شحمه
Break, crack, split	شدخ
Alcohol or other drinks and juice	شراب
Epigastrium, the upper central region of the abdomen	شراسيف
Scarification, scarifying	شرط
Aorta	شريان عظيم
Urticaria (yellow rash)	شري صفراوي
Artery	شريان
Semitertian	شطر الغب
Branch	شعبه
Dog star (Sirius)	الشعري

---

*Cacochymia referred to a depraved habit of body, replete with ill humors, from various causes.

†*Suewaiq* is an old dish in the Arabian culture made of barley, dates, butter, and cardamom. It is made from the flour of roasted wheat or barley.

‡Alum is both a specific chemical compound (hydrated potassium aluminum sulfate [potassium alum] with the formula $KAl(SO_4)_2 \cdot 12H_2O$) and a class of chemical compounds known as alums with the general empirical formula $AB(SO_4)_2 \cdot 12H_2O$.

Slit	شق
Splitting	شقاق
Migraine	الشقيقه
Alkanet (*Alkanna tinctoria*)	شنكال
Dates, a dense preparation of dates	شهربز، الشهربزاني
Appetite	شهوه
Sexual desire	شهوه جماع
Bulimia, canine appetite	شهوه كلبيه
Broth, soup	شورباج
Hemlock	الشوكران
Nigella (*Nigella sativa*)	شونيز، حبه البركه
Suppository	شيافه، تحميله
Grayness	شيب
Absinthe, wormwood (*Artemisia judaica*)	شيح
Elderly	شيخ
Oil of coriander	شيرج
Sesame oil, gingili oil	شيرج عذب
Exudate from *Atraphaxis cotoneaster*, manna	شيرخشت، المن
Darnel (*Lodoicea temulentum*)	شيلم، زوان

ص

Fasting person, jejunum	صائم
Great saphenous vein	الصافن
Aloe (*Aloe vera*)	صبر
Children	صبيان
Sardine	صحناه
Rift	صَدْع
Temple	صدغ
Ichor, pus	صديد
Mountain thyme (*Origanum* sp.)	صعتر جبلي
Peritoneum	صفاق
Yellow bile (*safra'*)	صفراء
Leek-green bile	صفراء كراثي
Bilious, choleric	صفراوي

Ear canal, external auditory meatus	صمـاخ
Occupation	صنـاعه
Red sandalwood (*Pterocarpus santalinus*)	صنـدل
Formative	صوريـه
Scepter	صولـجـان

ض

Laxation	ضانـه
Laxation induced by coldness	ضانـه برد
Anxiety	ضـجر
Pulsation, throbbing	ضـربـان
Trauma, blow	ضـربـه
Frosted, frostbite	ضـربـه البـرد
Bandage	ضمـاده
Dyspnea	ضيـق النـفـس

ط

Plague (*ta'oon*)	طـاعون
Rock salt	المـلح طبـرزد
Bat, or racket	طبـطـابـه، طبطاب
Natural, natural function	طبـع
Nature, body system	طبيـعـه
Naturals (*tabie'iat*)	طـبـيـعـيـا ت
Tamarisk (*Tamarix gallica*)	طـرفاء
Sweet lemon (*Citrus medica*)	طـرنـج
Liquid rub	طـلاء
Talcum powder*	طـلـق
Khrasani clay	طين خراسـاني
Sealed clay, Lemnian earth†	طـيـن مـخـتـوم
Partridge, grouse	طـيـهـوج

---

*Talc (from Persian *tālk* [تـالـك] via Arabic *talk* [تـلـك]) is a mineral composed of hydrated magnesium silicate ($H_2Mg_3(SiO_3)_4$ or $Mg_3Si_4O_{10}(OH)_2$). It is the widely used substance known as talcum powder.

†Lemnia sphragis was used as an astringent for snakebites and wounds and in the sixteenth century for the plague. This medicinal soil was dug ceremonially once a year from a mound on the island of Lemnos, Greece.

ظ

Goat's hooves	ظلف المعز

ع

Disturbance	عارض
Pellitory, Spanish chamomile, or Mount Atlas daisy (*Anacyclus pyrethrum*)	عاقرقرحا
Surging water	عُبُب
Bulky	عبل (ج:عبال)
Number	عدد
Accidental, nonessential, indirectly	عرضي، عرضيه
Milk vetch (*Astragalus gummifera*)	عرفج، القتاد
Dracunculiasis	العرق المديني
Vessel	عرق
Temporal vein	عرق الصدغ
Sciatica	عرق النسا
Popliteal vein	عرق مأبض الركبه
Two veins in the lachrymal angle of the eye, vena angularis	عرق الماقين
Parietal branch of the superficial temporal vein	عرق الهامه
Achilles' heel, hamstring, tendo calcaneous	عرقوب
Greater celandine (*Chelidonium majus*)	عروق صفر \ عروق الصباغين
Difficulty in urination	عسر البول
Night blindness	عشى
Organ, body part	عضو
Meningitis	عطاس
Permanent dysfunction, destruction	عطب
Sneezing	عطس
Astringent, pungent	عفص
Orbital nodes (ascending and descending)	العقدتين
Treatment	علاج
Treatment with absolute opposite, allopathy	علاج بالضد على الاطلاق

Signs (*'alamat*)   علامـات

Turpentine resin (*Pistacia terebinthus*)   علك الانبـاط، بـطـم

European black nightshade   عنـب الثعـلب
(*Solanum nigrum*)

Area between the lower lip and chin   عنفقه

Agarwood, or oodh (or just agar)   عود
(*Aquilaria agallocha*)

غ

Agaric, white agaric (*Polyporus officinallis*)   غـاريـقون

Extreme, maximum   الـغايـه

Nausea   غـثـي

Glands   غدد محـضـه

Morning   غُدوه، (ج. غُدوات)

Egg's outer white membrane   غرقئ

Abnormal   غريبه

Nature, metabolic vigor*   غريزه

Innate   غريزي

Innate nature   غريزه (الغريزيه)

Leucoma   غشـاوه

Fainting, syncope   غشـي

Cartilage   غضـروف

Wrinkle, crease, corrugation   غضـن (ج:غضـون)

Fresh   غضـين

Thickness   غلـظ

Pétrissage, gentle poking with fingers   غمـز

Depth   غمـوره

ف

Lukewarm   فـاتـر

Farsi word that means antidote to poison   فادزهري

White bryony (*Bryonia alba*)   فـاشـرا

Good, virtuous   فـاضـل

---

*Metabolic vigor mostly refers to the metabolic vigor as aided by respiration and oxidative phosphorylation that produces adenosine triphosphate (ATP), the energy fuel of the cells.

Active	فاعليه
Sugar, candy, brown sugar	فانيد
Palsy	فالج
Falouthaj or falouzaj, sweet jelly, Turkish delight*	فالوذج (حلقوم، راحه)
Peony (*Paeonia* sp.)	فاوانيا
Hernia	فتق
Suppository	فتيله
Immature humors, dregs	فجاجه
Filter	فدام
Open slits	فدغ
Euphorbia (*Euphorbia serrata*)	فربيون
Phrysimyos	فريسميوس
Chick (young chicken)	فروج
Degradation, contamination, corruption	فساد
Rip	فسخ
Superfluous, excess	فضل
Seed of wild celery	فطراساليون، بزر الكرفس الجبلي
Beer	فقاع
Displacement	فك
Pepper	فلافلي
Universe's orbit	الفلك
Cardia, stomach mouth	فم المعده
Hiccup	فواق
Pennyroyal (*Mentha pulegium*)	فودنج، فوتنج
Cat thyme, hulwort, mountain or felty germander (*Teucrium polium*)	فوليون، جعده

ق

Astringent	قابض
Red, saturated red	قاني
Contraction and relaxation	قبض وإنبساط
Malodorous	قتمه، قتام

---

*Turkish delight is a sweet made of sugar, starch, and water.

Armenian cucumber, curving cucumber (*Cucumis melo* var. *flexuosus*)	قثاء
Squirting (exploding) cucumber (*Ecballium elaterium*)	قثاء الحمار
Dryness	قحل
Sore, ulcer	قرحه
Safflower	قرطم، عصفر
Pumpkin	قرع
Beat, heartbeat	قرعه
Rumbling	قرقره، قراقر
Carnation (*Dianthus caryophyllus*), clove (*Eugenia caryophyllata*)	قرنفل
Horripilation, goose skin, goosebumps	قشعريره
Dry and cracked skin	قشف
Trachea	قصبه الريه
Stuntedness	قصر
Lean, emaciated	قضيف (قضاف)
Loin	قطن
Tar*	قطران
Blond psyllium (*Plantago ovata*)	قطونا، لسان الحمل
Stomatitis, thrush, aphtha	قلاع
Sleeplessness, worry	قلق
Red iron oxide used for polishing glass	قلقطار
Occiput, external occipital eminence, occipital bone	قمدوحه
Branching centaury (*Erythraea pulchella*)	قنطوريون، قنطريون
Galbanum (*Ferula galbaniflua*)	قنه
Texture, consistency	قوام
Ringworm	قوبا، قوابي
Nine *okas*	قوطول، طولون
Comprehensive statement	قول كلي
Colic	قولنج
Flatulent colic	قولنج ريحي

---

*Tar is modified pitch (resin) produced primarily from the wood and roots of pine by destructive distillation.

Biliary colic	القولنـج يرقانـي
Colon	قولون
Power (strength) or faculty, depending on the context, functional capacity*	قوه
Active pulling	قوه جـاذبـه
Expulsive faculty	قوه دافعـه
Retentive faculty	قوه مـاسكه
Forming faculty	قوه مصـوره
Discerning or discriminating faculty	قوه مميزه
Digestive faculty	قوه هاضمـه
Instinctual\imaginary faculty	قوه وهمـيه
Analogy, syllogism, to measure	قيـاس
Pus, ichor	قيـح
Carat, two hundred milligrams	قيـراط
Cerate	قيـروطي
Hot weather	قيـظ
Cephalic vein	قيـفـال
Hydrocele†	قيـلـه المـاء

ك

Paper	كـاغد
Pickles	كـامخ، كـوامـيخ
Upper back between the shoulders	كـاهل
Clew, hank, ball of thread	كبـه
Extract of milk vetch (*Astragalus gummifera*)	كثيراء تستخرج من عرفج، القتـاد
Turbid, turbidity	كدر
Leek (*Allium porrum*)	كراث
Leek-green	كراثي
Anxiety, distress	كرب
Roast, barbecue	كردناج

---

*Nowadays, functional capacity can be referred to as the metabolic health, especially in relation to energy and heat production. See the discussion on this in the chapter "Primer: Concepts of Unani Medicine."

†This hydrocele is a fluid-filled sack along the spermatic cord within the scrotum.

Ervil (*Vicia ervillia*)	كرسنـه
Common cabbage	كرنب نبطـي
Trismus, lockjaw	كزاز
Sluggishness, laziness	كسـل
Barley milk*	كشك الشـعير
Fullness and heaviness from food	كظ
Heel	كعب
Animal feet	كفشـير
Freckles (reddish)	كلف
Tiredness, weariness, fatigue	كَل، كلل
Cloudiness	كمـوده
Oliban (*Boswellia* gum)	كندر
Middle age	كهـوله
Cauterization	كـي
Quality	كيفيـه

ل

Labdanum, or ladanum (*Cistus ladanifer* and *C. creticus*, species of rockrose)	لادن
Persistent	لاذب
Biting, irritant	لاذع
Azure, azureous	لازوردي
Accompanying, associated with	لازمـه
Pith, core, inside	لبـاب
Frankincense (from *Boswellia*, particularly *Boswellia sacra*)	لبـان
Lablab purpureus (syn. *Dolichos lablab*)	لبلاب
Milk	لبـن، اللـبن
Lisping, stammering	لثغ
Good-smelling rubs	لخـالخ
Burn, sting	لذغ
Grand plantain (*Plantago major*)	لسـان الحمـل
Poultice, smear	لطـوخ

---

*To make barley milk, barley flour is fermented and then soaked in milk and dissolved in it.

Fascia	لفافه، لفائف
Facial paralysis	لقوه
Uvula	اللهاه
Insomnia, tossing about in bed	لملمه
Sleeping sickness, drowsiness, inflammation of the brain with confusion	ليثيارغوس
Looseness of bowels	لين الطبيعه

م

Glaucoma	ماء في عدسه العين
Aqueous (*ma'yeh*)	مائيه
Wrist, carpus	مأبض، رسغ
Substance	ماده
Physical	ماديه
Eel	مارماهج، مارماهى (فارسيه)
Alpine daphne, mezereon (*Daphne alpina* and *Daphne mesereum*)	مازريون
Mesentery*	ماساريقا
Yogurt (Persian)	ماست
Melancholia, melancholy	مالنخوليا
Hypochondriasis, hypochondria	ماليخوليا مراقئي
Grappling, a form of wrestling	مباطشه
Coolants	مبردات
Person with diarrhea	مبطون
Wobbly, loose	متخلخل
Successive, consecutive	متدارك
Relaxed	متراخي
Distant	متفاوت
Irregular	متقطع
Condensed	متكاثف
Frequent	متواتر
Excite	مثوره
Probe	مجس

---

*The mesentery is the peritoneal fold attaching the intestine to the posterior abdominal wall.

Dispersing, decomposing, resolvent	محلل
Mucus	مخاط
Cavities	مخانق
Compact	مدمجه
Myrrh (*Commiphora myrrha*)	مر
Yellow bile, bile	مرار
Gallbladder	مراره
Abdomen, belly	مراق البطن
Antares	المرتعش
Yellow and black biles	المرتين
Oil rub	مرخ
Relaxing, softening, resolvent	مرخي،مرخيه، مرخيات
Oregano	مرزنجوش
Esophagus	مرىء
al-muri, or *almorri*	مري
Temperament (*mizaj*)	مزاج
Clavi, corns	مسامير
Causes of disease (*mousabibat*)	مسببات
Deer musk	مسك
Sedative, soother, demulcent	مُسكن
Laxative	مسهل
Similarity (relationship of an organ to other organ or organs)	مُشاكله
Elderly	مشايخ
Mastic tree (*Pistacia lentiscus*)	مصطكي
Whey (from milk)	مصل
Moderate, equitable	معتدل
Sudden	مغافص
Armenian clay, reddish clay	مغرة، طين المغرة
Glutinous, gelatinous	مغريه
Gripes, gastrointestinal cramps	مغص
Scattering, scatter	مفرق
Curly	مفافله
Astringents	مقبضات

Quantity	مقدار
Forehead	مقدم البدن
Anus	مقعده
Black salt, Indian black salt (*kala namak*)*	ملح نفطي
Cicatrizant, healing medication	ملحم
Attenuate, soother	ملطف
Digestive	ممرئ
Nostril	منخار
Contracted	منضمه
Obstructed, constricted	منسده
Shoulder girdle	منكب
Effects	موجبات
People who have been cauterized	موسوم (ين)
Desert water	مياه قفريه
Alcoholic extract of lily	ميسوسن
Styrax tree (*Styrax officinalis*)	ميعه
Mistletoe	ميوزج

ن

Spikenard, jatamansi, nardin, nard (*Nardostachys jatamansi*)	ناردين
Fiery†	ناريه
Fistula	ناصور
Musk pod of the deer musk	نافجه مسك
Shivering	نافض
Bishop's weed (*Carum copticum*)	نانخواه
Sawlike pulse	نبض منشاري
Wavy pulse	نبض موجي
Beat	نبضه
Christ's thorn jujube (*Ziziphus spin-christi*)	نبق

Kala namak is a salty and pungent-smelling condiment composed largely of sodium chloride with several impurities lending the salt its color and smell. The smell is mainly due to sulfur content.

†A fiery condition is produced by oxygen deprivation and/or an anaerobic condition. See the discussion on this in the chapter "Primer: Concepts of Unani Medicine."

Burned copper (copper baked with sulfur and salt)	نحـاس محـرق
Slimness, leanness	نحـول
Husk, bran	نخـالـه
Bleeding, hemorrhage, hematorrhea	نزف، نـزف الـدم
Menorrhagia	نزف الحـيض
Hematochezia, anal bleeding	نزف المقـعده
Catarrh	نزلـه، نزلات
Natron, native sodium carbonate	نطـرون
Douche	نطـول (ج:نطولات)
Bullae of emphysema	نفـاخـات
Blisters	نفـاطـات
Expectoration, sputum	نفـث
Hemoptysis*	نفـث الـدم
Flatulence or emphysema	نفـخ
Distension	النفـخـه
"Spirit," breath (*nafas*)	نَفَـسْ
A being, a life-form (*nafs*)	نَفْـسْ
Orthopnea	نفس الانتصـاب
Absorption, penetration	نفـاذ، نفـوذ
Puerpera	نفسـاء
Pit, cavity, fossa, socket	نقـره
Quickly	نقـله
Injury, vanquish	نكـايـه
Relapse	نكـس
Mint or thyme	نمـام
Freckles (reddish-black)	نمـش
Herpes	نملـه
Relapse	نوائب علل
Young birds	نواهـض
Quicklime (calcium oxide, CaO)	نوره
Species	نوع

---

*Hemoptysis is coughing up of blood or of blood-stained sputum from the bronchi, larynx, trachea, or lungs (e.g., in tuberculosis or other respiratory infections or cardiovascular pathologies).

Half-boiled egg	نيمبرشت

ه

Excited, hyperactive	هـائـج
Noon	هاجـره (وقت)
Head	هـامـه
Tear, rip	هتك
Mashes	هـرائـس، هـريـسـه
Bone debris	هشـيم الـعـظـام
True endive (*Cichorium endivia*)	هنـدبـاء
Structure, shape	هيئـه
Cholera	هـيضـه

و

Tendon	وتر
Sprain	وثـى
Corroding pain	وجع آكـل
Tiring and/or fatigue (*a'ya'i*)	وجـع إعيـائـي
Boring (*thaqeb*)	وجـع ثـاقـب
Heavy (*thaqeel*)	وجـع ثقيـل
Itching (*hakak*)	وجـع حكـاك
Dull (*khader*)	وجـع خـد ر
Rough (*khashin*)	وجـع خشـن
Softening (*rakhou*)	وجـع رخـو
Pressing (*daghet*)	وجـع ضـاغـط
Throbbing (*dharabani*)	وجـع ضـربـانـي
Biting and/or incisive (*lathe'*)	وجـع لاذع
Piercing (*masalee*)	وجـع مسـلـي
Splitting (*moufasekh*)	وجـع مفسـخ
Breaking (*moukaser*)	وجـع مكـسـر
Flattening and/or extending (*moumaded*)	وجـع ممـد د
Stabbing (*nakhes*)	وجـع نـاخـس
Coxalgia	وجـع الـورك
External, outer, lateral	وحشـي
Jugular vein	وداج

Oblique, in an oblique position or direction	ورب (مورب)
Hip	ورك
Hydrocephalus	ورم القحف المائي
Vein	وريد
Sickness	وصب
Position	وضع
Need, desire	وطر
Muggy	وَمِد

ي

Mandrake (*Mandragora officinarum*)	يبروح، شُجاع
Euphorbia sp.	يتوع
Euphorbiaceous plants	يتوعات
Percolate	يَحْقُنْ
Diminishes	يُذهب
Deters, repels	يردع
Stops bleeding	يرقأ الدم
Jaundice	يرقان
Discharge, emptying, expulsion, release, secretion	يستفرغ
Causes constipation	يعقد
Coated, smeared, covered	يطلى
Ferments	يغلي
Pull, draw	يقلع
Rubbing	يمرخ
Burns, stings	يلذغ
Mashed	يمرس
Relapse	ينكس
Stretch out	يوتر

Bibliography

Abu-Asab et al. "Biomarkers in the Age of Omics: Time for a Systems Biology Approach." *OMICS* 15, no. 3 (March 2011): 105–12.

Afnan, Soheil M. *Avicenna: His Life and Works*. London: George Allen and Unwin, 1958. [This is a simplistic and Persian-centric summary where the author's interpretations and comments should be viewed as his skewed views.]

Amri, Hakima, and Mones Abu-Asab. "Physiology of Qi." In *Energy Medicine East and West: A Natural History of Qi*, edited by David F. Mayor and Marc S. Micozzi. Churchill Livingstone Elsevier, London, 2011.

Arikha, Noga. *Passions and Tempers: A History of the Humours*. 1st ed. New York: Ecco, 2007.

Bakhtiar, Laleh Mehree, trans. *Canon of Medicine*. Chicago, Ill.: Great Books of the Islamic World Kazi Publications, Inc., 1999.

Berman, Jules J., and G. William Moore. *Precancer: The Beginning and the End of Cancer*. Sudbury, Mass.: Jones and Bartlett, 2010.

Caggiati, A., and J. J. Bergan. "The Saphenous Vein: Derivation of Its Name and Its Relevant Anatomy." *Journal of Vascular Surgery* 35, no. 1 (January 2002): 172–75. PMID 11802151.

Chandel, N. S., and P. T. Schumacker. "Cellular Oxygen Sensing by Mitochondria: Old Questions, New Insight." *Journal of Applied Physiology* 88, no. 5 (May 2000): 1880–89.

Chishti, G. M. *The Traditional Healer's Handbook: A Classic Guide to the Medicine of Avicenna*. Rochester, Vt.: Healing Arts Press, 1991.

Dobzhansky, Theodosius. "Nothing in Biology Makes Sense Except in the Light of Evolution." *American Biology Teacher* 35 (March 1973): 125–29.

Dykens, James A., and Yvonne Will, eds. *Drug-Induced Mitochondrial Dysfunction.* Hoboken, N.J.: John Wiley and Sons, 2008. doi: 10.1002/978470372531. fmatter.

Gordon, David, Leif Christensen, Hans Karle, and Theanne Walters. "The Avicenna Directories—A New Tool in Quality Assurance of Medical Education." *World Medical Journal* 55, no. 1 (2009): 9–11.

Graz, B. "Prognostic Ability of Practitioners of Traditional Arabic Medicine: Comparison with Western Methods through a Relative Patient Progress Scale." *Evidence-Based Complementary and Alternatative Medicine* 7, no. 4 (2010): 471–76.

Gruner, O. C. "Avicenna's *Canon of Medicine* and Its Modern Unani Counterpart." *Medical Bulletin (Ann Arbor)* 22, no. 6 (1956): 239–48.

———, trans. *A Comprehensive Glossary of Avicenna's* Canon of Medicine. New Delhi: Institute of History of Medicine and Medical Research, 1967.

———, trans. *A Treatise on the* Canon of Medicine *of Avicenna: Incorporating a Translation of the First Book.* New York: AMS Press, 1973.

Hajdu, S. I. "Greco-Roman Thought about Cancer." *Cancer* 100, no. 10 (May 15, 2004): 2048–51.

Hauser, N. S., I. Manoli, J. C. Graf, et al. "Variable Dietary Management of Methylmalonic Acidemia: Metabolic and Energetic Correlations." *American Journal of Clinical Nutrition* 93, no. 1 (2011): 47–56.

Hirschberg, Julius, and Julius Lippert. *Die Augenheikunde de Ibn Sina.* Leipzig: Verlag von Veit & Comp., 1902.

Karpenko, Vladimir, and John A. Norris. "Vitriol in the History of Chemistry." *Chem. Listy* 96 (2001): 997–1005.

Lane, Nick. *Power, Sex, Suicide: Mitochondria and the Meaning of Life.* Oxford: Oxford University Press, 2006.

Mamtimin, B., and H. Upur. "Plasma Metabonomics Analysis of Tumor Patients of Phlegm-Stasis Syndrome." [In Chinese.] *Zhongguo Zhong Xi Yi Jie He Za Zhi* 3, no. 14 (April 2011): 492–95. PMID: 21608220.

Mamtimin, B., H. Upur, F. H. Hao, et al. "Plasma Metabonomic Analysis with ^{1}H Nuclear Magnetic Resonance Revealing the Relationship of Different Tumors and the Disease Homology Theory of Traditional Uyghur Medicine." *Integrative Medicine* 17, no. 2 (February 2011): 111–15.

Michalsen, Andreas, Manfred Roth, and Gustav Dobos, eds. *Medicinal Leech Therapy.* Thieme Publishers New York, 2007.

Nuland, S. B. "Bad Medicine." *New York Times Book Review,* July 8, 2007, p. 12.

Osborn, D. K. "Greek Medicine." 2008. www.greekmedicine.net. Accessed February 15, 2013.

Roukos, D. H. "Networks Medicine: From Reductionism to Evidence of Complex Dynamic Biomolecular Interactions." *Pharmocogenomics* 12, no. 5 (May 2011): 695–98.

Shah, Mazhar H. *The General Principles of Avicenna's* Canon of Medicine. Karachi, Pakistan: Naveed Clinic, 1966.

Smith, R. D. "Avicenna and the Canon of Medicine: A Millennial Tribute." *Western Journal of Medicine* 133 (1980): 367–70.

Welch, G. Rickey. "In Retrospect: Fernel's 'Physiologia.'" *Nature* 456 (November 27, 2008): 446–47.

Index